# ESSENTIALS OF SMALL ANIMAL ANESTHESIA AND ANALGESIA

# ESSENTIALS OF SMALL ANIMAL ANESTHESIA AND ANALGESIA

Edited by

**John C. Thurmon, DVM, MS, DACVA**
**William J. Tranquilli, DVM, MS, DACVA**
**G. John Benson, DVM, MS, DACVA**

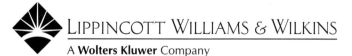

LIPPINCOTT WILLIAMS & WILKINS
A **Wolters Kluwer** Company

Philadelphia · Baltimore · New York · London
Buenos Aires · Hong Kong · Sydney · Tokyo

*Editor:* Donna Balado
*Managing Editor:* Jennifer Schmidt
*Marketing Manager:* Jennifer Conrad
*Project Editor:* Paula C. Williams

351 West Camden Street
Baltimore, Maryland 21201-2436 USA

227 East Washington Square
Philadelphia, PA 19106

The publisher is not responsible (as a matter of product liability, negligence or otherwise) for any injury resulting from any material contained herein. This publication contains information relating to general principles of medical care which should not be construed as specific instructions for individual patients. Manufacturers' product information and package inserts should be reviewed for current information, including contraindications, dosages and precautions.

*Printed in the United States of America*

**Library of Congress Cataloging-in-Publication Data**

Essentials of small animal anesthesia and analgesia / edited by John C.
  Thurmon, William J. Tranquilli, G. John Benson.
    p.     cm.
  ISBN 0–683–30107–1
    1. Veterinary anesthesia Handbooks, manuals, etc.   2. Analgesia
  Handbooks, manuals, etc.   3. Pets—Surgery Handbooks, manuals, etc.
  I. Thurmon, John C.   II. Tranquilli, William J.   III. Benson, G.
  John.
  SF914.E77   1999
  636.089'796—dc21                                                       99–14445
                                                                              CIP

*The publishers have made every effort to trace the copyright holders for borrowed material. If they have inadvertently overlooked any, they will be pleased to make the necessary arrangements at the first opportunity.*

To purchase additional copies of this book, call our customer service department at **(800) 638-3030** or fax orders to **(301) 824-7390**. International customers should call **(301) 714-2324.**

99  00  01  02  03
1  2  3  4  5  6  7  8  9  10

# Preface

This handbook is the product of several dedicated veterinary anesthesiologists who have made many outstanding contributions to the field of veterinary anesthesia over their careers. As the title indicates, the essential elements of veterinary anesthesia for commonly encountered small animal species is the focus of this text. To this end, the text provides an immediate source of usable facts and concepts necessary in performing anesthesia in a wide variety of species. In addition, important physiologic and pharmacologic principles are presented in a concise way to provide an understanding of how and why anesthetic drug administration and anesthesia alters normal body functions. The *Essentials* handbook can also can be used as a guide to the more comprehensive 3rd edition of *Lumb and Jones' Veterinary Anesthesia* textbook.

The editors wish to express their gratitude to the excellent contributing authors who worked so diligently toward the completion of this handbook. Thanks go to the University of Illinois anesthesiology residents (Dave Martin, John Tukey, Kurt Grimm, and Leigh Lamont) and the technical staff (Lucy Remillard, Ragenia Sarr, Richard Siemers, Deneen Cordell, and Glynis Reeves) who were so supportive of the editors during the completion of this project. Shirley Pelmore should also receive special thanks for her untiring efforts in processing the text.

# Contents

# Chapter 1

## General Considerations for Anesthesia

### Introductory Comments

*General anesthesia induces immobilization, relaxation, unconsciousness, and freedom from pain. By necessity, it must be reversible. Knowledge of underlying disease processes and other factors that may modify anesthesia and analgesia is essential to the success of the procedure. Marked variations in response to a standard dose of anesthetic result from the interplay of many factors, especially those related to the metabolic activity of the animal, existing disease or pathology, and the uptake and distribution of the anesthetic.*

**Patient Evaluation**
**Patient Preparation**
**Selection of Anesthetic**
**Pharmacology**
**Drug Interactions**
**Assessment of Anesthetic Action**
**Record Keeping**
**Recovery**

---

## I.   PATIENT EVALUATION

*For every mistake that is made for not knowing, a hundred are made for not looking.*

### A.   Purpose

The purpose of the preanesthetic evaluation is to determine the patient's physical status. Physical status is determined by (1) history; (2) inspection (attitude, condition, conformation, temperament); (3) palpation, percussion, and auscultation; and

1

(4) laboratory determinations and special procedures. The physical examination should include evaluation of the nervous, cardiopulmonary, hepatic, and renal systems and should be completed in the owner's presence to allow for questions and to communicate the risks of anesthesia (Table 1-1).

**B.  History**

The history should include current health, presenting complaint and its severity and duration, concurrent symptoms of disease (e.g., diarrhea, vomiting, exercise intolerance, cardiopulmonary dysfunction, ascites, rales, dyspnea, polyuria-polydipsia), pregnancy, a full or distended stomach, prior or current therapy, and anesthetic history (Table 1-2).

**C.  Laboratory Tests**

Preanesthetic laboratory test results must be carefully interpreted in light of the physical examination and history. Minimum evaluation should include assessment of packed cell volume, plasma protein concentration, and hemoglobin content. Additional laboratory tests may be indicated, including hematologic evaluations, serum chemistries, blood gases and pH, and coagulation times (Table 1-3). Fecal and/or filarial examination, electrocardiography, and imaging procedures may also be indicated.

**D.  Physical Status**

After the examination, the physical status of the patient should be classified in terms of its general state of health according to the American Society of Anesthesiologists (ASA) classification (Table 1-4). Classification of overall health is an essential part of any anesthetic record system. Guidelines for laboratory screening tests based on ASA physical status and age are presented in Table 1-5.

**E.  Operative Risk**

Operative risk refers to uncertainty and potential for misadventure or adverse outcome as a result of anesthesia and surgery. It should be emphasized that physical status, anesthetic risk, and operative risk are not one in the same. Anesthetic risk depends on the skill of the anesthetist and surgeon (may be one in the

*Text continued on p. 7.*

**Table 1-1. Preanesthetic Physical Examination**

   I. Body weight and body condition
     A. Obesity
     B. Cachexia
     C. Dehydration
  II. Cardiopulmonary
     A. Heart rate and rhythm (canine: 70–120; feline: 120–180)
     B. Auscultation
       i. Heart sounds and murmurs
       ii. Breath sounds
     C. Capillary refill time (< 1.5 s)
     D. Mucous membrane color
       i. Pallor
       ii. Cyanosis
     E. Pulse character
     F. Respiratory rate (15–25)
 III. CNS and special senses
     A. Temperament
     B. Seizure, coma, stupor
     C. Vision, hearing
 IV. Gastrointestinal
     A. Parasites
     B. Abdominal palpation
  V. Hepatic
     A. Icterus
     B. Abnormal bleeding
 VI. Renal
     A. Palpate kidneys, bladder
 VII. Integument
     A. Tumors
     B. Flea infestation
VIII. Musculoskeletal
     A. Lameness
     B. Fractures

**Table 1-2. Signalment and History**

I. Signalment
   A. Age
   B. Breed
   C. Sex
II. Body weight
III. Duration of complaint
IV. Concurrent medications
   A. Organophosphates
   B. $H_2$-blockers
   C. Antibiotics (aminoglycosides, chloramphenicol)
   D. Cardiac glycosides
   E. Phenobarbital
   F. NSAIDs
   G. Calcium channel blockers
   H. β-blockers
V. Signs of organ system disease
   A. Diarrhea
   B. Vomiting
   C. Polyuria-polydipsia
   D. Seizures, personality change
   E. Exercise intolerance
   F. Coughing, stridor
   G. Weight loss, loss of body condition
VI. Previous anesthesia, allergies
VII. Duration since last meal

## Table 1-3. Normal Reference Ranges for Standard Laboratory Tests

| Test | Canine | Feline |
|------|--------|--------|
| **NORMAL HEMATOLOGIC VALUES** | | |
| Hematocrit, % | 35–52 | 30–45 |
| Hemoglobin, g/dL | 12–18 | 8–15 |
| RBC count, $\times 10^6$ | 5.5–8.5 | 5–10 |
| Mean cell volume, fL | 60–77 | 39–55 |
| Mean cell hemoglobin, pg | 20–25 | 13–18 |
| Mean cell hemoglobin concentration, % | 32–36 | 30–36 |
| WBC count, $\times 10^3$ | 6–17.0 | 5.5–19.5 |
| Segment neutrophil, $\times 10^3$ | 3–11.5 | 2.5–12.5 |
| Band neutrophil, $\times 10^3$ | 0–300 | 0–300 |
| Lymphocyte, $\times 10^3$ | 1–4.8 | 1.7–7.0 |
| Eosinophil, $\times 10^3$ | 0.1–1.0 | 0–0.8 |
| Monocyte, $\times 10^3$ | 0.2–1.4 | 0–0.9 |
| Plate count, $\times 10^5$ | 2–9 | 3–7 |
| Fibrinogen, mg/dL | 150–300 | 150–300 |
| **NORMAL SERUM CHEMISTRY VALUES** | | |
| Albumin, g/dL | 2.1–4.3 | 2.7–3.8 |
| Calcium, mg/dL | 7.9–11.5 | 8.4–10.8 |
| Chloride, mEq/L | 104–125 | 112–124 |
| Cholesterol, mg/dL | 109–315 | 63–130 |
| Creatinine, mg/dL | 0.5–1.6 | 0–1.5 |
| Glucose, mg/dL | 65–127 | 65–129 |
| Phosphorus, mg/dL | 2.4–6.5 | 4.0–7.0 |
| Potassium, mEq/L | 3.9–5.7 | 3.8–5.4 |
| Sodium, mEq/L | 141–161 | 144–156 |
| Total carbon dioxide, mmol/L | 15–27 | 13–25 |
| Anion gap | 8–25 | 10–27 |
| Total bilirubin, mg/dL | 0.08–0.05 | 0–0.3 |
| Total protein, g/dL | 5.4–8.0 | 5.8–8.0 |
| BUN, mg/dL | 7.0–31 | 14–34 |
| Alkaline phosphatase, U/L | 12–110 | 6–93 |
| Alanine aminotransferase, U/L | 17–87 | 1–64 |
| Amylase, U/L | 223–1591 | 600–1500 |

*Continued*

**Table 1-3.** *(continued)*

| Test | Canine | Feline |
|------|--------|--------|
| Aspartate aminotransferase, U/L | | 0–34 |
| Complete alkaline phosphatase, U/L | 0–40 | |
| Creatine phosphokinase, U/L | 47–329 | 0–75 |
| γ-glutamyltransferase, U/L | 1–11 | 0–3 |
| Lipase, U/L | 25–534 | 3–125 |
| Pre-bile *acids,* mmol/L | 0–8 | 1–6 |
| Post-bile *acids,* mmol/L | 2–15 | 7–10 |
| **NORMAL COAGULATION VALUES** | | |
| Prothrombin time, s | 6–10 | 5–10 |
| Partial thromboplastin time, s | 16–24 | 19–22 |
| Activated coagulation time, s | 60–90 | < 65 |
| Fibrin split products, mg/mL | < 40 | < 8 |

**Table 1-4. ASA Classification of Physical Status**

| Category | Physical Status | Examples |
|----------|-----------------|----------|
| I | Normal healthy patient | No discernible disease; animal entered for ovariohysterectomy, ear trim, caudectomy, castration |
| II | Patient with mild systemic disease | Skin tumor, fracture without shock, uncomplicated hernia, cryptorchidectomy, localized infection, compensated cardiac disease |
| III | Patient with severe systemic disease | Fear, dehydration, anemia, cachexia, moderate hypovolemia |
| IV | Patient with severe systemic disease that is a constant threat to life | Uremia, toxemia, severe dehydration and hypovolemia, anemia, cardiac decompensation, emaciation, high fever |
| V | Moribund patient not expected to survive 24 h with or without operation | Extreme shock and dehydration, terminal malignancy or infection, severe trauma |

| | Age | | |
|---|---|---|---|
| **Physical Status** | **6 Months** | **6 Months–6 Years** | **> 6 Years** |
| I and II | Packed cell volume, total protein, glucose | Packed cell volume, total protein, BUN | Packed cell volume, total protein, BUN, creatinine, urinalysis, ECG |
| III | CBC, urinalysis, glucose, BUN, creatinine | CBC, urinalysis, surgery profile,[a] ECG | CBC, urinalysis, complete profile,[b] ECG |
| IV and V | CBC, urinalysis, complete profile | CBC, urinalysis, complete profile,[b] ECG | CBC, urinalysis, complete profile,[b] ECG |

**Table 1-5. Guidelines for Laboratory Screening Tests Based on Physical Status and Age**

[a]Glucose, BUN, creatinine, aspartate aminotransferase, alanine aminotransferase, and alkaline phosphatase.
[b]Surgery profile plus total protein, albumin, potassium, sodium, chloride, calcium, phosphorus, total carbon dioxide, anion, total bilirubin, and creatine phosphokinase.

same), the anesthetic to be employed, and the physical status of the patient. Anesthetic factors that can affect risk include the duration of anesthesia (fatigue increases risk) and the choice of anesthetic.

**F. Anesthetic Plan**

After conducting the patient evaluation; determining the ASA classification of physical status and the operative risk, the patient is prepared for anesthesia by developing the anesthetic plan (Table 1-6).

## II. PATIENT PREPARATION

**A. Food**

Food should be withheld for 12 h in most patients. Small mammals, birds, and neonates may become hypoglycemic with only a few hours of starvation. Vomiting and aspiration are more likely to occur in an animal with a full stomach.

## B.    Water

Water is allowed until preanesthetic drugs are given. Many old dogs suffer from nephritis. Even though they may remain compensated under ideal conditions, the stress of hospitalization, water deprivation, and anesthesia—even without surgery—may cause acute decompensation. Administering intravenous fluids before and during anesthesia helps maintain adequate blood pressure and urine production. The patient's serum electrolytes and acid–base status guide the type of crystalloid fluid administered.

## C.    Pre-Emptive Administration

Pre-emptive administration of antibiotics and analgesics enhances the effectiveness of therapy.

---

**Table 1-6. Considerations for Anesthetic Plan**

I. Procedure to be performed
   A. Duration
     i. < 15 min
     ii. 15–60 min
     iii. > 1 h
   B. Type of procedure
     i. Minor medical or surgical
     ii. Major invasive surgery
     iii. Anticipated postsurgical pain
II. Available assistance and equipment
   A. Assistance
     i. Anesthetic machine
     ii. Type of inhalation anesthetic
III. Temperament of the patient
   A. Quiet, relaxed, calm
   B. Nervous, excitable
   C. Vicious
   D. Moribund, comatose
IV. Physical status (ASA category, I–V)
V. Species and breed factors
   A. Sight hounds
   B. Brachycephalic
   C. Toy breeds

### D. Corrective Action

Anemia, hypoproteinemia, and hypovolemia should be corrected by administration of whole blood, blood components, colloids, and balanced electrolyte solutions. Patients in shock without blood loss or in a state of nutritional deficiency will benefit by administration of plasma or plasma expanders. Corticosteroids may also be indicated.

### E. Respiratory Concerns

In respiratory compromised patients, oxygen administration by nasal catheter or mask may be beneficial. A tracheotomy may be performed under local anesthesia before induction. Intrapleural air or fluid should be removed by aspiration. In laboratory animals (especially rats, guinea pigs, mice, and rabbits), chronic respiratory disease may be endemic, and in primates tuberculosis may be encountered. In these species, chamber oxygenation may be prudent before induction.

### F. Cardiac Concerns

Severe heart disease is a contraindication for general anesthesia. If such animals must be anesthetized, therapy with appropriate inotropes, angiotensin-converting enzyme (ACE) inhibitors, antiarrhythmic drugs, and diuretics should be given to stabilize the patient prior to anesthesia.

### G. Body Position

The patient should not be placed in a position (head-down tilt) that will further compromise vital physiologic functions (homeostasis).

## III. SELECTION OF ANESTHETIC

### A. Properties

Properties of the ideal anesthetic include the following: (1) not dependent on its metabolism for termination of its action; (2) rapid induction, controllable depth, quick recovery; (3) no cardiopulmonary depression and no side effects; (4) nonirritant to tissues; (5) inexpensive, stable, and nonflammable; and (6) no special equipment required for its use.

**B. Selection**

No one anesthetic drug possesses all of these properties; therefore, selection is a compromise, based on an appraisal of the following: (1) procedure to be performed, (2) duration of the procedure, (3) level of noxious stimuli anticipated (analgesic requirement), (4) muscle relaxation requirement, (5) species peculiarities (anatomic and physiologic), (6) patient disease or pathology (overall ASA physical status), (7) anesthetic history, (8) pharmacologic knowledge of anesthetics and analgesics, (9) personal experience with anesthetic drug or technique (expertise), and (10) protocol expense and equipment availability.

**C. Safety**

Safety of the patient is the overriding factor to consider when choosing the drugs and protocol to be used. In general, veterinarians are safest with anesthetic drugs they have used most frequently and with which they are most familiar. The art of administrating anesthesia comes with experience. Change from a familiar drug or anesthetic protocol to a new one is accompanied by a temporary increase in anesthetic risk. Nevertheless, a short-term increase in risk may be appropriate when there is compelling evidence of enhanced safety or patient care with the use of an unfamiliar drug or anesthetic technique. Generally, short procedures are done with short-acting, injectable drugs such as thiopental, propofol, and ketamine or combinations of these drugs with various tranquilizers, sedatives, and/or opioids. When anesthesia of longer duration is required, inhalation or balanced anesthetic techniques are preferable. Species differences may prevent the use of some drugs in some circumstances, but most anesthetics are efficacious in most species.

## IV. PHARMACOLOGY

**A. Definitions**

Pharmacology can be divided into pharmacokinetics and pharmacodynamics.

1. **Pharmacokinetics** is what the body does to a drug after its administration by any route (e.g., absorption, distribution, metabolism, and excretion).

2. **Pharmacodynamics** is what the drug does to the body and the mechanisms by which these responses occur (e.g., opioid receptor–mediated analgesia).

3. **Stereoselectivity** refers to the biologically active form of a molecule. Although most anesthetic drugs consist of racemic mixtures, drug stereoselectivity implies that only one isomer is active (e.g., D-ketamine is hypnotic and analgesic whereas L-ketamine produces unwanted side effects).

## B. Drug Response

Descriptions of drug responses are given in Table 1-7.

## C. Pharmacokinetics

The pharmacokinetics of injected drugs are characterized by the following factors.

1. **Two compartment models** illustrate the basic pharmacokinetics of anesthetic drugs after systemic administration (Fig. 1-1).

2. **Plasma concentration curves** characterize the distribution and elimination phases of a drug after its administration (Fig. 1-2).

### Table 1-7. Description of Drug Responses

| Response | Description |
| --- | --- |
| Hyperactivity | Unusually low dose produces the expected pharmacologic effect |
| Hypersensitivity | Allergy to a drug |
| Hyporeactivity | Unusually large dose is required to produce the expected pharmacologic effect |
| Tolerance | Hyporeactivity owing to chronic exposure to a drug; cross-tolerance is common between drugs that produce similar pharmacologic effects (alcohol and inhaled anesthetics) |
| Tachyphylaxis | Tolerance that develops acutely; reflects cellular tolerance |

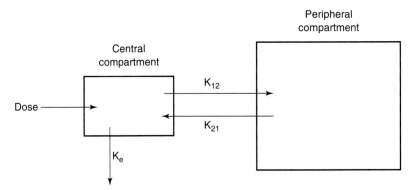

**Figure 1-1.** A two-compartment pharmacokinetic model derived from a biexponential plasma decay curve. $K_{12}$ and $K_{21}$, rate constants characterizing intercompartmental transfer of drugs; $K_e$, is the rate constant for overall drug elimination from the body.

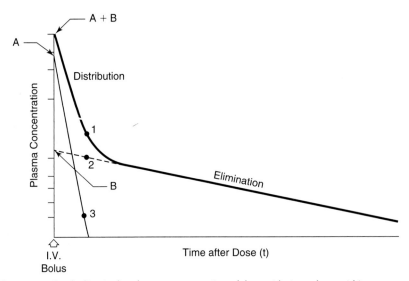

**Figure 1-2.** The decline in the plasma concentration of drug with time after rapid intravenous injection into the central compartment. The two distinct phases that characterize this (biexponential) curve are referred to as the distribution (*A*) and the elimination (*B*) phases.

3. **Rate of absorption** of a drug largely depends on its solubility and route of administration (Table 1-8).

4. **Drug distribution** is influenced by several factors: tissue perfusion, tissue solubility, tissue saturation, tissue permeability, protein binding, and drug ionization (Table 1-9).

**Volume of distribution** ($V_d$) is a mathematical expression of the distribution characteristics of a drug in the body as a function of plasma concentration. The value of $V_d$ is large for lipid-soluble drugs that are poorly bound to plasma protein (e.g., thiopental) and small for highly protein-bound drugs with low lipid solubility (e.g., nondepolarizing muscle relaxants).

5. **Drug clearance** occurs primarily by renal excretion and/or liver metabolism. Clearance of a drug in propor-

---

**Table 1-8. Route of Administration and Absorption**

| Route | Absorption Characteristics |
|-------|----------------------------|
| Gastrointestinal | Large surface area of the small intestine provides principal site of absorption; hepatic first-pass effect may decrease the amount of drug delivered to the systemic circulation |
| Oral transmucosal (sublingual, buccal, nasal mucosa) | Hepatic first-pass effect does not occur |
| Transdermal | Provides sustained therapeutic plasma concentrations |
| Parenteral (subcutaneous, intramuscular, intravenous) | Rapid and precise drug delivery is best achieved by intravenous administration |

---

**Table 1-9. Influence of Drug Ionization on Pharmacokinetic and Dynamic Actions**

| Characteristic | Non-Ionized | Ionized |
|----------------|-------------|---------|
| Pharmacologic effects | Active | Inactive |
| Solubility | Lipids | Water |
| Cross lipid barriers (gastrointestinal tract, blood–brain barrier, placenta) | Yes | No |
| Renal excretion | No | Yes |
| Hepatic metabolism | Yes | No |

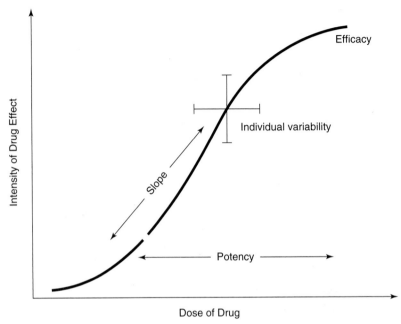

**Figure 1-3.** Dose–response curves are characterized by differences in potency, slope, efficacy, and individual response.

tion to the amount in the plasma is defined as first-order kinetics whereas clearance of a constant amount of drug from the plasma per unit of time is referred to as zero-order kinetics. Renal clearance of water-soluble compounds is more efficient than that for highly lipid soluble compounds.

6. **Drug metabolism** converts active lipid-soluble drugs into water-soluble and often inactive metabolites. Microsomal enzymes are largely responsible for this conversion and are located primarily in the liver.

7. The **dose–response curve** illustrates drug potency, receptor activity, efficacy, and individual response (Fig. 1-3). Drug potency makes little difference, as long as an effective dose can be administered conveniently (e.g., a reasonable volume). The efficacy of a drug (intrinsic activity) is important in determining the drug's safety margin and therapeutic index. Variability of a drug action

reflects differences in the pharmacokinetics and dynamics among individuals (e.g., genetic differences in metabolic pathways and receptor sensitivity) (Table 1-10).

## D. Pharmacodynamics

The pharmacodynamics of a drug is affected by the presence and action of receptors and the drug's concentration.

1. **Receptors** are protein macromolecules found in the lipid bilayer of cell membranes that are responsive to endogenous and/or exogenous substances. Exogenous molecules are temporary passengers for these receptors. Receptors can be classified on the basis of the antagonistic effect of specific molecules (e.g., naloxone) and the relative potencies of known agonists (e.g., opioids).

2. Receptor concentration in cell membranes is dynamic, increasing **(up-regulation)** or decreasing **(down-regulation)** in response to the degree and duration of stimuli.

3. **Plasma concentration** typically provides a direct relationship between dose administered and intensity of the drug effect (receptor concentration). Loading doses are usually necessary to produce effective plasma concentrations;

---

**Table 1-10. Factors Responsible for Variations in Drug Responses among Individuals of the Same Species or Breed**

I. Pharmacokinetics
   A. Bioavailability
   B. Renal function
   C. Liver function
   D. Cardiac function
   E. Patient age
II. Pharmacodynamics
   A. Enzyme activity
   B. Genetic differences
III. Drug interactions
   A. See page 18

these are followed by lower maintenance doses that match the plasma clearance of the drug. Intermittent dosing results in abrupt increases and decreases in plasma drug concentration and effect. Continuous rate infusion (CRI) maintains effective plasma concentrations and a more constant drug effect.

## E.    Mechanisms of Anesthesia

Several theories have been proposed to explain the mechanisms of anesthesia.

1.    *Meyer-Overton Theory (Critical Volume)*
Cell membrane expansion caused by dissolved anesthetic molecules distort channels, inhibiting sodium ion flux and damping the action potential necessary for synaptic transmission.

2.    *Protein Receptor Theory*
A crucial degree of protein receptor occupancy within the CNS may be responsible for the steep dose–response curve observed with inhaled anesthetics. Alternatively, activation of inhibitory guanine (G) protein may increase potassium conductance, resulting in membrane hyperpolarization.

3.    *GABA Receptor Activation Theory*
Inhaled and injectable anesthetics may activate γ-aminobutyric acid (GABA), glutamate, and calcium channels and as such share common cellular actions (Table 1-11), resulting in CNS depression and anesthesia.

4.    *Neurobiologic Theory*
A neurobiologic basis for the hypnotic and sedative effects of anesthetics results from activation of the GABA-receptor-chloride-ionophore complex, resulting in cell hyperpolarization and inhibition of neuronal transmission. Sedative-hypnotics or analgesics alone cannot induce anesthesia, whereas combinations of a benzodiazepine, propofol, or barbiturate with an opioid or $\alpha_2$-agonist produce anesthesia equivalent to that achieved with an inhalant (e.g., isoflurane) (Fig. 1-4).

| Table 1-11. Mechanisms of GABA Inhibition | |
| --- | --- |
| **Drug** | **Mechanism** |
| Benzodiazepines | Enhance inhibition by increasing binding of endogenously released GABA |
| Barbiturates, etomidate, propofol, volatile anesthetics | Enhance inhibition by modifying the receptor–chloride channel so that it remains open longer after binding endogenously released GABA |
| Volatile anesthetics | Inhibit GABA disposal |
| α-adrenergic agonists | Enhance presynaptic release of GABA |

Modified from Tanelin DL, Kosek P, Mody I, MacIver MB. The role of the GABA$_A$ receptor/chloride channel complex in anesthesia. Anesthesiology 1993;78:757–775.

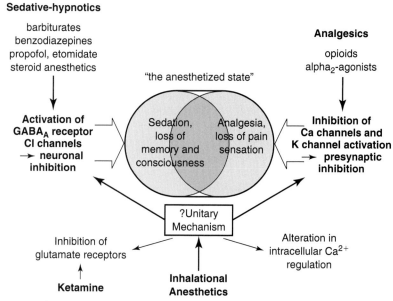

**Figure 1-4.** The major pathways for sedative-hypnotics and analgesics in generating the anesthetized state considered to be characteristic of volatile anesthetics. Reprinted with permission from Lynch C, Pancrazio JJ. Snails, spiders and stereospecificity—is there a role for calcium channels in anesthetic mechanisms? Anesthesiology 1994;81:1–5.

## V.   DRUG INTERACTIONS

### A.   Multiple Drug Administration

**Multiple drug administration** is frequently used to manage anesthesia (balanced anesthesia). First drugs may be given before induction to calm the patient, empty the gastrointestinal tract, reduce anesthetic requirements, or counteract side effects of the anesthetic drugs or surgery. Then one anesthetic drug or a combination of drugs may be administered to induce anesthesia and another drug may be used to maintain anesthesia. Neuromuscular blockers may be given, and other drugs may be administered intraoperatively to provide postoperative analgesia or protection from infection, or to maintain physiologic variables within a target range. The patient may also be receiving medications to treat diseases (e.g., bacterial infections, endocrine disturbances, cardiovascular and CNS disease, and endoparasitism or ectoparasitism).

### B.   Sources of Drug Interactions

**Drug interactions** result from the administration of (1) two drugs in one formulation, as a fixed-dose mixture; (2) two drugs in separate formulations; (3) a second drug during prolonged use of the first drug; or (4) two drugs given at specific time intervals. Drug interactions can be either pharmacokinetic or pharmacodynamic in nature. Pharmacokinetic interactions produce changes in drug concentration at the receptor site by altering absorption, elimination, or distribution. Pharmacodynamic interactions occur when one drug alters the response to another.

### C.   Pharmacokinetic Interactions

**Pharmacokinetic interactions** include pharmaceutic incompatibility, alteration of absorption, alteration of drug-biotransformation enzymes, alteration of protein binding, changes in renal or hepatic clearance, changes in excretion through the lungs, and changes in distribution.

1.   **Pharmaceutic incompatibility** occurs because one drug or drug vehicle reacts chemically or physically with another when two or more drug formulations are mixed. Differ-

ences in pH can cause the drugs to precipitate (e.g., ketamine combined with thiopental). Diazepam is in an organic vehicle and forms an emulsion when mixed with aqueous solutions (e.g., thiopental or ketamine). Mix drugs only when absolutely certain that no undesirable interaction will occur.

2.  **Alteration in absorption** may be influenced by a second drug. Epinephrine added to a local anesthetic prolongs the duration of action by decreasing blood flow and thus delaying local anesthetic absorption. In eutectic mixtures, neither drug is effective alone; but when combined, the eutectic mixture is effective (e.g., prilocaine and lidocaine surface analgesic).

3.  Alterations of drug **biotransformation enzymes** may either shorten or prolong the duration of action of a drug, depending on the importance of biotransformation in terminating the action of a drug, whether an active product is formed, and whether biotransformation is increased or decreased. Phenobarbital and phenytoin induce mixed-function oxidases that can shorten sleep time (e.g., hexobarbital) or increase the production of toxic products from drugs such as methoxyflurane (organofluorides). Chloramphenicol inhibits hepatic microsomal enzymes, prolonging the half-life of anesthetic drugs metabolized by this system, e.g., pentobarbital. Inhibition of plasma cholinesterase by organophosphorus compounds prolong the duration of action of succinylcholine.

4.  **Alterations in protein binding, blood flow, and ventilation** can result from concurrent drug administration. Many drugs are extensively bound to plasma albumin (acidic drugs) or $\alpha_1$-acid glycoprotein (basic drugs). Drug displaced from protein distributes rapidly into tissue and is available for biotransformation and excretion. Blood flow changes are most noted when the liver or kidney extracts a high fraction of drug. Lidocaine, meperidine, and morphine are examples of drugs relevant to anesthesia that have high hepatic extractions. Inhalational anesthetics, such as halothane, reduce hepatic blood flow. Drugs that

depress ventilation (e.g., opioids) may delay pulmonary excretion of inhalant anesthetics.

5.  **Changes in distribution** can affect the onset and duration of the action of a drug administered intravenously more profoundly than do changes in excretion and metabolism. Intravenous anesthetics such as the thiobarbiturates are typical examples. Thiopental given to a patient with low cardiac output results in the delivery of a higher-than-normal drug concentration to the brain and myocardium, further depressing cardiac function.

## D.  Pharmacodynamic Interactions

**Pharmacodynamic interactions** involve drug interactions at the same receptor sites or at different sites. These interactions can affect the cardiovascular, respiratory, and central nervous systems as well as the neuromuscular junction and metabolism. Agonist drugs, acting at specific receptor sites, induce a response. Antagonists bind to the same receptors and terminate the agonist's action. Examples include the opioids and benzodiazepines and their specific antagonists. Anticholinesterase compounds antagonize the action of nondepolarizing neuromuscular-blocking drugs by blocking the hydrolysis of endogenous acetylcholine (Ach), allowing Ach to accumulate and compete with the muscle relaxant drug for the receptor.

## E.  Nomenclature

The **nomenclature** commonly used to describe drug interactions are addition, synergism, potentiation, and antagonism. **Addition** refers to simple additivity of fractional doses of two or more drugs. For example, the minimum alveolar concentration (MAC) fractions of inhalant anesthetics are additive. **Synergism** refers to a response to fractional doses that is greater than the response to the sum of the fractional doses. **Potentiation** is enhancement of action of one drug by a second drug that has no detectable action of its own. **Antagonism** refers to the opposing action of two drugs. It may be competitive or noncompetitive. In competitive antagonism, the agonist and antagonist compete for the same receptor site. Noncompetitive antagonism occurs when the agonist and antagonist act via different receptors. Experimental approaches to determine these interactions include dose–response analysis (Fig. 1-5) and isobolographic analysis (Fig. 1-6).

**F.   Special Considerations**

The use of **anesthetic drugs** raises **special considerations** in regard to drug interactions; namely: (1) anesthetic drugs are rapidly acting; (2) the response to anesthetics is measured, often very precisely; (3) surgeons often rely on drug antagonism; and (4) anesthetic drugs are usually titrated to minimize the potential for overdose.

**G.   Complementary Pharmacodynamic Effects**

Anesthetic drugs frequently have **complementary pharmacodynamic effects** on the brain, but one agent may also antagonize an undesirable effect of another drug. Tiletamine produces sedation, immobility, amnesia, and marked analgesia; but it also may produce muscle rigidity and grand mal seizures. Zolazepam produces sedation, reduction of anxiety, and amnesia, and will prevent muscle rigidity and seizures. Other examples of drugs with complementary action include ketamine and diazepam or butorphanol and medetomidine. An example of an undesirable interaction is the response to neuromuscular blockers in patients receiving antibiotics or other drugs (e.g., aminoglycosides, polymyxin, or magnesium) that may enhance and prolong postoperative muscle paralysis.

# VI.   ASSESSMENT OF ANESTHETIC ACTION

**A.   General Anesthesia**

**General anesthesia** has been simply defined as complete unconsciousness but more accurately requires all of the following components: unconsciousness, insensitivity to pain, muscle relaxation, and absence of reflex response. Depth of anesthesia is often difficult to assess. Signs characterizing a continuum of progressive increases in CNS depression and analgesia may not occur with some drugs and drug combinations. For example, dissociatives do not induce the typical ocular signs of increasing CNS depression. Nevertheless, recognizing the signs characteristic of the four stages of

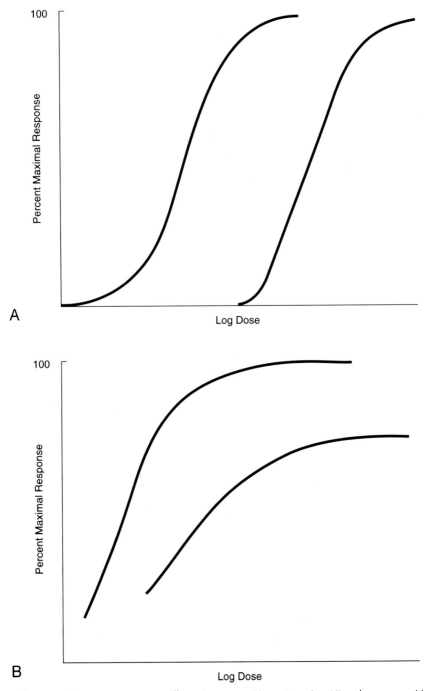

**Figure 1-5.** Dose–response curves illustrating competitive antagonism (A) and noncompetitive antagonism (B). Dose–response curve A is shifted to the right in the presence of an antagonist, but the shape of the curve is not changed. Dose–response curve B is shifted to the right in the presence of an antagonist, and the maximal response to the agonist is reduced.

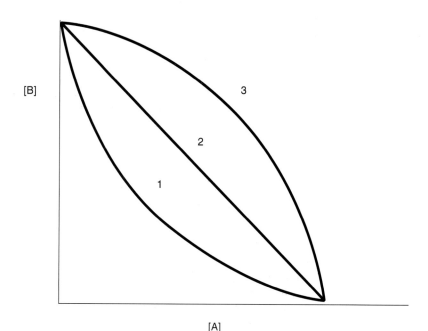

**Figure 1-6.** Isobolograms for the response to mixtures of drugs. The sets of concentrations of drugs *A* and *B,* which as a mixture produce an effect (e.g., 50% of a maximal response), are plotted. Strict *additivity,* which means [A] + [B] = a constant, results in a curve with a slope of −1 (*2*). If the curve is concave (*3*), some antagonism is present; if the curve is convex (*1*), synergism is present.

anesthesia induced by most anesthetics allows the veterinarian to determine whether the required intensity of CNS depression has been achieved or whether it is insufficient or too much.

### B.    Stages of General Anesthesia

For descriptive purposes, the levels of CNS depression induced by anesthetics have been divided into four stages, depending on a variety of respiratory, ocular, and neuromuscular signs exhibited by the patient (Fig. 1-7). These stages are best seen when slower acting inhalant anesthetics are administered, probably because considerable time is required for an anesthetic concentration to accrue in the CNS. This allows the signs to become apparent. With some intravenous anesthetics (e.g., dissociatives) or the concurrent use of preanesthetic sedatives, the assessment of anesthetic-induced depression is difficult, and these signs are not uniformly apparent. It should be emphasized that no clear division exists between the stages, one blends into the next. In addition, variation in response among species and patients is to be expected.

1. *Stage I*

   Stage I is termed the stage of voluntary movement and is defined as lasting from initial administration to loss of consciousness. Excited, apprehensive animals may struggle violently and voluntarily hold their breath for short periods. Epinephrine release causes a strong rapid heartbeat, and salivation is frequent in some species, as are urination and defecation. With the approach of stage II, the animal becomes progressively ataxic, loses its ability to stand, and assumes lateral recumbency.

2. *Stage II*

   Stage II is called the stage of delirium or involuntary movement. As the CNS becomes depressed, the patient loses all voluntary control. By definition, this stage lasts from loss of consciousness to the onset of a regular pattern of breathing. The patient reacts to external stimuli by violent reflex struggling, breath holding, tachypnea, and hyperventilation. Continued catecholamine release causes a fast, strong heartbeat, and the pupils may be widely dilated. Eyelash and palpebral reflexes are prominent. The larynx of cats is very sensitive

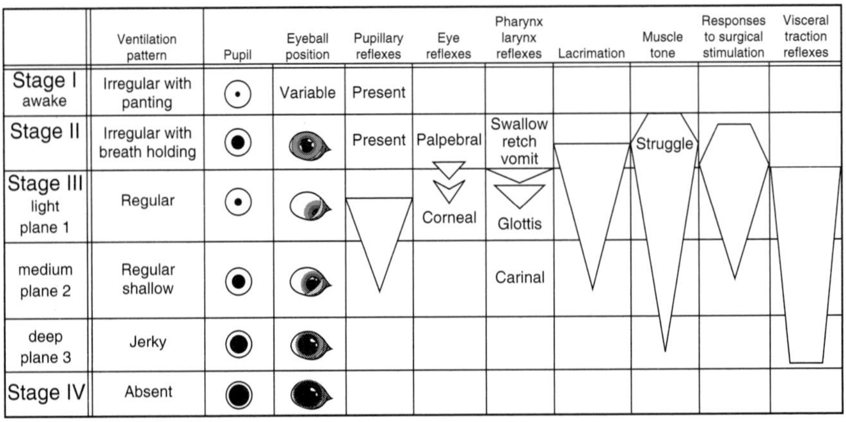

| | Ventilation pattern | Pupil | Eyeball position | Pupillary reflexes | Eye reflexes | Pharynx larynx reflexes | Lacrimation | Muscle tone | Responses to surgical stimulation | Visceral traction reflexes |
|---|---|---|---|---|---|---|---|---|---|---|
| Stage I awake | Irregular with panting | | Variable | Present | | | | | | |
| Stage II | Irregular with breath holding | | | Present | Palpebral | Swallow retch vomit | | Struggle | | |
| Stage III light plane 1 | Regular | | | | Corneal | Glottis | | | | |
| medium plane 2 | Regular shallow | | | | | Carinal | | | | |
| deep plane 3 | Jerky | | | | | | | | | |
| Stage IV | Absent | | | | | | | | | |

**Figure 1-7.** Signs associated with the stages of general anesthesia.

at this stage, and stimulation may result in laryngeal spasms. Jaw tone is still present, and attempts at endotracheal intubation are met with struggling and may initiate vomition.

3.  *Stage III*
    Stage III is the stage of surgical anesthesia and is characterized by unconsciousness with progressive depression of the reflexes. Muscular relaxation develops, and ventilation becomes slow and regular. Vomiting and swallowing reflexes are lost. This stage has been further divided into planes 1 to 4 to give finer differentiation. Other authors have suggested the simpler classification of light, medium, and deep. Light anesthesia persists until eyeball movement ceases. Medium anesthesia is characterized by progressive intercostal paralysis; and deep anesthesia, by diaphragmatic respiration. A medium depth of unconsciousness or anesthesia has traditionally been considered a light plane of surgical anesthesia (stage III; plane 2), characterized by stable respiration and pulse rate, abolished laryngeal reflexes, a sluggish palpebral reflex, a strong corneal reflex, and adequate muscle relaxation and analgesia for most surgical procedures. Deep surgical anesthesia (stage III; plane 3) is characterized by decreased intercostal muscle function and tidal volume, increased respiration rate, profound muscle relaxation, diaphragmatic breathing, a weak corneal reflex, and a centered and dilated pupil.

4.  *Stage IV*
    In stage IV, the CNS is extremely depressed, and respirations cease. The heart continues to beat only for a short time. Blood pressure is at the shock level, capillary refill of visible mucous membranes is markedly delayed, and the pupils are widely dilated. The anal and bladder sphincters relax. Death quickly intervenes unless immediate resuscitative steps are taken. If the anesthetic is withdrawn and artificial respiration is initiated before heart action stops, these effects may be overcome, and the patient will go through the stages in reverse order.

## VII. RECORD KEEPING

### A. Recorded Items

Among the **items recorded** on the anesthetic record are (1) species, breed, age, sex, weight, and physical status of the animal; (2) surgical procedure or other reason for anesthesia; (3) preanesthetic agents given; (4) anesthetic agents used and method of administration; (5) person administering anesthesia (veterinarian, technician, student, lay personnel); (6) duration of anesthesia; (7) supportive measures; (8) difficulties encountered and methods of correction.

### B. Anesthetic Record

An **anesthetic record** should be made on each patient to maintain a **legal record** of significant events and to enhance **recognition of trends** in monitored parameters. The record should include all drugs administered and the dose, time, and route of administration. Monitored parameters should be recorded on a regular basis (at least every 10 min) during anesthesia. If a veterinarian, technician, or other responsible person is unable to remain with the patient continuously, a responsible person should check the patient's status on a regular basis (at least every 5 min) during anesthesia and recovery. When the veterinarian is alone in the room, audible heart and respiratory monitors are suggested. In the best of situations, a person solely dedicated to managing and caring for the anesthetized patient remains with the patient continuously until the end of the recovery period.

## VIII. RECOVERY

### A. Early Recovery

During recovery, anesthesia lightens and excitement and motor activity may occur (stage II). Every effort should be made to avoid stimulation of the animal at this time. Coursing breeds, such as greyhounds, Russian wolfhounds, and Afghans, are particularly prone to this phenomenon. The use of **postoperative sedation** can do much to minimize excitement.

**B. Close Observation**

While the animal remains unconscious or immobile, vital signs should be recorded at 10-min intervals until the animal regains consciousness. **Close observation** is especially important until extubation and the return of coughing and swallowing reflexes. The patient should be covered to conserve body heat, because shivering increases oxygen and energy requirements, sometimes leading to hypoglycemia. Incubators are used in many laboratories in which birds, rodents, and primates are anesthetized. Birds should be housed at 100°F; mice, hamsters, and small primates at 95°F; rats, guinea pigs and rabbits at 90°F; and cats, dogs, and similar carnivores at 77 to 86°F. Fluids should be warmed to body temperature.

**C. Respiratory Precautions**

The tongue should be pulled forward to preclude its blocking the pharynx. In brachycephalic breeds and in animals in which respiratory function is compromised, an endotracheal tube should remain in place until upper airway reflexes and jaw movements return. Sternal recumbency is preferred. **Respiratory failure** may also result from: continuing drug-induced respiratory depression, postextubation spasm or glottic edema, diffusion hypoxia, mechanical splinting associated with pain and/or dressings, and persistent hypoventilation and/or atelectasis.

**D. Bandaging**

**Constrictive bandaging** of the head and throat must be avoided because of the danger of asphyxiation. Occasionally, cats that have been tightly bandaged around the abdomen show evidence of posterior paralysis on recovery.

**E. Pain Management**

A patient should not be returned to its owner until it is completely recovered from anesthesia and is demonstrating normal demeanor. Continued unusual behavior is often indicative of unrelenting pain. Analgesic drugs should be administered as needed in the recovery period and also dispensed for continued pain management when the patient is discharged.

# Chapter 2

---

## Perioperative Pain and Its Management

### Introductory Comments

*One of the essential goals of anesthesia is the control of pain and maintenance of homeostasis in the face of pain-inducing insults. Pain commonly arises from activation of a discrete set of receptors and neural pathways by noxious stimuli (nociception). It is an awareness of acute or chronic discomfort occurring in various degrees of severity resulting from injury or disease and is accompanied by fear, anxiety, and panic. Acute pain is the result of a traumatic, surgical, or infectious event that is abrupt in onset and relatively short in duration. Chronic pain persists beyond the usual course of an acute disease and may persist or recur for months or years. This type of pain is seldom permanently alleviated by analgesics, but may respond to tranquilizers or psychotropic drugs. Acute pain is a symptom of disease, whereas chronic pain is itself a disease. Acute pain leads to behavioral changes and limits of activity that are protective. Chronic pain does not serve a biologic function and imposes detrimental stresses on the patient. Veterinarians are becoming aware of the importance of pre-emptive analgesia as it relates to pain management even in the most routine and minor surgical procedures. It appears that the administration of analgesics before the onset of surgical stimulus decreases the analgesic requirements and intensity of postoperative pain and catabolic responses that accompany surgery.*

**Definitions**
**Classification of Pain**
**Nociception**
**Pain Management**

---

## I.  DEFINITIONS

**Allodynia:** Pain resulting from a stimulus that does not normally provoke pain.

28

**Analgesia:** Absence of pain in the presence of stimuli that would normally be painful.

**Anesthesia:** Absence of all sensory modalities; i.e., the inability to perceive painful stimuli.

**Anesthetics:** Drugs that induce regional anesthesia (i.e., in one part of the body) or general anesthesia (i.e., unconsciousness).

**Anxiety:** Emotional state that makes pain less tolerable; in the absence of pre-emptive analgesia, preoperative anxiety may predict the intensity of postoperative pain.

**Causalgia:** Syndrome of prolonged burning pain, allodynia, and hyperpathia after a traumatic nerve lesion, often combined with vasomotor and sudomotor dysfunction and later trophic changes.

**Central pain:** Pain associated with a lesion of the CNS.

**Central sensitization:** Increased excitability of neurones in the spinal cord to nociceptive afferent input.

**Deafferentation pain:** Caused by loss of sensory input into the CNS, as occurs with avulsion of the brachial plexus or other types of peripheral nerve lesions, or caused by pathology of the CNS.

**Dermatome:** Sensory segmental supply to the skin and subcutaneous tissue.

**Distress:** External expression of suffering through emotion or behavior (e.g, fear, anxiety, hyperactivity, aggression, or fractiousness).

**Hyperalgesia:** Increased response to a stimulation that is normally painful.

**Hyperesthesia:** Increased sensitivity to stimulation, excluding special senses.

**Hypoalgesia:** Diminished sensitivity to noxious stimulation.

**Hypoesthesia:** Diminished sensitivity to stimulation, excluding special senses.

**Neuralgia:** Pain in the distribution of a nerve or nerves.

**Neuritis:** Inflammation of a nerve or nerves.

**Neuropathy:** Disturbance of function or pathologic change in a nerve.

**Nociception:** Reception, conduction, and central nervous processing of nerve signals generated by the stimulation of nociceptors; it is the physiologic process that, when carried to completion, results in the conscious perception of pain.

**Nociceptor:** Naked afferent nerve ending preferentially sensitive to a noxious stimulus or to a stimulus that would become noxious if prolonged.

**Nociceptor threshold:** Minimum strength of a stimulus that will cause a nociceptor to generate a nerve impulse.

**Noxious stimulus:** Stimulus that is actually or potentially damaging to body tissue; its intensity and quality are adequate to trigger nociceptive reactions in an animal, including pain in people.

**Pain (detection) threshold:** Least experience of pain that a subject can recognize; the point at which a subject just begins to feel pain when a noxious stimulus is being applied in an ascending trial or at which pain disappears in a descending trial. Relatively constant among individuals and species; in most cases it is higher than the nociceptor threshold.

**Pain tolerance:** Greatest level of pain that a subject will tolerate. Varies considerably among individuals, both human and animal; influenced greatly by the individual's prior experience, environment, stress, and drugs.

**Pain tolerance range:** Arithmetic difference between the pain detection threshold and the pain tolerance threshold.

**Peripheral sensitization:** Decrease in the pain threshold at the site of injury and its surrounding tissues caused by the release of a variety of mediators (e.g., bradykinin, norepinephrine, histamine, cytokinins, and prostanoids); results in hypersensitivity to painful and nonpainful low-intensity stimuli, which causes hyperalgesia and allodynia, respectively.

**Pre-emptive analgesia:** Establishment of analgesia before the onset of pain stimuli to prevent central and peripheral sensitization processes that, if left unabated, results in hyperalgesia.

**Projected pain:** Unlocalized pain occurring in association with superficial pain that is often precisely localized.

**Reactions:** Combination of reflexes that do not involve the cerebral cortex and are designed to produce widespread movement in relation to the application of a stimulus; mass reflexes not under voluntary control. Even though pain thresholds may be similar, reactions may vary among individuals.

**Reflexes:** Involuntary, purposeful, and orderly responses to a stimulus. Anatomic basis for the reflex arc consists of a receptor; a primary afferent nerve fiber associated with the receptor; a region of integration in the spinal cord or brainstem (synapses); and a lower motor neuron leading to an effector organ, such as skeletal muscles (somatic reflexes), smooth muscles, or glands (visceral reflexes).

**Responses:** Willful movement of the body or parts of the body; cannot occur without involvement of the somatosensory cerebral cortex; a decerebrate animal can give a reaction but not a response.

**Somatic pain:** Usually used to describe input from body tissues other than viscera; sharp, stabbing, well-localized pain typically arising from skin, skeletal muscle, and the peritoneum. Examples include skin incision and peritoneal irritation.

**Suffering:** Unpleasant emotional state that is internalized; can be provoked by pain or by pain-free, non-tissue-damaging external stimuli, such as denial of the fulfillment of an animal's natural instincts or needs (e.g., maternal deprivation and absence of social contacts).

**Transcutaneous electric nerve stimulation (TENS):** Activation of large afferent fibers that produces a counterirritant effect through inhibition of smaller pain fibers; efficacy of this technique is based on the concept of the dorsal horn gate control theory.

**Visceral pain:** Originates from visceral tissues and is not well localized; receptors are sparsely distributed, so incision does not cause intense pain. It radiates, is often rhythmic, and may be referred to the body surface of the same dermatome.

## II.  CLASSIFICATION OF PAIN

### A.   Organic and Psychological Pain

Pain can be classified as **organic** or **psychological** in origin. Organic pain may be subdivided into two types of nociceptive responses (**somatic** and **visceral**). An additional type of organic pain associated with damage to, or changes within, the nervous system is commonly referred to as neuropathic pain. Nociceptive and **neuropathic pain** have similar physiologic characteristics, although nociceptive pain is usually quite responsive to opioid and NSAIDs, whereas neuropathic pain often is not.

### B.   Physiologic and Pathologic Pain

Pain can also be classified as either physiologic or pathologic in nature.

1.  **Physiologic pain** results from recognition of noxious amounts of heat, cold, or pressure and is protective to the animal.

    a.    **Fast pain** starts abruptly, is well localized, ends quickly when the stimulus is removed, and is conducted by A-δ fibers.

    b.    **Slow pain** produces throbbing, burning, or aching sensations, is poorly localized, continues after removal of the stimulus, and is conducted by unmyelinated C fibers.

    c.    **Fast and slow pain** are often referred to as **first** and **second** pain.

2.  **Pathologic pain** is the result of inflammatory or neuropathic processes.

    a.    **Inflammatory pain** results from tissue damage (burning, freezing, surgery, hypoxia, etc.) and is characterized by the following terms.

        i.    **Primary hyperalgesia** refers to the sensitization of nociceptors at the site of injury that occurs when inflammatory mediators (e.g., prostaglandins, histamine, bradykinins, leukotrienes, nitric oxide, and other cytokines) are released from the afferent nerve endings **(peripheral sensitization)**.

        ii.    **Secondary hyperalgesia** refers to changes in the sensory processing of the peripheral and central nervous systems, termed **facilitation** or **wind up.** This process is mediated by release of glutamate, substance P and other neuropeptides that activate $N$-methyl-D-aspartate (NMDA), α-amino-3-hydroxy-5-methly-4-isoxazoleproprionate (AMPA), and natural killer cell 1 (NK-1) receptors that promote gene induction within the dorsal horn of the spinal cord **(central sensitization)**. Table 2-1 organizes dorsal horn responses into four modes, mediated by incoming sensory stimuli. These modes describe the intensity and duration of acute pain when present for days or longer after surgery or trauma. Constant input from peripheral nociceptors induces a shift

| Table 2-1. State-Dependent Processing in the Dorsal Horn (Clinical Syndromes) | | |
| --- | --- | --- |
| Mode | State | Syndrome |
| 1 | Control | Physiologic sensitivity |
| 2 | Suppressed | Hyposensitivity |
| 3 | Sensitized | Postinjury hypersensitivity; inflammatory pain; peripheral neuropathic pain |
| 4 | Reorganized | Peripheral neuropathic pain; central neuropathic pain |

from mode 2 (**suppressed state**) to mode 3 (**sensitized state**). Structural reorganization of the dorsal horn and aberrant processing are characteristic of mode 4, in which **neuropathic pain** is both central and peripheral in origin.

iii. **Allodynia:** low threshold response.

iv. **Field plasticity:** poorly localized sensations and increases in the size of the receptive fields.

b. **Neuropathic pain** can be peripheral or central in origin (Table 2-1). The spinal cord displays a form of memory. Brief nociceptive stimuli elicit prompt, brief responses; whereas more prolonged input evokes analgesia through supraspinal (diffuse noxious inhibitory control; DNIC) inhibitory mechanisms. More persistent or suprathreshold stimuli transform the dynamic damping behavior of the dorsal horn from stable to underdamped (hypersensitization or wind up) and then finally to an unstable state. Thus the dorsal horn can evolve from a system that minimizes and attenuates noxious information (mode 2) to one that exaggerates and prolongs it (mode 3), even to the point of becoming self-sustaining (central neuropathic pain, or mode 4). In addition, damage to the autonomic nervous system (ANS) can evoke reflex efferent activity. Reflex sympathetic dystrophy (causalgia) is an example of this kind of extreme pain.

## III. NOCICEPTION

### A. Nociception Defined

**Nociception** is the transduction, conduction, and central nervous processing of nerve signals generated by the stimulation of nociceptors. It is the physiologic process that, when carried to completion, results in the conscious perception of pain. Because the anatomic structures and neurophysiologic mechanisms leading to the perception of pain (nociception) are remarkably similar in human beings and animals, it is reasonable to assume that a stimulus that is painful to people, is damaging or potentially damaging to tissues, and induces escape and behavioral responses in an animal must be considered to be painful to that animal. Further evidence that animals have the capacity to suffer from pain includes the facts that animals exhibit signs of distress and learned avoidance behavior and that they vocalize in response to noxious (painful) stimuli. Pain may not always be overtly expressed and may be evidenced only by subtle changes in behavior or posture. A degree of anthropomorphism is appropriate and desirable, especially in situations that are known to cause pain in people. Nociception consists of four physiologic processes that are subject to pharmacologic modulation (Fig. 2-1).

1. **Transduction** is the translation of physical energy (noxious stimuli) into electrical activity at the peripheral nociceptor. These receptors are considered mechanosensitive, thermosensitive, and chemosensitive.

2. **Transmission** is the propagation of nerve impulses through the peripheral nervous system. Afferent sensory fibers consist of myelinated A-δ fibers, which conduct fast pain, and nonmyelinated C fibers, which conduct slower, dull pain.

3. **Modulation** occurs through the endogenous descending analgesic systems, which modify nociceptive transmission. These endogenous systems (opioid, serotonergic, and noradrenergic) modulate nociception through the inhibition of stimuli processing within spinal dorsal horn cells. Figure 2-2 shows a model of pain transmission through

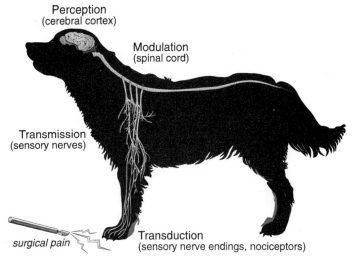

**Figure 2-1.** Nociception. The process of nociception consists of four physiologic processes, beginning at the end organ and ending in the cerebral cortex: transduction, transmission or conduction of nerve impulses, modulation within the spinal cord, and perception.

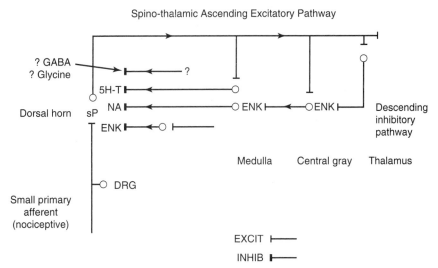

**Figure 2-2.** Pain transmission within the spinal cord. Primary afferent pain (nociceptive) signals travel through the dorsal root ganglion (*DRG*) to cells in the dorsal horn of the spinal cord, where substance P acts as the excitatory neurotransmitter. The endogenous endorphin (enkephalin; *ENK*) system is activated by pain signals that reach the thalamus. Activation of the descending inhibitory pain pathways by ENK results in inhibition of the dorsal horn neurons in the spinal cord through the release of inhibitory neurotransmitters, which may include serotonin (5-hydroxytryptamine; 5-HT), norepinephrine (*NA*), enkephalin (*ENK*), GABA, and glycine.

the peripheral and spinal pathways. Facilitatory pain receptors include substance P (NK-1 type), glutamate (NMDA type), and prostaglandin receptors. Spinal inhibitory receptors include γ-aminobutyric acid (GABA), opioid (μ, κ, δ), $α_2$ (types unknown), and adenosine ($A_1$ type) receptors.

4. **Perception** is the final process resulting from successful transduction, transmission, modulation, and integration of thalamocortical, reticular, and limbic function to produce the final conscious subjective and emotional experience of pain. Nociceptive input is modulated at every level of the sensory pathway, from the periphery to the cerebral cortex, where perception occurs. Deviations from normal behavior and altered physiologic responses are expressions of animal pain that must be appreciated in the absence of an animal's ability to communicate verbally. Deviations from normal can include (1) abnormal posture; (2) vocalization; (3) altered mentation (depression or aggression); (4) stereotypic behavior (licking, scratching, chewing); (5) altered ambulation (lameness, pacing); (6) tachycardia, tachypnea, and altered arterial blood pressure; (7) altered temperature; and (8) alterations in stress-related hormones (cortisol, norepinephrine, epinephrine), lactic acid, glucose, etc.

**B.    Strategies for Pain Management**

**Analgesia** in the strictest sense is an absence of pain, but clinically it is the reduction in the intensity of pain perceived. The goal should not be the complete elimination of pain but to make the pain as tolerable **(hypoalgesia)** as possible without undue depression of the patient. Analgesia in the clinical setting may be induced by obtunding or interrupting nociception at one or more points between the peripheral nociceptor and the cerebral cortex. Guidelines for accomplishing perioperative analgesia can be based on the following factors:

1. **Transduction** can be largely abolished by the use of local anesthetics infiltrated at the site of injury or incision or by an intravenous, intrapleural, or intraperitoneal injection. Systemically administered NSAIDs and intra-articular

opioid administration obtund transduction by decreasing the production of endogenous algogenic substances, such as prostaglandins, at the site of injury.

2.  **Transmission** can be abolished by local anesthetic blockade of peripheral nerves or nerve plexuses or by an epidural or subarachnoid injection.

3.  **Modulation** can be augmented by systemic or epidural injection of opioids and/or $\alpha_2$-adrenergic agonists. A novel method of systemic opioid administration is accomplished by a transdermal fentanyl patch delivery system that can effectively maintain analgesia from 48 to 72 h. Recent evidence also indicates that NSAIDs modulate spinal processing of painful stimuli. A single drug (tramadol) has been identified that simultaneously activates opioid receptors and aminergic (5-hydroxytryptamin and norepinephrine) descending inhibitory pathways within the spinal cord. Because of its rapid metabolism in animals, however, tramadol appears to be of limited value in nonhumans.

4.  **Perception** can be obtunded with general anesthetics or by systemic administration of opioids and $\alpha_2$-agonists either alone or in combination with other sedative–tranquilizers (see Fig. 1-4).

C.  **Pre-Emptive Analgesia**

**Preemptive analgesia** refers to the application of analgesic techniques before exposing the patient to noxious stimuli (surgical trespass). By so doing, the spinal cord is not exposed to the barrage of afferent nociceptive impulses that induce spinal hypersensitivity and the neuroplastic changes associated with the development of **allodynia** and **hyperalgesia.** This concept has gained acceptance as one of the most efficacious and cost-effective means of controlling postoperative pain and improving patient outcome.

D.  **Balanced Analgesia**

**Balanced** or **multimodal analgesia** is accomplished by administration of two or more classes of analgesic drugs that interfere

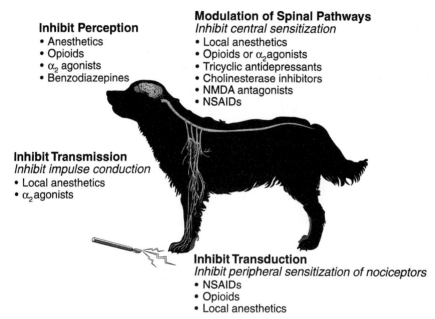

**Inhibit Perception**
- Anesthetics
- Opioids
- $\alpha_2$ agonists
- Benzodiazepines

**Modulation of Spinal Pathways**
*Inhibit central sensitization*
- Local anesthetics
- Opioids or $\alpha_2$ agonists
- Tricyclic antidepressants
- Cholinesterase inhibitors
- NMDA antagonists
- NSAIDs

**Inhibit Transmission**
*Inhibit impulse conduction*
- Local anesthetics
- $\alpha_2$ agonists

**Inhibit Transduction**
*Inhibit peripheral sensitization of nociceptors*
- NSAIDs
- Opioids
- Local anesthetics

**Figure 2-3.** Nociception—therapeutic intervention. A variety of drugs can be used to inhibit nociception by interfering with the processes of transduction, transmission, modulation, and/or perception. Classes of drugs commonly used to inhibit pain by altering each of these processes are shown. Multimodal analgesia can best be accomplished by pre-emptive administration of a combination of different classes of drugs that inhibit nociceptive processes at two or more sites. Pre-emptive analgesic administration can result in inhibition of both peripheral and central sensitization mechanisms. *NMDA,* N-methyl-D-Aspartate; *NSAIDS,* nonsteriodal anti-inflammatory drugs.

with nociception (Fig. 2-3). Transduction can be inhibited by NSAIDs, transmission obtunded by peripheral nerve block with a local anesthetic, and modulation enhanced (damping of somatosensory afferent pathways) by combined systemic or epidural opioids and/or $\alpha_2$-agonists. For example, butorphanol and medetomidine produce excellent sedation and analgesia, permitting many minor diagnostic and surgical procedures to be completed without injectable or inhalant anesthetics. Balanced multimodal analgesic techniques appear to offer several advantages. When used **pre-emptively,** analgesics can prevent or inhibit surgery-induced peripheral nociceptor sensitization (inflammation) and neuroplastic changes within the spinal cord (wind up); can prevent development of tachyphylaxis; can suppress the neuroendocrine response (stress) to pain and injury; and can shorten convalescence through improved tissue healing (decreased catabolic processes), maintenance of immune responses, (decreased infection), and improved patient mobility.

## IV. PAIN MANAGEMENT (DRUGS AND TECHNIQUES)

### A. Pre-Emptive Administration

It is appropriate to administer analgesics **pre-emptively.** The commonly stated reasons for withholding analgesics (e.g., to avoid opioid-induced respiratory depression or because pain relief would result in increased activity leading to self-injury) are seldom if ever valid. Accurate selection and dosing of analgesic drugs provides relief of pain without severe respiratory depression. Appropriate splinting, bandaging, or confinement prevent self-injury. Animals should not have to endure pain because of real or imagined sequelae to its relief. Pain-induced alterations in metabolism, endocrine balance, and cardiopulmonary function are well recognized and of serious consequence to the animal.

### B. Analgesics

Analgesics are drugs that primarily suppress pain or induce analgesia. Although actions and effects of most other drugs differ little among mammalian species, there are marked differences in responses to selected analgesics (e.g., **opioids**) that are independent of pharmacokinetics. The concentration of opioid receptors in the amygdala and frontal cortex of species that are depressed by opioids (e.g., dogs and primates) is nearly twice as great as in those species that become excited in response to opioids (e.g., horses and cats). By decreasing the dose, excitement can be avoided in species prone to bizarre reactions. Excitement may result indirectly from increased release of norepinephrine and dopamine, which may explain the mechanism whereby dopaminergic- and noradrenergic-blocking drugs, such as **phenothiazine** and **butyrophenone** tranquilizers, suppress clinical evidence of opioid-induced excitement. Because analgesia and excitement are mediated by different receptors (i.e., $\mu$ analgesia and phencyclidine excitement), they can occur concurrently and are not mutually exclusive.

## C.   Nonsteroidal Anti-Inflammatory Analgesics

Whereas opioids induce analgesia by interfering with nociceptive neural transmission centrally, the **nonsteroidal anti-inflammatory analgesics** (NSAIAs) act peripherally to decrease the production of algogenic substances, primarily prostanoids, which facilitate generation and conduction of impulses that give rise to pain. When administered before tissue damage, many NSAIAs suppress inflammation and the production and elaboration of kinins and prostaglandins. These drugs are effective primarily against pain of low to moderate intensity associated with inflammation. They are generally regarded as being useful for treating chronic pain of somatic or integumental origin but are less efficacious for visceral pain. In dogs, the pre-emptive administration of an injectable formulation of carprofen has been shown to induce superior postoperative analgesia with less sedation than meperidine administered after orthopedic surgery. The NSAIAs are generally not sufficient by themselves to relieve severe postoperative pain, but they can be used in combination with **opioids postoperatively** to good effect. Because NSAIAs and opioids have different mechanisms and sites of action, they can produce supra-additive or synergistic effects. Furthermore, they can be continued when opioids are no longer necessary.

## D.   $\alpha_2$-Adrenergic and Opioid Analgesics

$\alpha_2$-Adrenergic and opioid analgesics interact in ways that are not fully understood. They have been used to "rescue" opioid-induced analgesia that has waned after chronic opioid administration. The combination of an opioid and an $\alpha_2$-agonist enhances and prolongs analgesia in dogs and cats when given by systemic or epidural routes.

## E.   Dissociative-Induced Analgesia

**Dissociative**-induced analgesia is poorly understood, but it is believed that somatic analgesia results from the interruption or dissociation of ascending nociceptive input as it traverses the thalamoneocortical system. Low doses of dissociatives are often used for chemical restraint and immobilization of cats but may have to be supplemented with an analgesic for invasive visceral surgery. They are perhaps best viewed as antihyperalgesic drugs that interfere with central sensitization phenomena rather than primary analgesics. Ketamine may be particularly effective in obtunding pain arising from superficial surfaces (e.g., burn pain).

### F. Local Anesthetics

Analgesia can be induced by neural blockade of the sensory afferent nerves or tracts by local infiltration, by regional nerve blocks, or by epidural or intrathecal injection of **local anesthetics.** Analgesia so induced is complete in the area blocked. Intercostal nerve blockade and interpleural local anesthetic infusion have been advocated for relieving pain after a thoracotomy and may result in better alveolar ventilation postoperatively compared to opioid-induced analgesia.

### G. Injectable and Oral Analgesics

**Injectable analgesics** are given to control **acute pain,** whereas **oral** or **transdermal** preparations are preferred for **chronic pain** management. Generally, oral, rectal, and subcutaneous administration require longer onsets and result in lower plasma drug concentration than do intravenous or intramuscular injection. The advantage of more peripheral routes is to prolong drug actions via slower uptake; they are thus preferred for analgesic management of chronic pain. As with any therapeutic regimen, the response should be monitored, and when an adequate response—relief of pain—has not occurred, an additional drug or drugs should be given.

### H. Mechanisms of Action

**Drugs** commonly used to inhibit nociceptive processes in animals are divided into several classes, based on their **mechanisms of action** (Table 2-2).

### I. Techniques

Common analgesic **techniques** and the classes of drugs used to interfere with nociception are listed in Table 2-3. Nonpharmacologic methods of pain relief can also be used to good effect. These include immobilization and support with casts, splints, or bandages; appropriate use of hot and cold packs; and physical therapy, such as massage and stretching.

| Table 2-2. Classes of Analgesic Drugs and Mechanisms of Action | |
| --- | --- |
| **Class** | **Mechanism of Action** |
| Local anesthetics | Blocks nerve impulse transmission and nociceptor excitation |
| NSAIDs | Inhibition of sensitizing mediators peripherally and centrally |
| Opioids | Damping of peripheral and central afferent nociceptive processes |
| $\alpha_2$-Agonists | Activation of central descending inhibitory pathways |
| Dissociatives | NMDA antagonist (produces antihyperalgesic action) |

## J. Drugs and Dose Recommendations

Some drugs and **dose recommendations** from each class of analgesic drugs used in the management of pain in dogs and cats are presented in Tables 2-4 to 2-8.

## K. Selecting an Anesthetic Protocol

**Factors** considered in selecting an anesthetic protocol and controlling pain in healthy or stabilized patients (American Society of Anesthesiologists stage I to III) should be based on the anticipated degree of surgical trauma, duration of the procedure, required CNS depression, and both intraoperative and postoperative analgesic requirements. Table 2-9 provides **guidelines** for selecting anesthetic and analgesic protocols based on these factors. Several diagnostic and surgical procedures are listed in each of four categories. Table 2-10 provides examples of specific sedatives; pre-emptive analgesics; induction drugs; maintenance drugs; perioperative analgesic techniques; and dispensable, take-home analgesics that can be used in the dog and cat for each of these four categories. These tables are specifically designed to help the practitioner focus attention on perioperative pain management while performing anesthesia in a variety of situations.

## L. Critically Ill Patients

Critically ill patients (American Society of Anesthesiologists stage IV and V) are not included in the pain management recommendations found in Tables 2-9 and 2-10. These patients require special evaluation and appropriate therapy in addition to the factors considered in Table 2-9. Anesthetic protocols in these patients should induce minimal cardiopulmonary depression and usually consist of increased reliance on local and regional analgesic techniques (nerve blocks), pre-emptive NSAIAs, and the combined use of opioids (e.g., oxymorphone) with cardiopulmonary-sparing drugs (e.g., benzodiazepines).

**Table 2-3. Techniques and Classes of Drugs Used to Control Pain**

| Technique | Drug Class |
|---|---|
| Epidural or spinal injection (drugs from different classes can be combined) | Local anesthetics; opioids; $\alpha_2$-agonists |
| Peripheral nerve blocks (intercostal, brachial plexus, infraorbital, mandibular-alveolar, auricular, ulnar and median, fibular and tibial, sciatic and saphenous) | Local anesthetics; $\alpha_2$-agonists (prolong block) |
| Intraoperative systemic analgesic administration (alternative to increased inhalant concentration) | Opioids; local anesthetics; dissociatives |
| Interpleural–intraperitoneal infusion | Local anesthetics |
| Local infiltration | Local anesthetics |
| Intra-articular injection | Local anesthetics; opioids |
| Mucous membrane application | Local anesthetics (topical preparations) |
| Ocular application | Local anesthetics (topical preparations) |
| Transdermal delivery | Opioids (fentanyl patch); local anesthetics (eutectic mixture) |
| Wound application | Local anesthetics (splash block; with catecholamine) |
| Mentation alteration | Pheothiazines; benzodiazepines; $\alpha_2$-agonists; tricyclic antidepressants; corticosteroids; herbs |
| Acupuncture | |
| Bandaging; immobilization | |
| Massage | Salves; ointments |

**Table 2-4. NSAIAs and Corticosteroid Dose Recommendations**

| Drug | Class | Dosage | Major Toxicity | Comments |
|---|---|---|---|---|
| Aspirin (many brands) | NSAIA | 10–25 mg/kg q 12 h PO in food (canine) / 10–20 mg/kg PO q 48–72 h in food (feline) | Gastrointestinal irritation, ulcers, kidney damage. | Appropriate for mild analgesia and anti-inflammatory therapy; gastrointestinal side effects are likely at higher doses |
| Phenylbutazone (many brands) | NSAIA | 15–20 mg/kg q 8–12 h PO (canine) (max: 800 mg/day) | Gastrointestinal irritation, kidney damage, bone marrow suppression | Approved for use in felines in the UK at 25 mg/kg q 12 h for 5 days |
| Carprofen (Rimadyl) | NSAIA | 2.2 mg/kg q 12 h PO (dog) (feline max: 2 days) | Toxicity associated with chronic use in felines; minimal in canines | Recently approved for long-term use in canines in 25-, 75-, and 100-mg tablets; recommended for pain and inflammation of osteoarthritis by the FDA |
| Etodolac (Etogesic) | NSAIA | 10–15 mg/kg PO q 24 h | Selective cyclooxygenase 2 inhibitor reduces toxicity potential | Available in 150- and 300-mg tablets |
| Ketoprofen (Orudis-KT; Ketofen; Anafen) | NSAIA | 1–2 mg/kg q 24 h PO for 5 days or 1–2 mg/kg q 24 h IV, SC, IM for 5 days (canine, feline) | Gastrointestinal irritation, ulcers, kidney damage | Tablet is 12.5 mg Orudis-KT; injectable form is approved for horses; tablets are approved for small animals in Canada |

| Meloxicam (Metacam) | NSAIA | 0.2 mg/kg loading dose PO then 0.1–0.5 mg/kg q 24 h placed in food (canine) | Selective cyclooxygenase 2 inhibitor reduces toxicity potential | Available in Europe and Canada at this time as oral suspension |
|---|---|---|---|---|
| Piroxicam (Feldene; generic) | NSAIA | 0.3 mg/kg q 48 h PO in food (canine) Cancer dose: q 24 h (canine) Dose not established in feline | Gastrointestinal irritation, ulcers, kidney damage | Potent NSAID; available only in 10-mg capsules |
| Naproxen (Naprosyn; Naxen; Aleve) | NSAIA | 5 mg/kg loading dose Then 2 mg/kg q 48 h PO in food (canine) | Narrow margin of safety; gastrointestinal irritation, ulcer, kidney damage | Aleve available as 220-mg OTC tablets; Naproxyn available in large tablets and a 25-mg/mL oral suspension |
| Meclofenamic acid (Arquel) | NSAIA | 1 mg/kg q 24 h PO in food (canine) (max: 5 days) | Gastrointestinal irritation, ulcers, kidney damage | Tablets not available in the United State; granules available for horses |
| Ketorolac tromethamine (Toradol) | NSAIA | 0.3–0.5 mg/kg q 8–12 h IV, IM for 1–2 doses; 5–10 mg/dog (10 mg > 30 kg) PO (canine) 0.25 mg/kg q 8-12 h IM for 1–2 doses (feline) | Similar effects to other NSAIDs | Do not use for > 3 consecutive days; effective for acute pain in canines at the 0.5 mg/kg IV or IM dose |
| Flunixin meglumine (Banamine) | NSAIA | 1.1 mg/kg q 24 h IV, IM, SC, PO for 3 days (canine) | Similar effects to other NSAIDs | Limit to 3 days; tablets not available in the United State; granules and paste (50 mg/g) available for horses |

Continued

**Table 2-4. (continued)**

| Drug | Class | Dosage | Major Toxicity | Comments |
|---|---|---|---|---|
| Acetaminophen (Tylenol) | NSAIA | 15 mg/kg q 8 h PO (canine) Contraindicated in felines | *Toxic to felines* | Appropriate for minor pain; has low anti-inflammatory effects |
| Prednisolone (many brands) | Cortico-steroids | 0.5–1 mg/kg q 12–24 h PO (canine) 2.2 mg/kg q 12–24 h PO (feline) Taper to q 48 h for both canines and felines | Gastrointestinal irritation, polydipsia, polyphagia, weight gain | Co-administration with NSAIA greatly enhances the toxicity hazards of the NSAIA |

**Table 2-5. Commonly Used Local Anesthetic Drugs[a]**

| Local Anesthetic | | Usual Doses, mg/kg | | | Toxic Doses, mg/kg | | Approximate Onset of Block, h | Approximate Duration of Block, h |
|---|---|---|---|---|---|---|---|---|
| Generic | Trade Name (Manufacturer) | Concentration | With Epinephrine | Without Epinephrine | Convulsive | Lethal | | |
| Lidocaine[b] | Xylocaine (Astra) | 0.5–2 | 7 | 5 | 11–20 | 16–28 | 10–15 | 1–2 |
| Mepivacaine | Carbocaine (Breon) | 1–2 | 7 | 5 | 29 | | 5–10 | 2–2.5 |
| Bupivacaine[c] | Marcaine (Breon) | 0.25–0.5 | 3 | 2 | 3.5–4.5 | 5–11 | 20–30 | 2.5–6 |
| Ropivacaine | LEA 103 (Breon) | 0.5 | 5 | 3 | 4.9 | | 5–15 | 2.5–4 |
| Etidocaine | Duranest (Astra) | 0.5–0.75 | 5 | 3 | 4.5 | 20 | 5–10 | 2–5 |

[a]Drugs listed can be used for both peripheral and epidural analgesia. Only lidocaine and bupivacaine are safely administered into the subarachnoid space. Local anesthetics used for topical analgesia include tetracaine (Pontocaine), proparacaine (Ophthaine), and Cetacaine (Benzocaine). A preparation of lidocaine and prilocaine (EMLA) in a cream formulation produces transdermal analgesia.

[b]Dose of lidocaine for constant infusion is 30–50 µg/kg/min in the canine. When used for local infiltration, the total dose should not exceed 12 mg/kg in canines and 4 mg/kg in felines. Epinephrine should be used with 1% lidocaine when infiltrating large areas, to retard systemic absorption and toxicity. Epidural dose of lidocaine is 3–5 mg/kg of 2% solution in both canines and felines.

[c]Dose of bupivacaine (0.2% solution) should not exceed 3 mg/kg in the canine and 1.5 mg/kg in the feline when infiltrating large areas. When administered into the pleural space, a 0.25% concentration is used at a dose not to exceed 3 mg/kg in canines and 2 mg/kg in felines. Can be diluted with saline (10–30 mL) to provide additional volume to enhance spread throughout the pleural cavity. Preservative-free bupivacaine (0.5% solution) should be used for epidural administration at a dose of 1.5–2.5 mg/kg in both canines and felines. To reduce the potential for motor blockade, reduce concentration to 0.125% and dose at 0.1–0.5 mg/kg. Both bupivacaine and lidocaine can be combined with opioids in the epidural space to enhance and prolong analgesia. Bupivacaine requires a longer time for onset of blockade, but its duration of action may be twice that of lidocaine.

**Table 2-6. Opioid Analgesics**

| Drug | Dose, mg/kg and Route of Administration | Dose Interval, h | Comments |
|---|---|---|---|
| **Injectables** | | | |
| Morphine (Duramorph is preservative free) | Canine: 0.1–0.5 IV | 1–4 | Titrate IV dose to effect (0.1–0.5 mg/kg) |
| | Canine: 0.5–1.0 IM, SC | 2–6 | IM administration less histamine release |
| | Feline: 0.05–0.3 IV, IM, SC | 2–6 | Stop titration if mydriasis occurs in felines |
| | Canine: 0.1–0.3 epidural | 4–8 | Dilute in saline (2 mg/mL concentration) |
| Oxymorphone (Numorphan) | Canine: 0.02–0.2 IV | 2–4 | Titrate to effect to control pain as for morphine |
| | Feline: 0.02–0.05 IV | 2–4 | |
| | Canine: 0.05–0.2 IM, SC, epidural | 2–6 | Epidural dose same as morphine dose |
| | Feline: 0.05–0.1 IM, SC | 2–4 | Combine with tranquilizer |
| Fentanyl (Sublimaze) | Canine: 0.02–0.04 IV, IM | 1 | Can be given with other analgesics or as a continuous infusion alone |
| | Feline: 0.02–0.04 IV, IM | 1 | |
| Butorphanol (Torbutrol) | Canine: 0.2–1.0 IM, IV, SC | 1–2 | Sedation lasts longer than analgesia; inadequate for severe pain; potential to antagonize full agonist |
| | Feline: 0.1–0.8 IM, IV, SC | 2–6 | |
| Meperidine (Demerol) | Canine: 5–10 IM | ³⁄₄ | Short duration of action and causes histamine release with IV injection; used primarily as a preanesthetic for its sedative actions |
| | Feline: 3–5 IM | ³⁄₄ | |
| Buprenorphine (Buprenex) | Canine: 0.05–0.02 IM, IV, epidural | 4–8 | Partial agonist with longer duration than agonists; produces a more localized analgesic action when placed into the epidural space than does morphine |
| | Feline: 0.05–0.01 IM, IV, epidural | 4–8 | |

**Oral and Transdermal**

| | | | | |
|---|---|---|---|---|
| Morphine | Canine: 0.3–1.0 PO | 4–8 | Tablets: 15, 30 mg | All scheduled medications require appropriate security, record keeping, and inventory |
| | Feline: 0.1–1.0 PO | 4–8 | Solution (Roxane): 4, 20 mg/mL; suppository (Roxane): 5, 10, 20, 30 mg | Long-lasting opioids may result in gastrointestinal stasis |
| Morphine (oral) sustained release | Canine: 1.5–3.0 PO | 8–12 | MS Contin (Purdue Frederick): 15, 30, 60, 100 mg; Oramorph SR (Roxane): 30, 60, 100 mg tablets | Long-lasting opioids may result in gastrointestinal stasis |
| Codeine | Canine: 0.5–2.0 PO | 4–8 | Tablets: 15, 30, 60 mg | Chronic use may result in tolerance |
| Codeine with acetaminophen | Canine: 1.0–2.0 PO | 6–8 | Tablets: 60 mg codeine/300 mg acetaminophen (dose is mg/kg codeine); *toxic to Feline* | Administer based on NSAIA dose |

*Continued*

**Table 2-6.** (*continued*)

| Drug | Dose, mg/kg, and Route of Administration | Dose Interval, h | Formulation | Comments |
|---|---|---|---|---|
| Fentanyl transdermal patch (Duragesic Patch) | Canine:<br>< 10 kg: 25 µg<br>10–20 kg: 50 µg<br>20–30 kg: 75 µg<br>> 30 kg: 100 µg<br>Feline: 25 µg | 72–120 | Duragesic (Janssen): 25, 50, 75, 100 µg patches | Latency of 6–12 h in feline and 12–24 h in canine; variation in transdermal uptake may be quite large; many factors influence rate and efficacy of absorption and duration of action; feline < 3.5 kg can be treated with partially covered patches; sometimes therapeutic concentrations not reached; other opioids can be co-administered |
| Butorphanol | Canine and Feline:<br>0.2–1.0 PO | 4–6 | Tablets (Torbutrol; Ft. Dodge): 1, 5, 10 mg | Gastrointestinal stasis can result from chronic use |
| Pentazocine | Canine: 2.0–10 PO | 4–6 | Tablets (Talwin Nx; Sanofi Winthrop): 50 mg pentazocine/0.5 mg naloxone | Has been used to control stereotypic behavior in canines |

**Table 2-7. $\alpha_2$-Agonists Analgesics**

| Drug | Dose, mg/kg, and Route of Administration | Comments |
|---|---|---|
| Xylazine (Rompun) | Canine: 0.2–1.0 IV, IM, SC<br>Feline: 0.2–1.0 IV, IM, SC | Analgesia will wane before sedation Use low end of dose range when giving IV; increased incidence of vomiting following IM or SC injection; expect increased urine production |
| Medetomidine (Domitor) | Canine:<br>0.01–0.04 IV, IM, SC<br>0.005–0.01 epidural<br>Feline: 0.01–0.05 IV, IM, SC | Bradycardia commonly occurs when an anticholinergic is not used; duration is dose dependent; relatively low systemic dose in combination with an opioid will prolong and enhance analgesia in both species; has been used in combination with morphine (0.1 mg/kg) in the epidural space to prolong analgesia for 6–12 h |

**Table 2-8. Adjuvant Drugs Used to Prolong and Improve Analgesia**

| Drug | Class | Dosage | Comments |
|---|---|---|---|
| Amitriptyline (Elavil, generics) | Tricyclic antidepressant | Canine: 1–2 mg/kg q 12–24 h PO<br>Feline: 0.5–1.0 mg/kg q 24 h PO | Sedation, nausea, cardiac conduction disturbances, dry eye, dry mouth, constipation, urinary retention |
| Imipramine (Tofranil) | Tricyclic antidepressant | Canine: 0.5–1 mg/kg q 8 h PO<br>0.25–0.4 mg/kg q 12 h PO | |
| Desipramine (Norpramin, generics) | Tricyclic antidepressant | 1–4 mg/kg PO q 24 h or divided BID | Taste terrible: give with food or in gel capsule |
| Nortriptyline (Pamelor, Aventyl, generics) | Tricyclic antidepressant | 1–4 mg/kg PO q 24 h or divided BID | Give at bedtime to decrease sedative side effects |
| Lidocaine infusion in low doses | Local anesthetics | Canine: 0.05 µg/kg/min IV<br>Feline: 0.025 µg/kg/min IV | Lidocaine infusion during or after anesthesia reduces anesthetic and postoperative analgesic requirements; duration: 3–5 h after drug termination |

| | | | |
|---|---|---|---|
| Ketamine | Dissociatives and other NMDA antagonists such as memantine are being developed for neuropathic pain syndromes | Canine: 0.1 mg/kg IM, SC<br>Feline 0.1 mg/kg IM, SC | Low doses of ketamine may potentiate analgesia and interfere with the development of central sensitization (hyperalgesia); low doses can be given with an opioid or $\alpha_2$-agonist to prolong effects |
| Acepromazine | Phenothiazines | Canine: 0.05–0.2 mg/kg IM, SC<br>Feline: 0.1–0.3 mg/kg IM, SC | Duration of effect may be as long as 8–12 h; usually given with an opioid |
| Diazepam | Benzodiazepines | Canine: 0.25–1 mg/kg PO<br>Feline 0.25–1 mg/kg PO | Duration after oral medication may be 12–24 h; usually given with an opioid |
| St. John's wort, willow, thyme, arnica (many others) | Herbal remedies | Dosing is empirical based on anecdotal evidence and reports | Herbs can produce a variety of actions including anti-inflammatory, muscle relaxing, antidepressant, and anti-anxiety effects. These effects may be beneficial in some chronic pain conditions but are inadequate for acute trauma or surgical pain |

**Table 2-9. Factors Considered in the Selection of an Anesthetic Protocol and Pain Management (Healthy or Stabilized Patients)**

| Anticipated Procedure | Heavy Sedation | Minor Surgery | Moderate Surgery | Major Surgery |
|---|---|---|---|---|
| **Duration of Procedure** | Variable | < 15 min | 15–45 min | > 1 h |
| Surgical trauma | None | Minimal trauma | Moderate trauma | Severe trauma |
| Intraoperative noxious stimuli (pain) | None to minimal | Minimal pain | Moderate to severe pain | Profound pain |
| Intraoperative analgesic requirement | None | Minimal | Moderate | Major |
| Type of procedure | • Physical examination and restraint<br>• Radiography<br>• Suture removal<br>• Casting<br>• Bandage change<br>• Grooming<br>• Nail trimming | • Suturing laceration<br>• Wound debridement<br>• Urinary catheterization<br>• Dental cleaning<br>• Ear examination and cleaning<br>• Abscess lancing<br>• Removal of foreign bodies (e.g., foxtails) | • Neuter<br>• Ovariohysterectomy<br>• Feline declaw<br>• Cystotomy<br>• Anal sacculotomy<br>• Cutaneous mass removal<br>• Dental extractions<br>• Caesarean section<br>• Severe lacerations | • Fracture repair<br>• Thoracotomy<br>• Limb amputation<br>• Gastric dilatation volvulus<br>• Cruciate repair<br>• Ear ablation<br>• Laminectomy<br>• Exploratory laparotomy<br>• Perineal urethrostomy |

| | | | | |
|---|---|---|---|---|
| Sedation, anesthesia and analgesic requirement | Moderate to heavy sedation (chemical versus physical restraint); analgesic requirement none | Heavy sedation with analgesic or short anesthesia ± local anesthetic; opioid agonist–antagonists recommended with $\alpha_2$-agonists or phenothiazine (PTZ) tranquilizer | Analgesic premedications; general anesthesia with attention to postoperative pain management; $\alpha_2$-agonist–opioid agonist–antagonist combination or full opioid agonist ± NSAIA recommended | Analgesic premedications; general anesthesia with postoperative pain management a must; full opioid agonists or $\alpha_2$-agonist–full opioid agonists combination ± NSAIA recommended |
| Postoperative pain and reversal options | Reversal acceptable when no pain is anticipated upon arousal | Reversal depends on postoperative analgesic requirement; reversal of $\alpha_2$-agonist when pre-emptively combined with opioid or local anesthetic is acceptable | Reversal not recommended unless indicated for a medical reason or excessive depression is of concern | Reversal not recommended unless indicated for medical reason or excessive CNS depression is of concern |

Continued

**Table 2-9.** *(continued)*

| Anticipated Procedure | Heavy Sedation | Minor Surgery | Moderate Surgery | Major Surgery |
|---|---|---|---|---|
| **Duration of Procedure** | Variable | <15 min | 15–45 min | >1 h |
| Dispensable pain medication | Usually none required | Usually minimal | Indicated for short period (1–2 days) with most routine procedures; PO medications preferred; opioid agonist–antagonists ± NSAIA recommended | Highly recommended; pain medication may be necessary for several days. Drug preparations that provide longer durations of activity preferred (e.g., PO or transdermal delivery systems); opioids with longer durations of action ± NSAIA drugs dosed at 12–24-h intervals |

**Table 2-10. Sedation, Pre-Emptive Analgesia, Anesthesia, and Intraoperative and Postoperative Analgesic Options in the Canine and Feline[a]**

| Anticipated Procedure | Heavy Sedation | Minor Surgery | Moderate Surgery | Major Surgery[b] |
|---|---|---|---|---|
| Trauma / Duration / Analgesia | None / Variable / None | Minimal / Short / Minimal Need | Moderate / 30–45 min / Moderate Need | Severe / >1 h / Large Need |
| Sedative and pre-emptive analgesic medications[c] | • $\alpha_2$-agonist alone[d]<br>• $\alpha_2$-agonist[e] + butorphanol 0.2 mg/kg IM (both species) Acepromazine 0.1 mg/kg + butorphanol 0.2 mg/kg IM (both species)<br>• Diazepam 0.2 mg/kg IV + butorphanol 0.2 mg/kg IV (older animal; both species)<br>• Sedative doses of propofol 2.0–3.0 mg/kg IV (both species)<br>• Ketamine 5.0 mg/kg + diazepam 0.2 mg/kg IV (both species) | • Medetomidine 10–15 µg/kg + butorphanol 0.2 mg/kg IM (both species)<br>• Acepromazine 0.1 mg/kg + butorphanol 0.2 mg/kg IM (both species)<br>• Butorphanol 0.2–0.4 mg/kg IV or IM; can be co-administered with ketamine 5.0 mg/kg and diazepam 0.2 mg/kg IV (both species) or telazol 3–5 mg/kg IM (both species) to enhance analgesia of these mixtures | • Medetomidine 10 µg/kg IM (canine) / 20–30 µg/kg IM (feline) + butorphanol 0.2 mg/kg IM<br>• Acepromazine 0.1 mg/kg + butorphanol 0.2 mg/kg IM (both species)<br>• Telazol 2–4 mg/kg IV or IM ± $\alpha_2$-agonist (Table 2-7) (both species)<br>• TKX[f] 0.1 mL/5 kg (feline)<br>• Ketamine 6–12 mg/kg IM + xylazine 1.0 mg/kg IM or medetomidine 30–50 µg/kg IM (both species) | • Medetomidine 10 µg/kg + morphine 0.5 mg/kg (canine) or oxymorphone 0.2 mg/kg IM (both species)<br>• Oxymorphone (0.1 mg/kg) IV, IM or morphine 0.5 mg/kg IM alone (canine)<br>• Acepromazine 0.05 mg/kg IM + oxymorphone 0.1 mg IM (feline) or + morphine 0.5 mg/kg IM (canine)<br>• Fentanyl patch[g] placement 12–24 h before induction (both species) |

Continued

**Table 2-10. (continued)**

| Anticipated Procedure | Heavy Sedation | Minor Surgery | Moderate Surgery | Major Surgery[b] |
|---|---|---|---|---|
| Trauma / Duration / Analgesia | None / Variable / None | Minimal / Short / Minimal Need | Moderate / 30–45 min / Moderate Need | Severe / > 1 h / Large Need |
| | | | | • After induction, a variety of local anesthetic techniques can be used to pre-empt surgically induced pain; see Table 2–5 and perioperative analgesics, below |
| Anesthetic induction drugs[h] | Usually unnecessary | All induction drugs (thiopental, propofol, ketamine, telazol) should be given slowly to effect to reduce the likelihood of excessive depression when premedication has already produced heavy sedation and analgesia; mask or chamber induction with inhalants can be achieved with reduced concentrations | | |
| Anesthetic maintenance drugs | Usually unnecessary | When using injectables and inhalants that produce minimal analgesia unrelated to the unconscious state, additional analgesics or techniques should be pre-emptively incorporated into the anesthetic protocol; if pre-emptive analgesics are *not* given, postoperative analgesic requirements will likely increase; patients rendered sedate and analgesic before induction will often require much lower inhalant concentration (by 0.5–0.75%) to maintain anesthesia | | |

| Perioperative analgesic techniques | None required | Topical or infiltrative local anesthetic can be used to provide additional analgesia intraoperatively and postoperatively; be aware of toxic doses of local anesthetics when infiltrating large areas, especially in smaller animals (Table 2–5) | Local anesthetics can be used for infiltrative or regional anesthesia; specific nerve blocks include mandibular nerve for dental procedures, median and ulnar nerve blocks for declaw procedure; immediate postoperative analgesics should be given as needed | • Epidural with bupivacaine 1 mL/5 kg or lidocaine 1 mL/5 kg or with morphine 0.2 mg/kg + 5.0 µg/kg medetomidine qs to 1 mL/4.5 kg with saline<br>• Intra-articular morphine 0.2 mg/kg or intra-articular bupivacaine 0.1 mL/kg<br>• Fentanyl or lidocaine infusion intraoperatively and postoperatively.<br>• Protective bandaging |

*Continued*

**Table 2-10.** *(continued)*

| Anticipated Procedure | Heavy Sedation | Minor Surgery | Moderate Surgery | Major Surgery[b] |
|---|---|---|---|---|
| **Trauma / Duration / Analgesia** | None / Variable / None | Minimal / Short / Minimal Need | Moderate / 30–45 min / Moderate Need | Severe / > 1 h / Large Need |
| Postoperative dispensable pain medications | None needed | NSAIAs may be adequate (Table 2-4); if additional analgesia is needed opioid agonist–antagonist drugs are a good choice (Table 2-6) | • Torbutrol tablets or syrup preparation<br>• NSAIA (Table 2-4)<br>• Opioid agonist oral preparations (Table 2-6)<br>• Opioid–NSAIA combinations (Table 2-6) | • Opioid agonist oral preparations<br>• NSAIAs + opioid preparations<br>• Fentanyl patch[g] (Table 2-6)<br>• Adjuvant drugs when necessary for chronic management of pain (Table 2-8)<br>• NMDA antagonists (memantine) |

[a]Specific dosages of local anesthetics and analgesics not included in this table can be found in Tables 2-4 to 2-8.

[b]Full opioid agonists are recommended for major procedures; opioid agonist–antagonists are likely not adequate to control this level of pain.

[c]Drugs and combinations listed based on pre-emptive analgesic properties, sedative effects, and anesthetic-sparing actions.

[d]Medetomidine dose: 10–20 μg/kg IM (canine), 20–30 μg/kg IM (feline); xylazine dose: 0.5 mg/kg IM (canine), 0.7–1.0 mg/kg IM (feline); if heart rate decreases by 30% or more, anticholinergic administration is warranted.

[e]Medetomidine dose: 5–10 μg/kg IM (canine), 10–20 μg/kg IM (feline); xylazine dose: 0.25–0.5 mg/kg IM (canine), 0.5–0.75 mg/kg IM (feline); clinical experience indicates that the sedative–analgesic actions of medetomidine with butorphanol exceed those produced by xylazine–butorphanol.

[f]Telazol–ketamine–xylazine mixture.

[g]Fentanyl patches should not be dispensed if young children are in the household or if the patient is an outside pet; schedule II drugs listed in Table 2-6 should not be dispensed if there is any suspicion that the pet owner is not responsible and trustworthy.

[h]Lower end of dose range of injectable anesthetics should be used when premedications produce heavy sedation and analgesia; typical dose requirements are 2–10 mg/kg thiopental, 1–6 mg/kg propofol, 1–4 mg/kg ketamine, and 2–3 mg/kg telazol.

# Chapter 3

## Anesthesia and the Cardiovascular, Respiratory, and Central Nervous Systems

### Introductory Comments

*The importance of cardiovascular function to patient well-being and the diverse effects of drugs used in the practice of anesthesia emphasize the importance of having a working knowledge of the effects of anesthetics on cardiovascular function. The uptake, delivery, distribution, redistribution, metabolism, and clearance of anesthetic drugs depends on blood flow. Similarly, maintenance of adequate respiratory function is a prime requirement for safe anesthesia. Inadequate tissue oxygenation may lead to acute cessation of vital organ function, especially of the brain or the myocardium, and an anesthetic fatality. Because anesthetics preferentially affect the nervous system, a general knowledge of its parts and function is also essential for safe administration of analgesics and anesthetics.*

**Cardiovascular System**
**Respiratory System**
**Nervous System**

---

## I. CARDIOVASCULAR SYSTEM

*W. W. Muir and Diane Mason*

The cardiovascular system is composed of the **heart, blood vessels,** and **blood volume** and is designed to supply a continuous flow of blood and nutrients to all tissues of the body. Oxygenated blood

61

returning from the lungs enters the left atrium and subsequently the left ventricle; it is then ejected into the aorta, which, through major arteries, distributes blood to all the tissues of the body. The end branches of these major arteries, the arterioles, give rise to a vascular bed of exchange vessels, the capillaries, in which oxygen and nutrients are exchanged for the by-products of cellular metabolism. The capillaries, in turn, reunite to form venules and veins that return blood to the right atrium, the right ventricle, and via the pulmonary artery, the lungs (Fig. 3-1). The continuous circulation of blood depends on a functional heart, normal blood vessels, and adequate blood volume, serving to maintain a constant internal environment for all living cells.

## A.   Heart Anatomy

The heart, as one key component of the cardiovascular system, functions to pump blood throughout the body. The heart is composed of four chambers: two thin-walled **atria** separated by an interatrial septum and two thick-walled **ventricles** separated by an interventricular septum.

## B.   Blood Vessels

The **aorta** and other large arteries make up the high-pressure portion of the systemic circulation and are relatively stiff compared to veins and possess a high proportion of elastic tissue compared to smooth muscle and fibrous tissues. The highly elastic vessel architecture of the aorta facilitates the continuous, albeit nonuniform, flow of blood to the peripheral tissues throughout the cardiac cycle (contraction–relaxation–rest) and has been termed the *Windkessel effect*. The most distal small arteries—**terminal arterioles** and **arteriovenous anasto-moses**—contain a predominance of smooth muscle, are highly innervated, and function as sphincters that regulate the distribution of blood flow, aid in the regulation of systemic blood pressure, and modulate tissue perfusion pressure. The **capillaries** are the functional exchange sites for oxygen, nutrients, electrolytes, cellular waste products, and other substances. Postcapillary **venules** are composed of an endothelial lining and fibrous tissue and collect blood from capillaries. Some venules act as postcapillary sphincters, and all venules merge into small **veins.** Between 60 and 70% of the blood volume may be stored in the venous vasculature during resting conditions (Fig. 3-2).

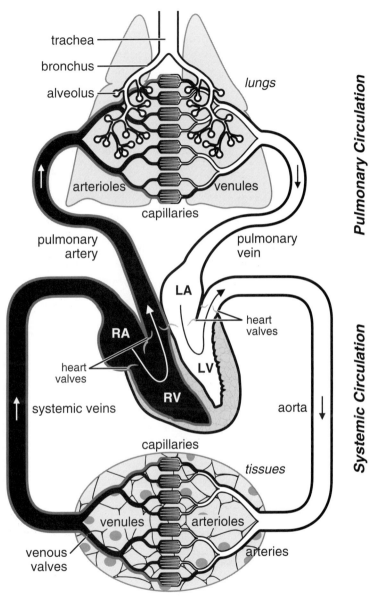

**Figure 3-1.** The cardiovascular system includes the heart, blood, and two parallel circulations (pulmonary, systemic). In the pulmonary circulation, the pulmonary artery carries blood from the right ventricle (*RV*) to the lungs, where carbon dioxide is eliminated and oxygen is taken up. Oxygenated blood returns to the left atrium (*LA*) via pulmonary veins. In the systemic circulation, blood is pumped by the left ventricle (*LV*) into the aorta, which distributes blood to the peripheral tissues. Oxygen and nutrients are exchanged for carbon dioxide and other by-products of tissue metabolism in the capillary beds, after which the blood is returned to the right atrium (*RA*) through venules and large systemic veins. Modified from Shepherd JT, Van Houtte PM. The human cardiovascular system: facts and concepts. New York: Raven, 1979.

### C.　Blood

**Blood** is the fluid (approximately 60% plasma and 40% cells) responsible for carrying oxygen, nutrients, and other blood-borne substances to all the tissues of the body and for delivering carbon dioxide, the by-products of cellular metabolism, and foreign substances (e.g., anesthetic drugs) to the appropriate organs of elimination. This suspension of red and white blood cells and platelets in plasma is also responsible for prevention of hemorrhage (clotting). Red blood cells contain **hemoglobin,** which binds and carries oxygen to peripheral tissue sites.

　　Binding of oxygen to hemoglobin depends on the partial pressure of oxygen ($P_{O_2}$) and the shape of the oxyhemoglobin

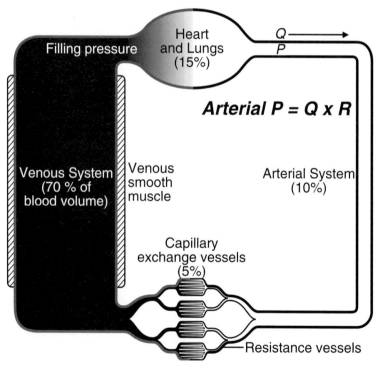

**Figure 3-2.** Blood is unevenly distributed throughout the circulatory system. The largest portion of the blood volume is contained within the systemic veins. Relatively small changes in venous capacity can alter the heart's filling pressure dramatically, resulting in predictable changes in cardiac output ($Q$), peripheral vascular resistance ($R$), and arterial blood pressure ($P$). Decreases in filling pressure, for example, decrease Q and P and increase R. Modified from Shepherd JT, Van Houtte PM. The human cardiovascular system: facts and concepts. New York: Raven, 1979.

dissociation curve. The oxyhemoglobin dissociation curve is generally sigmoid and is influenced by pH, $P_{CO_2}$, temperature, and 2,3-diphosphoglycerate (2,3-DPG) concentration. Increases in pH and decreases in $P_{CO_2}$, temperature, and 2,3-DPG in the lung all shift the oxyhemoglobin dissociation curve to the left, increasing oxygen binding to hemoglobin and decreasing oxygen availability. The opposite changes occur in peripheral tissues, where hemoglobin divests itself of oxygen in proportion to the decrease in $P_{O_2}$. Once the amount of deoxygenated hemoglobin (unsaturated hemoglobin) exceeds 5 g/100 mL, the blood changes from red to blue (cyanosis). Carbon dioxide produced by metabolizing tissues binds to deoxygenated hemoglobin and is eliminated by the lung during the oxygenation process, before the blood returns to the systemic circulation and the cycle repeats itself.

The **plasma** is composed of about 90% water by weight, plasma proteins (7%), and other organic (carbohydrates, fats) and inorganic (sodium, potassium, chloride, etc.) substances. Although there are molecules, including electrolytes, in the plasma that contribute to the total osmotic pressure, their importance in the exchange of water between the circulation and the tissues is minimized by their small size and their relatively free permeability across capillaries. The relevant osmotic pressure influencing water exchange between capillaries and tissues is the **colloidal osmotic pressure** (COP), which is primarily caused by the relatively large molecular weight of plasma proteins. The COP is approximately 25 mm Hg, and it and the capillary hydrostatic pressure are the two key forces that govern water exchange in the capillaries, the acute maintenance of the plasma volume, and thus blood volume.

### D.   Electrophysiology of the Heart

1.   Normal **cardiac electric activity** is essential for normal cardiac contractile function (excitation–contraction coupling). Indeed, myocardial contraction is preceded by and will not occur without electric activation, although normal or near-normal electric activity is possible without myocardial contraction (electric–mechanical uncoupling, electric–mechanical dissociation). The cardiac cell membrane (sarcolemma) is a highly specialized lipid bilayer that contains protein-associated channels, pumps, en-

zymes, and exchangers in an architecturally sophisticated yet fluid (reorganizable, movable) medium. Most drugs and many anesthetic drugs produce important direct and indirect effects on the cell membrane and intracellular organelles, ultimately altering cardiac excitation–contraction coupling.

2. **Ion transport** and membrane-associated electric properties are determined by the molecular composition and fluidity of the cardiac membranes. The unequal distribution of different ions—especially sodium, potassium, and chloride—is responsible for the development of the resting membrane potential of cardiac cells. It should be noted that in the presence of many anesthetic drugs, particularly local anesthetics (lidocaine, mepivacaine), and inhalation anesthetics (halothane, isoflurane), use-dependent block may occur. Use-dependent block is the phenomenon exhibited by cardiac cells wherein, in the presence of a drug, increases in stimulation rate (e.g., heart rate) produces a more pronounced drug effect on the electric properties of the heart than during slower stimulation.

3. **Excitability** or the ability of the cardiac cell membrane to generate an electric potential (action potential) is a fundamental intrinsic property of cardiac cells. The action potential of cardiac muscle varies considerably from that of nerves and skeletal muscle. The cardiac action potential arises from a more negative membrane potential (90 versus 65 mV), is greater in magnitude (130 versus 80 mV), and is much longer in duration (150 to 300 versus 1 ms). Five characteristic phases of the cardiac action potential are discernible in most cardiac cells:

   a. **Phase 0,** or the phase of rapid depolarization, is the result of the rapid flux of sodium ions (fast inward current) into the cell.

   b. **Phase 1,** the early phase of repolarization, is caused by the transient outward movement of potassium ions.

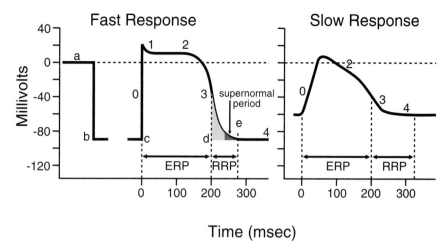

**Figure 3-3.** Cardiac transmembrane potential changes associated with fast- and slow-response action potentials. Note that slow-response action potentials originate from a less negative resting membrane potential and have a much slower rate of rise (phase 0). During the supernormal period, a subthreshold stimulus can elicit a normal action potential. See text for explanation of phases 1 through 4. *ERP,* effective refractory period; *RRP,* relative refractory period.

      c.    **Phase 2,** the plateau phase, is attributed to the continued but decreased entry of sodium ions and a large but slow influx of calcium ions (slow inward current) into cells.

      d.    **Phase 3** is the phase of repolarization during which the membrane potential returns to its resting value owing to potassium efflux (outward current) from the cell.

      e.    **Phase 4** is a resting phase in atrial and ventricular muscle cells before the initiation of the next action potential (Fig. 3-3).

  4.  **Arrhythmias** develop if there are large disparities or inhomogeneities in the action potential duration and refractoriness of adjacent cardiac cells owing to re-entry of electric impulses and re-excitation of the heart. Re-entry is one mechanism whereby the ultra-short-acting barbiturates and inhalation anesthetics are known to produce cardiac arrhythmias.

5. **Diastolic depolarization** (pacemaker potential) occurs in the sinoatrial and atrioventricular nodes and atrial and ventricular (Purkinje network) specialized tissues. Diastolic depolarization imparts the unique property of **automaticity** to the heart. The resting membrane potential depolarizes toward a threshold potential in tissues with this property; when the threshold is reached the development of an action potential is triggered. The cardiac tissue with the most rapid rate of phase 4 depolarization (normally the sinoatrial node) is termed the *pacemaker* and determines the heart rate. The cardiac pacemaker normally depresses the automaticity of slower or subsidiary pacemakers (overdrive suppression), preventing more than one pacemaker from controlling the heart rate. Automaticity is influenced by heart rate and local factors, including temperature, pH, blood gases ($P_{O_2}$, $P_{CO_2}$), extracellular potassium concentration, catecholamines, and various hormones (Fig. 3-4).

6. The **electrocardiogram** is the algebraic sum of all the action potentials produced by each cardiac cell after activation by the sinoatrial node (Fig. 3-5). Initiation of an electric impulse in the sinoatrial node is followed by rapid electric transmission of the impulse through

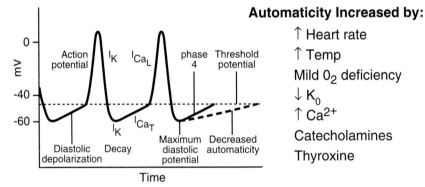

**Automaticity Increased by:**

↑ Heart rate
↑ Temp
Mild $O_2$ deficiency
↓ $K_0$
↑ $Ca^{2+}$
Catecholamines
Thyroxine

**Figure 3-4.** The transmembrane potential of cardiac tissue within the sinoatrial node (pacemaker tissue) is characterized by a less negative maximum diastolic potential, which depolarizes toward the threshold (phase 4 diastolic depolarization), a slow phase 0 caused primarily by activation of $I_{Ca-L}$ and a relatively rapid repolarization owing to $I_K$. The rate of phase 4 diastolic depolarization (automaticity) can be increased by increases in the heart rate, temperature, calcium, catecholamines, and thyroxine and decreases in oxygen tension and extracellular potassium concentration.

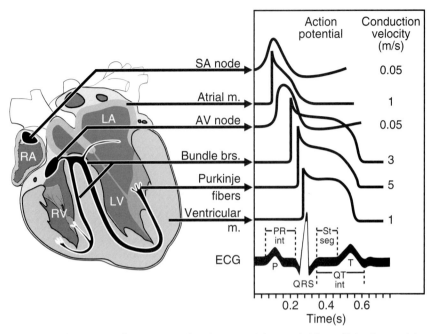

**Figure 3-5.** The transmembrane potential (action potential) recorded from all the tissues of the heart (specialized tissue and muscle) summate to produce the P-QRS-T complex (ECG) recorded at the body surface. *SA*, sinoatrial; *AV*, atrioventricular.

the atria, giving rise to the P wave. Once the wave of depolarization reaches the atrioventricular node, conduction is slowed because of the atrioventricular node's low resting membrane potential (approximately −60 mV) and the relatively depressed rate of phase 0 (decremental conduction). Increased parasympathetic tone can produce a marked slowing of atrioventricular nodal conduction, leading to first-, second-, and third-degree heart block. Many drugs used in anesthesia, including opioids, $\alpha_2$-agonists, and occasionally acepromazine, increase parasympathetic tone, causing heart block and bradyarrhythmias. The anticholinergic drugs atropine and glycopyrrolate are generally effective therapy in these situations.

Once the electric impulse has traversed the atrioventricular node, it is rapidly transmitted to the ventricular muscle by specialized muscle cells, commonly referred to as Purkinje fibers. **Ventricular depolarization** (activation) produces the QRS complex of the ECG and is immediately followed by **ventricular repolarization,** giving rise to the T wave. The configuration and magnitude of the T wave vary considerably among species and are influenced by changes in heart rate, blood temperature, and the extracellular potassium concentration. Hyperkalemia, for example, produces T waves that are large in magnitude, generally spiked or pointed, and short in duration (short QT interval).

7. **In summary,** the cardiac cell membrane possesses both active (ion movement) and passive (resistive, capacitive) properties that determine the heart's excitability, automaticity, rhythmicity, refractoriness, and ability to conduct an electric impulse. **Anesthetic drugs,** via their effects on both the active (e.g., lidocaine, a sodium channel blocker; barbiturates, and inhalants suppress calcium currents) and the passive (e.g., halothane and isoflurane change membrane fluidity and depress gap junctions) properties of the heart, can produce significant alterations in cardiac excitability and conduction of the electric impulse, predisposing the patient to cardiac arrhythmias and mechanical contraction abnormalities.

## E.    Cardiac Cycle

Historically, the **cardiac cycle** has been used as a diagrammatic attempt to describe the electric (ECG), mechanical (pressure, volume, flow) and acoustic (heart sound) events associated with cardiac contraction and relaxation as a function of time (Fig. 3-6).

## F.    Determinants of Cardiac Output

The ultimate goal of the heart's pumping activity is to deliver adequate quantities of oxygenated blood to the peripheral tissues. This is accomplished by the continuous adjustment of cardiac output (CO), which is the product of heart rate (HR) and stroke volume (SV):

$$CO = HR \times SV$$

Stroke volume is the amount of blood ejected from the ventricle during contraction and, therefore, represents the difference

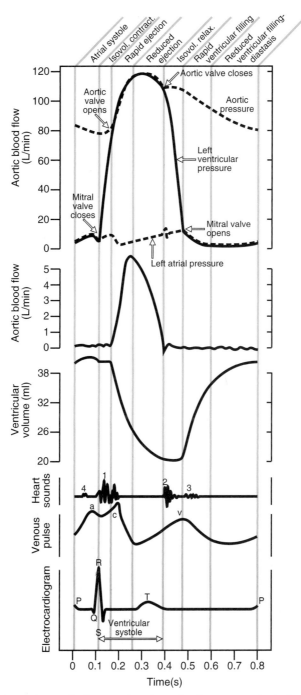

**Figure 3-6.** The cardiac cycle illustrates the relationship between mechanical, acoustical, and electrical events as a function of time. Modified from Berne RM, Levy MN. Principles of physiology. St. Louis: Mosby, 1990.

between the end-diastolic and end-systolic ventricular volumes. Traditionally, stroke volume has been considered to be primarily determined by one intrinsic property **(cardiac contractility)** and two vascular-coupling factors **(preload and afterload).** The refinement and development of more descriptive methods for assessing cardiac function, however, have led to the consideration of relaxation (lusitropic) effects on stroke volume. **Lusitropic** properties are responsible for ventricular chamber stiffness ($dP/dV$) or its inverse, compliance ($dV/dP$). It should be remembered that changes in preload, afterload, or myocardial contractile (inotropic) and relaxant (lusitropic) properties can influence each other and thus influence stroke volume. These factors in turn are all influenced by heart rate, leading to a complex interplay of variables that collectively determine cardiac output (Fig. 3-7).

1.  Cardiac **contractility** (inotropy) is the intrinsic ability of the heart to generate force and as such relates directly to

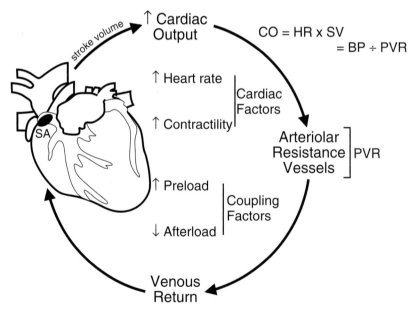

**Figure 3-7.** Cardiac output is equal to heart rate (*HR*) times stroke volume (*SV*), or arterial blood pressure (*BP*) divided by peripheral vascular resistance (*PVR*). Increases in heart rate, cardiac contractility, and preload and decreases in afterload increase cardiac output. Preload and afterload are considered to be coupling factors, because they depend on vascular resistance, capacitance, and compliance.

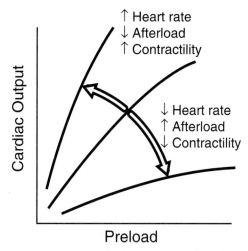

**Figure 3-8.** Cardiac output increases as preload increases (Frank–Starling effect). The steepness of the Frank–Starling curve is also affected by changes in heart rate, cardiac contractility, and afterload.

physicochemical processes and the availability of intracellular calcium. Contractility is generally described by shifts in the ventricular function curve (e.g., shifts in the Frank–Starling relationship) (Fig. 3-8). It is generally believed that a decrease in cardiac contractility is the key cause of heart failure in patients with cardiac disease or after the administration of potent negative inotropic drugs (e.g., anesthetics).

2. **Preload** in the intact animal is usually explained in terms of the Frank–Starling relationship or as heterometric autoregulation; increases in myocardial fiber length (ventricular volume) increase the force of cardiac contraction and cardiac output (Fig. 3-8). The Frank–Starling relationship serves as an important compensatory mechanism for maintaining stroke volume when ventricular contractility and afterload are acutely changed.

3. **Afterload** describes the force opposing ventricular ejection. One major reason for the great interest in this physiologic determinant of cardiac function is its inverse relationship with cardiac output and its direct correlation with myocardial oxygen consumption (Fig. 3-7).

4. **Diastole** is divided into four phases: isovolumic relaxation, early rapid ventricular filling, slow ventricular filling (diastasis), and atrial systole (during sinus rhythm). Mechanical factors, loading factors, inotropic activity, heart rate, and asynchronicity (patterns of relaxation) are the major determinants of diastole. Drugs used as preanesthetic medication or for intravenous or inhalation anesthesia can produce profound effects on indices of cardiac performance and are often much more complex in their actions than once surmised (Table 3-1).

## G.    The Vascular System

Originating from the heart, the circulatory system consists of two separate circulations connected in series (Fig. 3-1). The **pulmonary circulation** receives its blood supply from the right ventricle, perfuses the lung, and empties into the left atrium. The systemic circulation receives its blood supply from the left ventricle, perfuses most of the body's organs and tissues, and empties into the right atrium. More specifically, the systemic circulation (and the pulmonary) undergoes repeated division into smaller and smaller parallel vascular beds that terminate in the arterioles (the smallest arteries), which further subdivide to form the capillary bed. During this process of repeated division, the overall cross-sectional area of the circulation increases dramatically, reaching a maximum in the capillaries (Fig. 3-9).

1. **Blood pressure** in arteries (arterial pulse pressure and blood pressure), whether obtained directly or indirectly, is frequently assessed during anesthesia. Arterial blood pressure measurement in particular is one of the fastest and most informative means of assessing cardiovascular function; and when done correctly, it frequently provides an accurate indication of drug effects, surgical events, and hemodynamic trends. The most important vascular determinant of arterial blood pressure is arteriolar tone, which can be modified by almost all drugs used to produce anesthesia. The factors that determine arterial blood pressure are heart rate, stroke volume (HR × SV = CO), vascular resistance, arterial compliance ($dV/dP$), and blood volume. Most drugs used to produce anesthesia decrease cardiac output and peripheral vascular resis-

**Table 3-1. Common Hemodynamic Effects of Anesthetic Drugs in Intact Animals**

| Drug | Heart Rate | Cardiac Output | Contractility | Blood Pressure | Right Atrial Pressure | Myocardial Oxygen Consumption |
|---|---|---|---|---|---|---|
| Anticholinergics | ↑ | ↑ | ↑ | NC-↑ | → | ↑ |
| Phenothiazines | ↑ | ↑ | → | → | → | NC-↑ |
| Butyrophenones | ↑ | NC-↑ | → | Slight ↓ | NC | NC-↑ |
| Benzodiazepines | NC | NC | NC | NC | ↑ | → |
| $\alpha_2$-Agonists | → | → | NC-↓ | Initial ↑, then ↓ | ↑ | ↑ |
| Opioids | → | → | NC-↓ | NC-↓ | NC | NC |
| Barbiturates | ↑ | → | → | → | → | NC-↑ |
| Propofol | NC-↑ | → | → | → | → | NC-↑ |
| Etomidate | NC-↑ | NC-↓ | NC-↓ | NC-↓ | NC-↓ | NC-↑ |
| Dissociative drugs | ↑ | ↑ | ↑ | ↑ | ↑ | ↑ |
| Inhalation anesthetics | → | → | → | → | → | → |
| Skeletal muscle relaxants | | | | | | |
| Pancuronium | ↑ | ↑ | NC | ↑ | NC | ↑ |
| Atracurium | NC-↑ | NC | NC | May ↓ (histamine) | NC | NC |
| Vecuronium | NC | NC | NC | NC | NC | NC |

↑, increase; ↓, decrease; NC, no change.

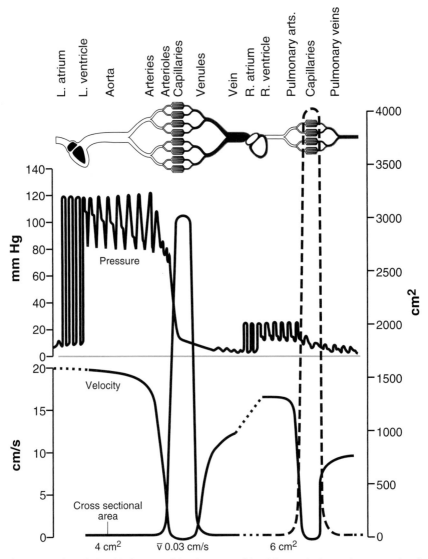

**Figure 3-9.** The relationship between blood pressure, blood flow velocity, and cross-sectional area of the cardiovascular system. Note that as blood approaches the capillaries, blood pressure and blood flow velocity decrease and cross-sectional area increases. Modified from Witzleb E. Functions of the vascular system. In: Schmidt RF, Thews G, eds. Human physiology. New York: Springer-Verlag, 1983:408.

tance. It should be remembered that if peripheral vascular resistance is elevated, the arterial blood pressure may be within normal limits, regardless of low blood flow to peripheral tissues. Several anesthetic drugs (ketamine, low doses of thiobarbiturates) can increase peripheral vascular resistance (producing no change or increase in arterial blood pressure) while decreasing cardiac output (Table 3-1).

2. **Arterial pulse pressure** (Ps − Pd) and pulse pressure waveform can provide valuable information regarding changes in vascular compliance and vessel tone. Generally, drugs (phenothiazines) or diseases (endotoxic shock) that produce marked arterial dilating effects increase vascular compliance, causing a rapid rise, short duration, and rapid fall in the arterial waveform while increasing the arterial pulse pressure. Situations that produce vasoconstriction decrease vascular compliance, resulting in a longer duration pulse waveform and a slower fall in the systolic blood pressure to diastolic values. The pulse pressure may contain secondary and sometimes tertiary pressure waveforms, particularly if the measuring site is in a peripheral artery some distance from the heart. Secondary and tertiary pulse waves indicate normal or elevated vascular tone in response to sympathetic nervous system stimulation or the vascular effects of drugs (ketamine, catecholamines).

## H.    Nervous, Humoral, and Local Control

**Regulatory control** of the cardiovascular system is integrated through the combined effects of the central and autonomic nervous systems, the influence of circulating (humoral) vasoactive substances, and local tissue mediators that modulate vascular tone (Fig. 3-10). These regulatory processes maintain blood flow at an appropriate level while distributing blood flow to meet the needs of tissue beds that have the greatest demand.

1. **The autonomic nervous system** exerts a major influence on the regulation of cardiovascular function. Peripheral receptors—including baroreceptors, mechanoreceptors, and chemoreceptors—respond to changes in blood pres-

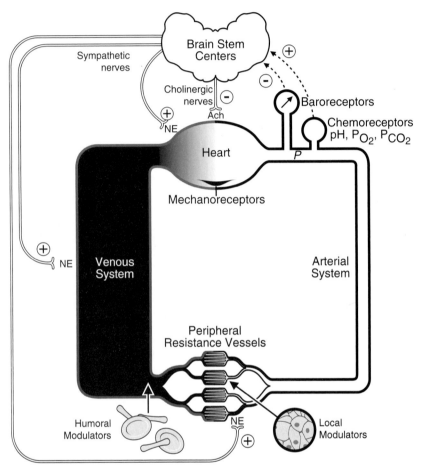

**Figure 3-10.** Nervous, humoral, and local (tissue) regulatory factors ensure that blood flow and pressure are maintained within physiologic limits. Mechanoreceptors and chemoreceptors sense changes in wall tension (stretch) and changes in pH and blood gases ($Pao_2$, $Paco_2$), respectively. Substances produced in peripheral tissues and released into the circulation by endocrine glands also modulate blood vessels and the distribution of blood flow. Nervous impulses generated by the heart, vasculature, and peripheral sensors are transmitted to and integrated in the brainstem, which alters sympathetic and parasympathetic tone to make appropriate adjustments. The release of norepinephrine (NE) by sympathetic nerves stimulates the heart and constricts the blood vessels. The release of acetylcholine (Ach) by parasympathetic nerves depresses the heart. +, stimulatory; –, inhibitory. Modified from Shepherd JT, Van Houtte PM. The human cardiovascular system: facts and concepts. New York: Raven, 1979.

sure, volume, and gas tensions, respectively, and send information to the CNS through afferent nerves. These sensory signals are integrated in control centers located in the hypothalamus, pons, and medulla into responses carried by efferent sympathetic or parasympathetic nerves to the periphery (Fig. 3-11). In addition, the vascular endothelium is known to modulate both local and neural control mechanisms through the release of prostaglandins and endothelial-derived factors, such as nitric oxide (NO). Anesthetic drugs can and do interfere with the sensory (input), neural integration (processing), and effector (output) mechanisms that control cardiovascular function.

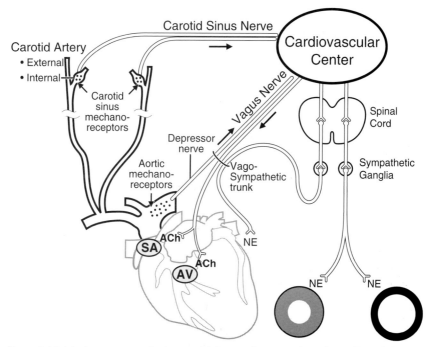

**Figure 3-11.** Mechanoreceptors in the carotid sinus and aortic arch send impulses via the carotid sinus nerve (a branch of the glossopharyngeal nerve) and the vagosympathetic trunk, respectively, to the solitary tract nucleus in the brainstem (cardiovascular centers). Changes in the activity of these mechanoreceptors caused by changes in arterial blood pressure result in adjustments in sympathetic and parasympathetic outflow to the heart and resistance (arterial) and capacitance (veins) vessels. *SA,* sinoatrial node; *AV,* atrioventricular node; *NE,* norepinephrine; *Ach,* acetylcholine. Modified from Shepherd JT, Van Houtte PM. The human cardiovascular system: facts and concepts. New York: Raven, 1979.

2. **Humoral mechanisms** produce sustained changes in cardiopulmonary function. The adrenal medulla is a modified sympathetic ganglion innervated by preganglionic sympathetic fibers and is part of the sympathetic nervous system. The "neuronal" cells of the adrenal medulla, rather than sending axons to target organs, release the neurotransmitters **epinephrine** and **norepinephrine** into the circulation. Precipitating factors for the release of catecholamines from the adrenal medulla include pain, trauma, hypovolemia, hypotension, hypoxia, hypothermia, hypoglycemia, exercise, stress, and fear (fight or flight).

The kidney is the major site for activation of the **renin–angiotensin** system. Renin is produced in the kidney during sodium depletion, decreases in the extracellular fluid volume, and increases in sympathetic output. Secretion of renin into the systemic circulation converts circulating angiotensinogen, produced by the liver, to angiotensin I. Angiotensin I is converted to angiotensin II by an angiotensin-converting enzyme that is present in pulmonary vascular endothelium. Angiotensin II produces arteriolar constriction, resulting in increases in blood pressure, and stimulates the adrenal cortex to release aldosterone, a hormone that causes renal reabsorption of sodium and water, effectively increasing the extracellular fluid volume (Fig. 3-12).

**Arginine vasopressin (antidiuretic hormone; ADH)** is produced in the hypothalamus and is transported through nerve cell axons to the posterior pituitary. Under normal circumstances, the pituitary releases vasopressin in response to increases in plasma solute, resulting in an increase in circulating vasopressin. Vasopressin acts on the collecting ducts of the kidney, where it stimulates water conservation, thereby returning plasma osmolality (and volume) to normal. Vasopressin is a vasoconstrictor, especially in mesenteric vessels; therefore, the presence of circulating vasopressin is influential in the redistribution of systemic blood flow. Examples of non-osmotic stimuli that cause the release of vasopressin are pain, stress, hypoxia, heart failure, and volume depletion. A number of anesthetic drugs are associated with increased circulating levels of arginine vasopressin, including opioids (morphine, meperidine) and barbiturates.

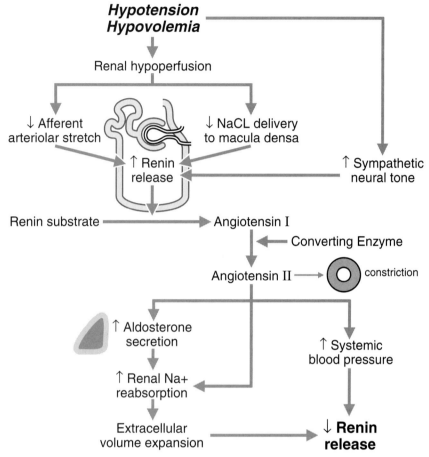

**Figure 3-12.** The renin–angiotensin system. Note that either hypotension or hypovolemia can result in renal hypoperfusion and activation of the sympathetic nervous system, increasing renal renin release.

   3.   **Autoregulation** is the ability of blood vessels to adjust blood flow in accordance with metabolic need and to maintain blood flow despite extreme changes in tissue perfusion pressure. Most tissues are capable of regulating their own blood flow by release of local tissue mediators.

**I.   Cardiovascular Disease**

**Heart disease** from any cause usually progresses through three phases: **overload (excessive work), compensatory,** and **patho-**

**logic.** Whatever the inciting cause, ventricular overload brought about by excessive work leads to increases in both the oxygen and nutrient requirements of the heart. Initial compensatory changes include increases in sympathetic tone and a variety of neurohumoral responses that act to sustain or increase cardiac inotropy and promote the retention of salt and water (Fig. 3-13). These responses are usually followed by compensatory ventricular hypertrophy associated with decreases in both the rate of ventricular pressure development and the rate of relaxation. The pathologic phase of heart failure exists when an abnormality in cardiac function is responsible for a decrease in cardiac output to a degree that is insufficient to meet the oxygen and nutrient requirements of metabolizing tissues. It is important to realize that this definition incorporates situations in which the heart may be contracting normally or be hypercontractile. For example, cardiac output may be decreased during sinus tachycardia or bradycardia, cardiac arrhythmias, and the initial stages of valvular insufficiency (mitral insufficiency). Decrease in cardiac contractile performance is only one potential cause for a decrease in cardiac output and should be differentiated from other potential causes of heart failure to provide appropriate therapy and prevent drug-induced complications.

1. **Heart failure** is ultimately caused by pressure overload, volume overload, or primary myocardial disease (cardiomyopathy). The **cardiomyopathies** have been further categorized as hypertrophic, dilated, restrictive (infiltrative myocardial disease), and constrictive (pericardial disease). The signal for ventricular hypertrophy, although uncertain, is probably multifactorial, involving stretch-activated ion channels, increased ventricular tension, adrenergic factors, increased oxygen consumption (oxygen supply–demand imbalance) and ATP use, and/or increases in the quantity of metabolic breakdown products.

2. **Cardiac arrhythmias** include abnormalities in cardiac rate, rhythm, site of origin of the cardiac impulse, and pattern of atrial or ventricular depolarization. The cause for cardiac arrhythmias in intact hearts is attributed to abnormalities in automaticity, conduction, or both (Table 3-2). Abnormal heart rhythm resulting from abnormal

conduction and random or ordered re-entry can be caused by spatial differences in membrane refractory periods or discontinuous anisotropic (dissimilar in all directions) propagation (Fig. 3-14). The latter electro-

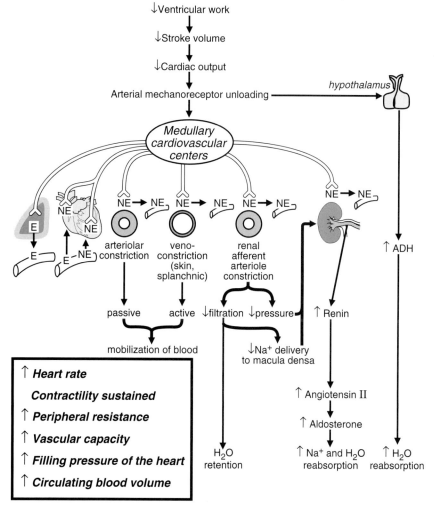

**Figure 3-13.** Reflex adjustments to heart failure and decreased ventricular work include increases in heart rate, peripheral vascular resistance vascular capacity, filling pressure of the heart, and circulating blood volume. Cardiac contractility is sustained by increases in sympathetic tone. These changes help maintain cardiac output. Modified from Shepherd JT, Van Houtte PM. The human cardiovascular system: facts and concepts. New York: Raven Press, 1979.

**Table 3-2. Classification of Arrhythmogenic Mechanisms at the Cellular Level in Terms of Vulnerable Parameters**

| Mechanisms of Arrhythmia | Vulnerable Parameter (Antiarrhythmic Effect) | Ionic Currents Most Likely to Modulate Vulnerable Parameter |
| --- | --- | --- |
| Automaticity | | |
| Enhanced normal automaticity | Phase 4 depolarization (decrease) | $I_f$, $I_{Ca-T}$ (block) |
| Abnormal automaticity | Maximum diastolic potential (hyperpolarize) or phase 4 depolarization (decrease) | $I_{KACh}$ (activate); $I_K$, $I_{KACh}$ (activate); $I_{Ca-L}$; $I_{Na}$ (block) |
| Triggered activity based on | | |
| EAD | Action potential duration (shorten) or EAD (suppress) | $I_X$ (activate) |
| DAD | Calcium overload (unload) or DAD (suppress) | $I_{Ca-L}$, $I_{Na}$ (block); $I_{Ca-L}$ (block); $I_{Ca-L}$, $I_{Na}$ (block) |
| Conduction: re-entry depends on calcium channels | | |
| Primary impaired conduction (long excitable gap) | Excitability and conduction (decrease) | $I_{Na}$ (block) |
| Conduction encroaching on refractoriness (short excitable gap) | Effective refractory period (prolong) | $I_K$ (block) |
| Other | | |
| Re-entry depends on calcium channels | Excitability and conduction (decrease) | $I_{Ca-L}$ (block) |
| Other mechanisms | | |
| Reflection | Excitability (decrease) | $I_{Na}$, $I_{Ca-L}$ (block) |
| Parasystole | Phase 4 depolarization (decrease) | $I_f$ (block) (if MDP high) |

Modified from The Task Force of the Working Group on Arrhythmias of the European Society of Cardiology. The "Sicilian gambit": a new approach to the classification of antiarrhythmic drugs based on their actions on arrhythmogenic mechanisms. Eur Heart J 1991;12:1112–1131. *EAD*, early after depolarizations; *DAD*, delayed after polarizations.

physiologic abnormality can occur as a result of cellular uncoupling, owing to a decreased number of effective cellular connections (gap junctions) caused by fibrosis, ischemia, or drug therapy. Regardless of cause, changes in either the active (ion current movements) or passive (membrane characteristics) properties of the cardiac cell membrane can result in a wide array of cardiac rate or rhythm disturbances, which are recordable at the body

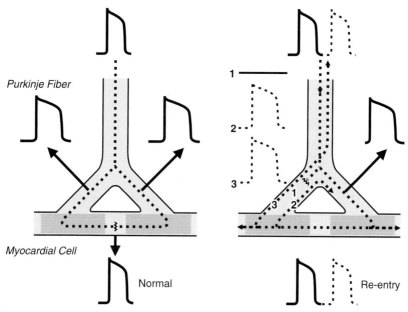

Purkinje Fiber

Myocardial Cell

Normal

Re-entry

**Figure 3-14.** Re-entry. During normal conditions, the cardiac action potential is transmitted through modified muscle fibers (specialized fibers) to the atrial and ventricular muscle cells, resulting in depolarization followed by repolarization. The action potential is not perpetuated, because the surrounding tissues at the end point of activation remain refractory to reactivation (normal). *1,* During various disease processes (ischemia, hypoxia, inflammation, fibrosis) and in the presence of some drugs (intravenous and inhalation anesthetics), the action potential may be blocked (unidirectional block) as it travels in an antegrade direction through cardiac tissue. If the electrical impulse is delayed (conduction delay) as it travels through adjacent tissue, it may re-enter and be conducted in a retrograde direction (retrograde conduction), thereby reactivating the same tissue segment (*2*) or more peripheral tissue segments (*3; left*). The longer the conduction delay, the more likely the electric impulse will find the tissue to be re-entered excitable (not refractory) and the greater the likelihood for re-entry (*dotted lines*). Continuous re-entry of cardiac tissue is called circus movement and can lead to sustained cardiac rhythm disturbances, including ventricular fibrillation. Re-entry involving a small amount (several square millimeters) of cardiac tissue is called micro re-entry, and re-entry that incorporates the specialized conducting system of the heart is called macro re-entry.

**Table 3-3. Cardiac Arrhythmias Produced by Preanesthetic and Anesthetic Drugs**

| Drugs | Arrhythmia |
|---|---|
| Anticholinergics | |
| Atropine | Sinus tachycardia |
| Glycopyrrolate | Sinus tachycardia |
| Phenothiazine | |
| Acepromazine | Sinus tachycardia; sinus bradycardia (rarely) |
| $\alpha_2$-Agonists | |
| Xylazine | Sinus bradycardia; first- and second-degree atrio- |
| Detomidine | ventricular block; third-degree atrioventricular |
| Medetomidine | block (rarely); sinus arrest (rarely) |
| Opioids | |
| Morphine | Sinus bradycardia; first- and second-degree atrio- |
| Oxymorphone | ventricular block |
| Fentanyl | |
| Butorphanol | |
| Benzodiazepines | |
| Diazepam | Arrhythmias rarely observed; sinus bradycardia, |
| Midazolam | temporary cardiac arrest |
| Intravenous anesthetics | |
| Thiobarbiturates (Thiamylal, Thiopental) | Bradyarrhythmias; premature ventricular depolar-izations; ventricular tachycardia; sinus tachycar-dia; ventricular arrhythmias, sinus tachycardia, bradyarrhythmias (rarely) |
| Inhalation anesthetics | |
| Methoxyflurane | Sinus bradycardia; bradyarrhythmias; premature ventricular depolarizations; ventricular tachycar- |
| Halothane | dia; ventricular fibrillation or cardiac arrest (halothane and methoxyflurane sensitize the |
| Isoflurane | myocardium to catecholamines) |

surface. Anesthetic drugs and various anesthetic techniques produce marked changes in cardiac cellular active and passive electrophysiologic properties, resulting in the development of cardiac arrhythmias (Table 3-3). The inhalation anesthetics in particular are known to shorten the action potential duration and decrease refractoriness, thereby predisposing the patient to conduction abnormalities and re-entry. Halothane and, to a lesser extent, methoxyflurane, enflurane, and isoflurane sensitize the myocardium to catecholamines. Both $\alpha_1$- and $\beta_1$-adrenoceptors are involved in the cardiac sensitization phenomena. Finally, most anesthetic drugs can produce pronounced effects on cardiac rate and rhythm because of their general membrane depressant effects.

3. **Adequate oxygen delivery** ($DO_2$) is of the utmost importance, because reduced oxygen consumption ($VO_2$) is known to be the common denominator in all forms of **shock,** including hemorrhagic and anemic shock. Oxygen transport is the major function of the cardiovascular system. Oxygen is the most flow-dependent blood constituent, because it has the highest extraction ratio of any substance carried in the blood and cannot be stored. Mortality is virtually 100% when the cumulative $VO_2$ deficit following hypoxemia, hemorrhage, or anemia exceeds 140 mL/kg. Reductions in $VO_2$, therefore, can be viewed as the ultimate regulatory factor responsible for cardiovascular compensatory responses, including increases in heart rate, cardiac contractility, cardiac output, and vascular tone. Other changes in cardiovascular function are determined by the primary precipitating event. Hemodilution, for example, produces increases in stroke volume, a redistribution of blood flow to the coronary and cerebral blood vessels, and a marked decrease in blood viscosity. The last effect—decrease in blood viscosity—facilitates capillary blood flow and can increase cardiac output by decreasing afterload. These hemodynamic changes have resulted in the clinical use of mild to moderate normovolemic hemodilution before anesthesia and surgery to improve cardiac output, peripheral perfusion, and $DO_2$.

## II.   RESPIRATORY SYSTEM
*Wayne McDonell*

**Respiration** is the total process whereby oxygen is supplied to and used by body cells and carbon dioxide is eliminated by means of gradients. **Ventilation** is the movement of gas in and out of the alveoli. The ventilatory requirement for homeostasis varies with the metabolic requirement of the animal; and it thus varies with body size, the level of activity, body temperature, and the depth of anesthesia. Pulmonary ventilation is accomplished by expansion and contraction of the lungs. Several terms are used to describe the various types of **breathing** that may be observed.

**Apnea:** Transient (or longer) cessation of breathing.
**Apneustic respiration:** Long, gasping inspirations with several subsequent ineffective exhalations.
**Biot respirations:** Sequences of gasps, apnea, and several deep gasps.
**Bradypnea:** Slow, regular respiration.
**Cheyne–Stokes respirations:** Increase in rate and depth, then become slower, followed by a brief period of apnea.
**Dyspnea:** Labored breathing.
**Eupnea:** Ordinary quiet breathing.
**Hyperpnea:** Fast and/or deep respiration, indicating over-respiration.
**Hypopnea:** Slow and/or shallow breathing, indicating under-respiration.
**Kussmaul respirations:** Regular, deep respirations without pause.
**Polypnea:** Rapid, shallow, panting type of respiration.
**Tachypnea:** Increased respiratory rate.

To describe the events of pulmonary ventilation, air in the lung has been classified into volumes and capacities (Fig. 3-15). Pulmonary capacities allow the clinician to consider two or more volumes together. Only tidal volume and functional residual capacity can be measured in conscious noncooperative animals.

**Expiratory reserve volume** (ERV): Amount of air that can be expired by forceful expiration after a normal expiration.
**Functional residual capacity** (FRC): Expiratory reserve volume plus the residual volume; the amount of air remaining in the lungs after a normal expiration.
**Inspiratory capacity** (IC): Tidal volume plus the inspiratory reserve volume; the amount of air that can be inhaled starting after a normal expiration and distending the lungs to the maximum amount.

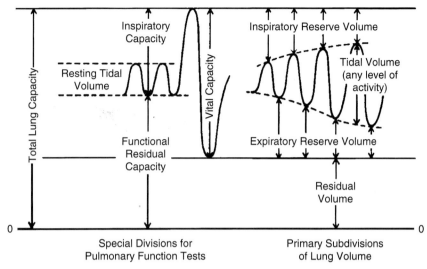

**Figure 3-15.** Lung volumes and capacities. Reprinted with permission from Standardization of definitions and symbols in respiratory physiology. Fed Proc 1950;9:602.

**Inspiratory reserve volume** (IRV): Volume of air that can be inspired over and above the normal tidal volume.

**Minute respiratory volume** ($\dot{V}_E$): Also referred to as minute ventilation; equal to tidal volume times the respiratory frequency.

**Residual volume** (RV): Air remaining in the lungs after the most forceful expiration.

**Tidal volume** ($V_T$): Volume of air inspired or expired in one breath.

**Total lung capacity** (TLC): Inspiratory reserve volume plus the tidal volume plus the expiratory reserve volume plus the residual volume; the maximum volume to which the lungs can be expanded with the greatest possible inspiratory effort.

**Vital capacity** (VC): Inspiratory reserve volume plus the tidal volume plus the expiratory reserve volume; the maximum amount of air that can be expelled from the lungs after first filling them to their maximum capacity.

## A.    Ventilation

It is useful to consider the ventilatory system in terms of its major components: **neural control,** the **bellows mechanism** (chest wall and diaphragm), **upper airway,** and **lung parenchyma** (Fig. 3-16). Alterations in the neural control of ventilation by sedative, opioid, or anesthetic depression; changes in the upper or lower airway patency by muscle relaxation or spasm; and variations in the bellows mechanism of the thorax through neuromuscular paralysis, space-occupying lesions of the thorax, or a change in the diaphragm (shape, location, or function) may all appreciably affect ventilatory adequacy and the efficiency of gas exchange. Within the parenchyma less than optimum matching of fresh alveolar gas with pulmonary capillary blood will produce blood gas alterations, particularly in regard to $Pao_2$.

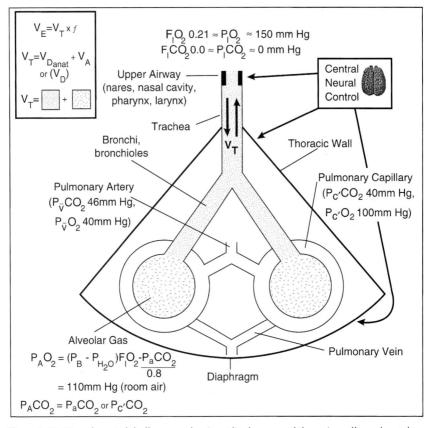

**Figure 3-16.** Neural control, bellows mechanism (diaphragm and thoracic wall), and matching of pulmonary artery blood and alveolar gas in the lung. $F_I$, fraction of inspired gases; $f$, respiratory frequency; $V_T$, tidal volume; $V_{Ds\ anat}$, anatomic dead space; $V_A$, alveolar volume. Also shown are partial pressures of oxygen and carbon dioxide in inspired air ($P_I$), alveolar air ($P_A$), pulmonary arterial blood ($P_{pa}$), and pulmonary end-capillary blood ($P_C$). See text for detailed explanation.

1. **Control of respiratory function** occurs in the central respiratory centers, central and peripheral chemoreceptors, pulmonary reflexes, and nonrespiratory neural input. Control of respiration has been described as an integrated feedback control system. Sedatives, analgesics, anesthetics, and the equipment used for inhalational anesthesia may profoundly alter respiration and the ability of the animal to maintain cellular homeostasis.

2. **Transfer of gases** to and from the lungs depends on developing a pressure gradient between the atmosphere and the alveoli and is modified by the resistance to flow between these two regions and the elasticity of the lungs and chest wall. During spontaneous inspiration, active muscular effort enlarges the pleural cavity through expansion of the thoracic wall and contraction of the diaphragm (Fig. 3-16). The factors that contribute to these pressure gradients and the measurement of their magnitude are referred to as pulmonary mechanics.

3. During **assisted** or **controlled ventilation,** atmospheric to alveolar pressure gradients also occur, but mouth pressure is more positive than is alveolar pressure on inspiration; hence the term *positive pressure ventilation.* This has important circulatory consequences. If the lungs and/or chest wall are less compliant than normal (i.e., stiffer), then higher transthoracic pressures are required to deliver a given tidal volume. The experienced anesthetist can often sense this change, because an increased force is required to mechanically squeeze a set volume from a rebreathing bag by hand. This may provide the first clue that an animal is developing a space-occupying problem in the thorax or abdomen (e.g., accumulation of air or blood), or that the end of the endotracheal tube has become repositioned in one main bronchus and is inflating only one lung.

4. **Airway resistance** during anesthesia can be minimized by using an airway that is as wide as possible and in which sudden alterations in direction or diameter are minimized. The caliber of the airway and the rate and pattern of airflow contribute to the pressure gradient along the

airway. Airway resistance increases with the rate of respiration and with narrowing of the airway by reflex contraction of the bronchiolar muscles, with small airway disease in which there is edema of the airway wall and mucous accumulation, and with a reduction in lung volume or through aspiration of foreign material.

5. **Pulmonary ventilation** is the rate at which alveolar air is exchanged with atmospheric air. This is not equal to the minute ventilation volume, because a large portion of inspired air is used to fill the respiratory passages, rather than alveoli, and no significant gaseous exchange occurs in this air (Fig. 3-16). Representative normal ventilation, blood gas, and acid–base values for some small species are shown in Tables 3-4 and 3-5.

6. **Matching** of **alveolar gas** and **pulmonary capillary blood flow** is influenced by gravitational factors and the fact that the pulmonary artery circulation is a low-pressure system. The major effect of gravity on the lung is to produce a vertical perfusion gradient in the pulmonary circulation; the lower region is more perfused. The distribution of these gravitational effects on lung perfusion is commonly divided and functionally described as a three- or four-zone system (Fig. 3-17).

7. For any given metabolic output, $Pa_{CO_2}$ and alveolar ventilation are directly and inversely related: If ventilation falls by 50%, $Pa_{CO_2}$ doubles; whereas if alveolar ventilation is increased by 100% (say by intermittent positive-pressure ventilation) $Pa_{CO_2}$ levels fall by 50% once equilibrium is established. This explains how good approximations about the resultant $Pa_{CO_2}$ level can be made when an animal is put on a volume-limited ventilator at a particular f and $V_T$ setting. For instance, in most anesthetized dogs with a body weight that is average for the breed, $Pa_{CO_2}$ will be near eucapnic levels when f is set at 8 to 10/min and $V_T$ at 20 mL/kg.

8. The interrelationship between a lower **hemoglobin** level (e.g., 10 g/dL) and **blood oxygen content** with altered ventilatory homeostasis is important (Fig. 3-18). The

**Table 3-4. Breathing Frequency (f), Tidal Volume ($V_T$), and Minute Ventilation ($V_E$) of Various Species**

| Species | Conditions | Mean Body Weight, kg | n | f, breaths/min | $V_T$ mL | $V_T$ mL/kg | $V_E$ mL/min | $V_E$ mL/kg/min |
|---|---|---|---|---|---|---|---|---|
| Mice | Awake, prone | 0.02 | NS | 163.4 | 0.15 | 7.78 | 24.5 | 1239 |
| | Anesthetized | 0.032 | NS | 109 | 0.18 | 5.63 | 21.0 | 720 |
| Rats | Awake, prone | 0.113 | NS | 85.5 | 0.87 | 7.67 | 72.9 | 646 |
| | Awake, pleth | 0.305 | NS | 103 | 2.08 | 6.83 | 213 | 701 |
| Cats | Unanesthetized, pleth | 3.8 | 4 | 22 | 30 | 7.9 | 664 | 174 |
| | Anesthetized | 3.7 | NS | 30 | 34 | 9.2 | 960 | 310 |
| Dogs | Awake, prone, chronic trach, intubated | 18.6 | 6 | 13 | 309 | 16.6 | 3818 | 205 |
| | Awake, standing, chronic trach, intubated | 18.8 | 8 | 16.5 | 314 | 16.9 | 4963 | 264 |

*NS, not specified; pleth, whole body plethysmograph; trach, tracheostomy.*

**Table 3-5. Arterial Blood Gas and Acid–Base Values for Various Species**

| Species | Conditions | Body Weight, kg | n | pH | $Paco_2$ | $Pao_2$ | $HCO_3^-$ |
|---------|-----------|-----------------|---|-----|----------|---------|-----------|
| Rats | Awake, chronic catheter | 0.207 | 10 | 7.44 | 32.7 | | 21.5 |
| | Awake, prone, chronic catheter | 0.305 | 8 | 7.467 | 39.8 | | 28.7 |
| Rabbits | Awake, catheter | 3.1 | NS | 7.388 | 32.8 | 86 | 21 |
| | Awake, catheter | 3.5 | 20 | 7.47 | 28.5 | 89.2 | 20.2 |
| Cats | Unsedated, chronic catheter, prone | 2.5–5.1 | 8 | 7.41 | 28.0 | 108 | 18 |
| | Unsedated, not restrained, chronic catheter | 3–8 | 10 | 7.426 | 32.5 | 108 | 22.1 |
| Dogs | Chronic tracheostomy, catheter, unsedated, standing | 18.8 | 8 | 7.383 | 39.0 | 103.8 | 22.1 |
| | Chronic catheters lateral recumbency | 12.2 | 22 | 7.40 | 35 | 102 | 21 |

*NS*, not specified.

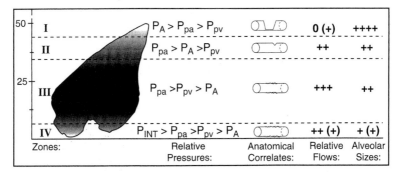

**Figure 3-17.** Pulmonary artery ($P_{pa}$), pulmonary vein ($P_{pv}$), pulmonary interstitial ($P_{INT}$) and alveolar ($P_A$) pressure–flow relationships in the lung. See text for detailed explanation. Modified from Porcelli RJ. Pulmonary hemodynamics. In: Parent RA, ed., Treatise on pulmonary toxicology. Boca Raton, FL: CRC Press, 1992:243.

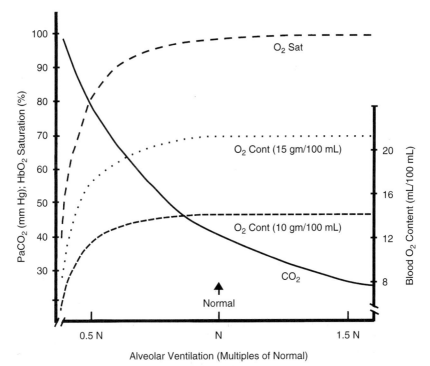

**Figure 3-18.** Effect of altered alveolar ventilation on hemoglobin saturation, blood oxygen content, and $Paco_2$ levels. As alveolar ventilation is halved, the $Paco_2$ level doubles, illustrating the inverse and direct relationship between alveolar ventilation and carbon dioxide clearance. Note the difference in oxygen content with anemia (hemoglobin 10 g/100 mL instead of 15 g/100 mL) and the eventual sharp drop in hemoglobin oxygen saturation and oxygen content as alveolar ventilation decreases to < 50% of the normal value. See text for further explanation.

blood oxygen content is reduced by nearly 7 mL/dL with a decrease in hemoglobin from 15 to 10 g/dL, even when hemoglobin saturation is 100%; dangerously low blood oxygen contents occur with further ventilatory depression.

9. **Hypoxia** refers to any state in which the oxygen in the lung, blood, and/or tissues is abnormally low, resulting in abnormal organ function and/or cellular damage. Hypoxemia refers to insufficient oxygenation of blood to meet metabolic requirement. Resting $Pa_{O_2}$ in domestic species generally ranges from 80 to 100 mmHg in healthy, unsedated animals (Table 3-5). The clinical significance of blood oxygen tension varies in relation to the rate of tissue metabolism (e.g., hypothermic anesthetized patients require less oxygen).

## B.    Oxygen Transport in Blood

1. **Gas exchange** occurs across both the alveolar and capillary membranes. The total distance across which exchange takes place is $< 1$ μ; therefore, it occurs rapidly. Equilibrium almost develops between blood in the lungs and air in the alveolus, and the $P_{O_2}$ in the blood almost equals the $P_{O_2}$ in the alveolus. At complete saturation, each gram of hemoglobin combines with 1.36 mL oxygen. The ability of hemoglobin to combine with oxygen depends on the partial pressure of oxygen in the surrounding environment. The degree to which it will become saturated at various partial pressures of oxygen varies considerably. There is relatively little change in saturation between 70 and 250 mm Hg partial pressure of oxygen; a marked change occurs between 10 and 40 mm Hg (as is illustrated by the **oxyhemoglobin dissociation curve**), a partial pressure characteristic of actively metabolizing tissues (Fig. 3-19). Thus as hemoglobin is exposed to tissues with partial pressures of oxygen within this range, it must yield its oxygen to the tissues. The lower the $P_{O_2}$ of the tissues, the greater the amount of oxygen that hemoglobin must give up. The degree to which hemoglobin gives up its oxygen is influenced by environmental pH, $P_{CO_2}$, and temperature—all mechanisms that protect the metabolizing cell.

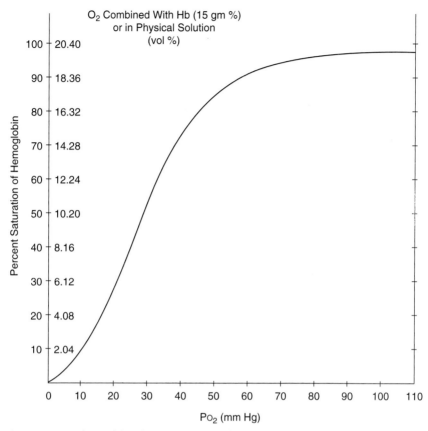

**Figure 3-19.** Oxyhemoglobin dissociation curve of canine blood at pH 7.40. The percentage of Hb saturation and $O_2$ content changes little when the $Po_2$ changes from 100 (normal) to 60 mm Hg, as may occur during cardiopulmonary dysfunction or disease. Reprinted with permission from Gillespie JR, Martin DB. Long-term oxygen cage therapy for hypoxemic dogs. J Am Vet Med Assoc 1970;156:717.

2.  The **enzyme 2,3-DPG** enhances dissociation of oxygen from hemoglobin by competing with oxygen for the binding site. Lowered levels of this enzyme increase the affinity of hemoglobin for oxygen, causing the curve to shift to the left.

3.  With **100% oxygen administration,** the partial pressure of oxygen in the alveoli is raised from 100 to almost 650 mm Hg. Plasma oxygen is thus elevated almost 7 times; i.e, from 0.3 to 1.8 mL/100 mL blood. The result is an

increase of about 10% in oxygen content of the blood. This is of some importance, because oxygen transfers from blood to tissues by diffusion, and the process occurs at a rate proportional to the difference in oxygen tension between plasma and body tissues.

4.  **Factors increasing the availability of oxygen to tissues** are increased circulation (up to five times as much blood as normal may flow through the tissues), increased respiratory rate (the carbon dioxide tension of the blood regulates the respiratory center), and increased deoxygenation of a given volume of blood. Increased deoxygenation may be caused by lowered oxygen tension in the cells; increased temperature with increased dissociation; and increased amounts of metabolic by-products, such as carbon dioxide and lactic acid. These factors favor local vasodilation with the consequent benefit of increased oxygen supply in instances of increased tissue metabolism. When combined, these factors can increase oxygen availability to tissues over the resting state by a factor of 10. The rate of muscular activity is not limited by oxygen supply, because muscle can incur an oxygen deficit.

## C.  Carbon Dioxide Transport in Blood

1.  **Carbon dioxide** is an end product of glucose oxidation. During severe exercise, the production of carbon dioxide is increased enormously; whereas during anesthesia, production likely decreases. In the tissues, carbon dioxide in the presence of carbonic anhydrase reacts with water to form carbonic acid. Because of the blood buffer systems, transport of carbon dioxide to the lungs for excretion is effected with little change in blood pH. The importance of the lungs in excreting this volatile acid is illustrated by the fact that, in humans, the kidneys eliminate 40 to 80 mEq/day, whereas the lungs eliminate 13,000 mEq/day.

2.  The **carbon dioxide dissociation curve** is more or less linear. Just as the amount of oxygen transported by the blood depends on the partial pressure of oxygen to which the blood is exposed, so is carbon dioxide transport likewise affected. In contrast to the minimal effects on

oxygen content (Fig. 3-18), hyperventilation and hypoventilation may have marked effects on the carbon dioxide content of blood and tissues.

### D.   Anesthetic Alterations of Respiration

1.   **Anesthetics** and **preanesthetic drugs** alter the central and peripheral chemoreceptor response to carbon dioxide and oxygen in a dose-dependent manner. This has important clinical implications in terms of maintaining homeostasis during the perioperative period. There will also be a **diminution in external signs** in an hypoxemic or hypercarbic anesthetized animal. Whereas unsedated animals usually demonstrate obvious tachypnea and an increase in $V_T$ or respiratory effort in response to serious hypoxemia or hypercapnia, these external signs of an impending crisis may well be absent or greatly diminished in the anesthetized animal.

   a.   **General anesthetics** in current use produce a dose-dependent decrease in the response to carbon dioxide. With the commonly used inhalant agents (enflurane, halothane, isoflurane), the carbon dioxide response is almost flat in deep anesthesia. **Barbiturates, propofol,** and the **cyclohexamines** (ketamine, phencyclidine, tiletamine) cause dose-related alteration of the carbon dioxide response. In the case of barbiturates, the alteration may outlast the period of anesthesia. Ketamine is not as much of a respiratory depressant as the barbiturates; however, clinically effective doses of ketamine may induce apnea in some susceptible animals. When injectable anesthetics are used before inhalations, the respiratory depressant effects of both drugs are at least additive.

   Although the control of ventilation during anesthesia is primarily determined by central carbon dioxide responsiveness (albeit reduced), during very deep barbiturate anesthesia $CO_2$ ventilatory drive may disappear, and the drive becomes hypoxic. Hypoxic drive sensitivity is also lessened appreciably by general anesthetics (at least **inhalants**) in a dose-related manner. The inspired oxygen levels used in most inhalant regimens appear to contribute somewhat to depression of ventilation while helping ensure that the level of oxygenation is adequate.

b. **Opioids** shift the carbon dioxide response curve to the right with little change in slope, except at very high doses. This means that the resting $Paco_2$ level might be a little higher in an animal receiving a therapeutic dose of an opioid for premedication or postoperative recovery, but that the response to further carbon dioxide challenge (from metabolism, airway obstruction, etc.) will not be abolished. Clinically, when opioids are used at high doses as part of a balanced anesthetic regimen, there is an additive effect of the opioid depression of the respiratory center and the general anesthetic, and apnea may be produced. In addition, the μ opioids (e.g., oxymorphone) in particular tend to produce rapid, shallow breathing in dogs, which may interfere with the subsequent uptake of an inhalant anesthetic.

c. **Phenothiazine** and **benzodiazepine** sedatives often reduce the respiratory rate, especially if the animal is somewhat excited before administration; but they do not appreciably alter arterial blood gas tensions.

d. **The $\alpha_2$-adrenoceptor agonists** produce a more complicated effect on respiration. In cats, xylazine sedation does not appear to produce hypercapnia or hypoxemia. In dogs, xylazine's respiratory effects have not been definitively documented.

## E.  Changes in Ventilation and Perfusion

1. **Hypoxic pulmonary vasoconstriction** (HPV) may occur in the conscious, unsedated animal if regional ventilation is decreased and there is a local vasoconstriction that tends to divert blood flow away from underventilated areas of the lung. There is an apparent difference in the strength of the HPV response to whole-lung hypoxia in various species. Under normal conditions, even species with a

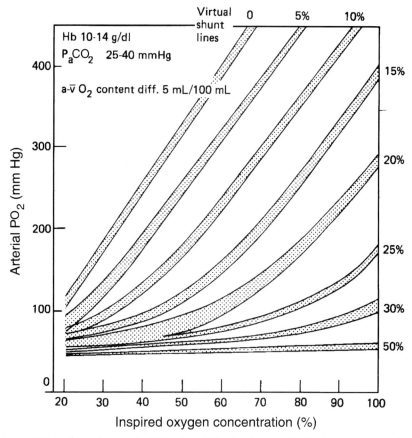

**Figure 3-20.** Isoshunt diagram depicting the relationship between inspired oxygen concentration, Pao2, and various degrees of venous admixture or pulmonary shunt. Shunt flow is expressed as a percentage of cardiac output. The arteriovenous oxygen content difference is assumed to be 5.0 mL/100 mL blood, reflecting a normal cardiac output. The shunt bands have been drawn to include the range of hemoglobin, and Paco2 levels shown. Modified from Benetar SR, Hewlett AM, Nunn JF. The use of iso-shunt lines for control of oxygen therapy. Br J Anaseth 1973;45:713.

weak hypoxic pulmonary reflex are capable of considerable blood flow diversion in response to regional areas of low alveolar $O_2$ content. It is possible to use an **isoshunt diagram** to provide a reasonably accurate estimate of pulmonary shunt flow if inspired oxygen concentration and Pao2 are known (Fig. 3-20). Such a diagram illustrates the poor response to increasing Pao2 with increased inspired oxygen concentrations when shunt flows exceed 30%.

a.  **Inhalant anesthetics reduce HPV.** None of the examined injectable agents (narcotics, barbiturates, and benzodiazepines) has any detectable effect on HPV. The onset of the interference with HPV is rapid with inhaled anesthetics and persists throughout the duration of the anesthetic. The end result of this interference with HPV is that, for any given level of altered intrapulmonary gas distribution caused by reduced lung volume, intermittent airway closure, or regional atelectasis, a greater degree of hypoxemia exists.

b.  **Atelectasis,** increased thoracic or abdominal blood volume, and loss of some inherent tone in the diaphragm at end-exhalation all seem to reduce FRC. There is little information regarding FRC changes in dogs and cats. The onset of general anesthesia appears not to alter FRC significantly in sternal, lateral, or dorsally recumbent dogs.

c.  Whether **chest wall** (including diaphragm) **and lung mechanical factors** influence $PAo_2$–$Pao_2$ during anesthesia is unclear, because the evidence is often conflicting. It appears that most dog breeds (and probably cats) have a compliant lateral chest wall that tends to contribute relatively little to the inspiratory effort compared to the diaphragm with clinical doses of most anesthetics. In all species, dangerously deep planes of anesthesia are commonly associated with flaccidity of the thoracic wall and paradoxical inward movement during inspiration (paradoxical inspiration). This same type of respiration may be seen in cats, ferrets, and other small mammals, even with light levels of anesthesia.

## F.  Clinical Implications

In healthy dogs and cats the **$PAo_2$–$Pao_2$ gradient and the degree of venous admixture** is small compared to other species. Perhaps this is owing to the smaller lungs in these species or to the difference in the chest wall changes during anesthesia or perhaps because there is excellent collateral pulmonary ventilation in these species. A high degree of collateral ventilation means that if an alveolus is not ventilated via the airway, it may well receive gas exchange through passages (pores of Kohn) leading to other alveoli that are ventilated.

1.  **A minimum inspired oxygen of 30 to 35% is recommended,** despite the relatively favorable situation in regard to $\dot{V}/\dot{Q}$ mismatch in these species. Oxygen supplementation is needed nearly as much in deeply sedated animals as in those receiving a general anesthetic (intravenous or inhalant). As can be seen in Figure 3-21, increasing the inspired oxygen level also provides protection against hypoxemia caused by hypoventilation; and adequate protection is generally achieved with 30 to 35%. This is why simple maneuvers, such as placing a face mask with oxygen on a high-risk patient before and during

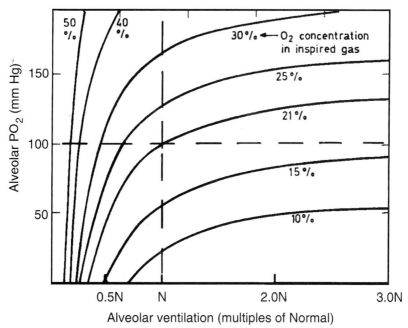

**Figure 3-21.** Protective effect of increased inspired oxygen concentrations with various degrees of alveolar hypoventilation and hyperventilation. With 30% inspired oxygen, $PA_{O_2}$ levels are above 100 mm Hg, even when alveolar ventilation is half normal. Modified from Nunn JF. Applied respiratory physiology. 3rd ed. London: Butterworth, 1987.

induction or use of a nasal oxygen catheter in the postoperative period, are beneficial.

2.  When **100% oxygen is used** with the common inhalant anesthetics in dogs and cats free of serious cardiopulmonary disease, the $Pao_2$ level is generally 450 to 525 mm Hg, whether the animal is breathing spontaneously or being ventilated. With such high inspired oxygen levels, hypoxemia usually only occurs through disconnection of the animal from the anesthetic machine, or with faulty placement of the endotracheal tube, cardiac arrest, or total apnea for over 5 min.

3.  The decision to institute **assisted or controlled intermittent positive-pressure ventilation** (IPPV) is generally made to prevent or treat hypercapnia, rather than to achieve oxygenation. Nearly all spontaneously breathing dogs and cats show some degree of hypoventilation and hypercapnia ($Paco_2$ = 45 to 55 mm Hg). The clinical importance of this in the non-neurologic case is open to debate. Dogs and cats do not have atherosclerosis, and over the years hundreds of thousands of dogs and cats have been successfully anesthetized in practice while breathing spontaneously.

4.  Minimal **guidelines** for respiratory support during anesthesia include the following. Anesthesia is better done in dogs with an endotracheal tube in place, and in many situations cats should be intubated. Use at least 30 to 35% inspired oxygen in all anesthetized dogs and cats. Inflate the lungs to 30 cm $H_2O$ airway pressure (i.e., "sigh" the lungs) periodically and at the end of anesthesia.

## III.  NERVOUS SYSTEM

### A.  Central Nervous System

Anatomically, the nervous system can be divided into **central and peripheral divisions.** The central division, composed of the brain and spinal cord, contains all of the important nerve centers or nuclei. The peripheral division is made up of nerves and ganglia that supply the different organs and tissues.

1.  The **brain** can be divided into the **cerebrum** and the **brainstem.** The basal ganglia (corpus striatum, amygdaloid, and claustrum) are large masses of gray matter at the base of each cerebral hemisphere. Their primary function appears to be inhibition of motor function and maintenance of balance between opposing muscles at both the cortical and brainstem levels. Dopamine and γ-aminobutyric acid (GABA) are the primary inhibitory neurotransmitters released. The central core of the cerebrum consists of the thalamus, subthalamus, epithalamus, and hypothalamus and is positioned between the cerebrum and the brainstem. The **thalamus** receives fibers from all sensory systems, except the olfactory, and projects to sensory areas of the cerebral cortex. The cerebral cortex is an outgrowth of the lower centers, especially the thalamus. As a result, for each area of the cortex, there is a smaller corresponding area within the thalamus.

    a.  The **hypothalamus** is the primary center for integrative control of the autonomic nervous system. Parasympathetic responses, including slowing of the heart rate, vasodilation, decreased blood pressure, salivation, increased gastrointestinal peristalsis, contraction of the urinary bladder, and sweating, are elicited by stimulation of the anterior hypothalamus. Stimulation of the posterior and lateral hypothalamus elicits sympathetic responses, including increased heart rate and blood pressure, cessation of gastrointestinal peristalsis, dilation of the pupils, and hyperglycemia. The hypothalamus plays a major role in maintaining homeostasis through control of temperature, thirst, and appetite.

    b.  The **brainstem** consists of the midbrain, pons, and medullar oblongata. The cerebellum is connected to the midbrain by the superior cerebellar peduncles.

Caudal to the pons is the medulla oblongata and posterior to it is the spinal cord. In addition to nerve tracts, the medulla oblongata contains vital nerve centers that regulate respiration and circulation.

   c.   The **cerebellum** lies dorsal to the brainstem and is formed by two hemispheres separated by a central portion, the vermis. The cerebellum receives input from the sensory systems and the cerebral cortex. The cerebellum integrates muscle tone in relation to equilibrium, locomotion, posture and nonstereotyped movements based on experience. It is chiefly concerned with muscle coordination.

2.   **Cranial nerves** consist of a peripheral portion, a nuclear center in the brainstem (except olfactory and optic nerves), and central connections with other parts of the brain (Fig. 3-22). All twelve cranial nerves are paired.

3.   The **spinal cord** runs posteriorly in the vertebral canal. In the dog and cat, the spinal cord terminates at the level of the last lumbar vertebra. The caudal portion of the vertebral canal contains the cauda equina, which is composed of descending spinal nerves. The cord is surrounded by the meninges, which support and protect it. From without inward, they are the dura mater, arachnoid, and pia mater. The spinal fluid is found in the subarachnoid space. The cord has an H-shaped central core of **gray matter,** which contains nerve cell bodies. The gray matter is surrounded by the **white matter,** the myelinated axons of intermediate longitudinally running nerve fibers. The spinal cord is much more complex than a mere cable or conduit, and it plays a much larger role in regulating CNS function than was once thought.

   a.   The **meninges** surround the spinal cord. Various spaces are associated with the meninges and are important in understanding spinal anesthetics and nomenclature. The **dura mater** has two layers within the cranial vault, an inner or visceral layer and an outer layer adherent to the cranial periosteum. The inner or visceral layer invests the spinal cord and

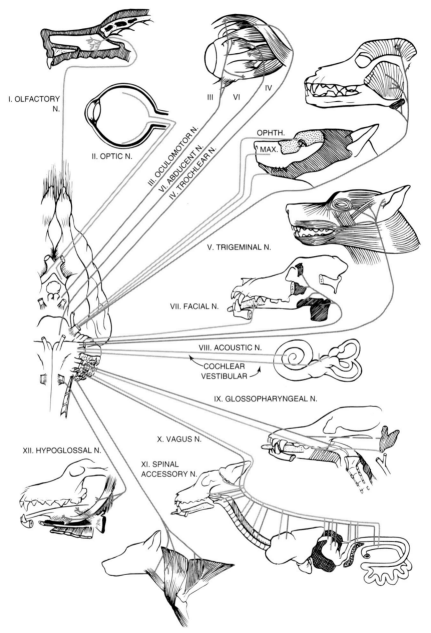

**Figure 3-22.** The origin and major distribution of the cranial nerves in the dog. Reprinted with permission from Hoerlein BF. Canine neurology, diagnosis and treatment. 3rd ed. Philadelphia: Saunders, 1978.

ventral and dorsal nerve root; the outer layer is absent in the vertebral canal of some species. The epidural space is the space within the spinal canal outside the visceral layer of the dura mater. It has also been referred to as the extradural space and, in species having both layers of dura, the intradural space.

b. The **subarachnoid space** is located between the arachnoidea and pia mater. It contains cerebrospinal fluid (CSF) and is continuous between the cranial and vertebral segments. There is no direct communication between the epidural and subarachnoid spaces. The **pia mater** is one cell layer thick and lies directly on the brain and spinal cord.

4. The **CSF** is found in both an internal (ventricular) system and an external (subarachnoid) system. CSF is produced by the choroid plexus, a fringe-like fold of pia mater found on the floor of both lateral ventricles and in the fourth ventricle and also by the ependymal epithelium lining the ventricles. The central canal of the spinal cord is continuous with the fourth ventricle. The external or subarachnoid system overlies the brain and spinal cord. Cerebrospinal fluid cushions the brain within the cranial vault. It is formed from the blood by secretory and filtration processes. Normal pressure of the CSF is 10 mm Hg.

## B. Peripheral Nervous System

1. **Spinal nerves** supply motor and sensory innervation to most of the body (somatic nervous system), with the exception of the head and viscera. They also form part of the ANS, which controls visceral functions. Spinal nerves vary in number, depending on species. Anatomically, the spinal nerves are formed by a combination of dorsal and ventral spinal roots arising from the spinal cord. These join and leave the spinal canal through the intervertebral foramina. Large, heavily myelinated fibers have the highest conduction velocities, whereas small, nonmyelinated fibers have lower conduction rates (Table 3-6).

**Table 3-6. Classification of Nerve Fibers**

| Fiber | Terminology | | Diameter | Conduction Speed, m/s |
|---|---|---|---|---|
| Myelinated somatic fibers | A | α | 20 μ | 120 |
| | | β | | |
| | | γ | ↓ | ↓ |
| | | δ | ↓ (3–4 μ) | ↓ (6–30) → pain fibers |
| | | ε | 2 μ | 5 |
| Myelinated visceral fibers (preganglionic autonomic) | B | | < 3 μ | 3–15 |
| Nonmyelinated somatic fibers | C | | < 2 μ | 0.5–2 → pain fibers |

Reprinted with permission from Wylie WD, Churchill-Davidson HC. A practice of anaesthesia. London: Lloyd-Luke, 1966; and Gasser HS. Pain producing impulses in peripheral nerves. Assoc Res Nerv Dis Proc 1943;22:44.

a.  The spinal cord is divided into segments for descriptive purposes; in the dog there are 8 cervical, 13 thoracic, 7 lumbar, 3 sacral, and 4 or 5 coccygeal segments. The segmental distribution of the motor roots in the dog is set forth in Table 3-7.

b.  Branches from several spinal nerves may combine to form plexuses, such as the brachial plexus, or major nerves, such as the sciatic nerve.

c.  **Rami communicantes** branch off the spinal nerves in the thoracic and lumbar areas. They connect the spinal nerves with a chain of ganglia lying lateral to the vertebral bodies, termed the vertebral sympathetic ganglia (Fig. 3-23).

## C.  Autonomic Nervous System

The **ANS** is often called the vegetative, visceral, or involuntary nervous system, because its action requires no conscious control. In this respect, it contrasts with the somatic nervous system supplying the striated muscles. The autonomic nervous system is made up of the efferent and afferent nerves innervating the viscera. Thus its primary efferent role is in maintenance of homeostasis through control of circulation, breathing, excretion, and maintenance of body temperature. The autonomic system can be further subdivided into the craniosacral or **parasympathetic** division and the thoracolumbar or **sympathetic** division (Figs. 3-24 and 3-25). A characteristic of the ANS is that both divisions are constantly active, resulting in a basal level of sympathetic and parasympathetic tone.

1.  The **parasympathetic nervous system** conserves and restores energy. Acetylcholine is the neurotransmitter at both preganglionic and postganglionic neurons. Each preganglionic fiber synapses with one to three postganglionic neurons, which terminate on a limited number of effector cells. Acetylcholine is rapidly inactivated by acetylcholinesterase at the synapse, resulting in a short duration of discharge. Thus parasympathetic activity is highly localized.

**Table 3-7. Segmental Distribution of Motor Roots in the Dog**

| Segment | Description |
| --- | --- |
| C3–5 | Distributed in segmental manner to most of the neck musculature |
| C5 | May send a branch to the phrenic nerve |
| C6 (usually 7) | Phrenic nerves to the diaphragm |
| C6–8, T1 (occasionally 2) | Brachial plexus to the forelimb |
| T2–8 | Intercostal nerves to the thorax |
| T9–13 | Nerves to the muscles of the ventral and lower lateral parts of the abdominal wall |
| L1–2 (occasionally 3) | Nerves to the muscles of the caudolateral abdominal wall and the thigh in the region of the stifle |
| L4–7, S1–3 | Lumbosacral plexus to the hindlimb |
| L4–6 (occasionally 3) | Femoral nerve to extensors of the stifle |
| L5–6 (occasionally 4) | Obturator nerve, the abductor of the hip |
| L6–7, S1 | Sciatic nerve supplying all other muscles of the hindlimb |

Reprinted with permission from McGrath JT. Neurologic examination of the dog. 2nd ed. Philadelphia: Lea & Febiger, 1960.

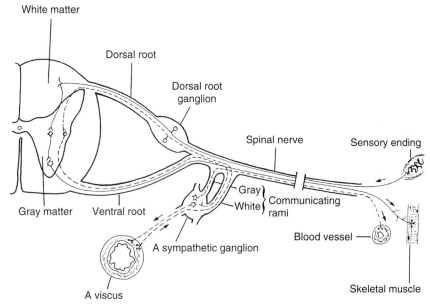

**Figure 3-23.** Components of a spinal nerve between the first thoracic and second or third lumbar segments. Reprinted with permission from Barr ML. The human nervous system: an anatomic viewpoint. Hagerstown, MD: Harper & Row, 1979.

a. The **vagus nerves** contain approximately 80% of the parasympathetic nerve fibers in the body. The preganglionic fibers are long and synapse in small ganglia that lie directly on or in the viscera of the thorax and abdomen. Fibers are supplied to the heart, lungs, esophagus, stomach, small intestine, proximal colon, liver, gallbladder, pancreas, kidneys, and upper ureters. In the heart, they are distributed to the SA and AV nodes, and to a lesser extent to the atria. There are few or no vagal parasympathetic fibers in the ventricles. In the intestinal wall, they form the plexuses of Meissner and Auerbach. The vagus also carries afferent fibers, arising from the nodose ganglion, that produce visceral reflexes but apparently not pain.

b. The **sacral outflow** originates in the second, third, and fourth sacral segments of the spinal cord. Preganglionic fibers form the pelvic nerves (nervi

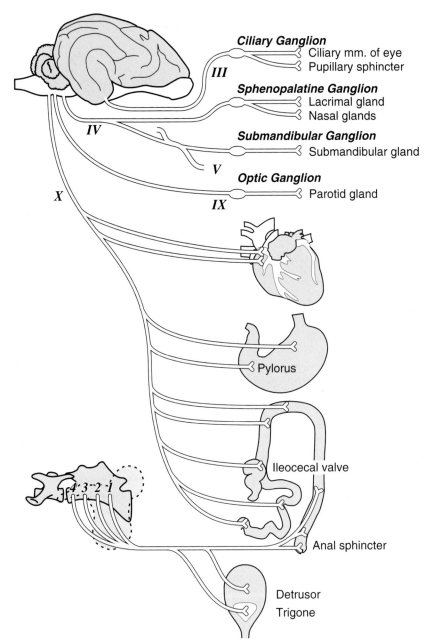

**Figure 3-24.** The parasympathetic nervous system. Note the distribution of cranial nerves III, IV, V, IX, and X. Modified from Guyton AC. Textbook of medical physiology. 8th ed. Philadelphia: Saunders, 1991.

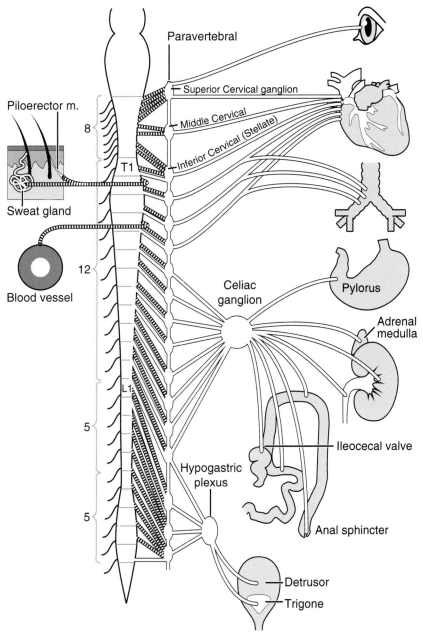

**Figure 3-25.** The sympathetic nervous system. Note the location of the stellate and hypogastric ganglia. Modified from Guyton AC. Textbook of medical physiology. 8th ed. Philadelphia: Saunders, 1991.

erigentes) which synapse in ganglia near the bladder, distal colon, rectum, and sexual organs. The vagus and pelvic nerves thus provide secretory, vasodilator, and motor fibers for the thoracic, abdominal, and pelvic organs.

2. The **sympathetic nervous system** mediates activities that accompany expenditures of energy. Thus sympathetic activity is greatest during stress or times of emergency. Sympathetic activity is necessary for normal responses to stimuli in the external environment (stressors). As in the parasympathetic system, acetylcholine is the neurotransmitter between preganglionic and postganglionic neurons. The neurotransmitter between postganglionic neurons and effector cells is norepinephrine. An exception is the sweat gland, whose sympathetic terminals are cholinergic. In contrast to the parasympathetic division, strong sympathetic stimulation produces generalized effects. This occurs because each preganglionic neuron synapses with 20 to 30 postganglionic neurons, each of which terminates on many effector cells. In addition, norepinephrine at postganglionic synapses and norepinephrine and epinephrine secreted by the adrenal medulla in response to sympathetic stimulation are deactivated rather slowly.

a. The **adrenal medulla** is unique in that it is embryologically, anatomically, and functionally homologous to the sympathetic ganglia. Chromaffin cells within the medulla originate from the neural crest and are innervated by preganglionic fibers. Activation of the sympathetic nervous system results in release of epinephrine and norepinephrine (80 and 20%, respectively), which act as systemic hormones, from the adrenal medulla. Circulating epinephrine has greater cardiac and metabolic effects than does norepinephrine and, because of $\beta_2$-receptor activity, induces vasodilation in skeletal muscle. In addition, circulating norepinephrine and epinephrine have generalized metabolic effects in tissues that do not receive sympathetic innervation.

### D.   Function of Neurons

1.   **Nerve impulses** are electric currents. They pass along the axon to the presynaptic membrane. From a pharmacologic standpoint, there is an important distinction between electric conduction of a nerve impulse along an axon and chemical transmission of this signal across the synapse. Local anesthetic agents block conduction, whereas a much larger group of drugs, including local anesthetics, alter transmission. When a resting axon is stimulated electrically, a nerve action potential (NAP) is produced that will travel the full length of the neuron in either direction (Fig. 3-26). Most general anesthetics (isoflurane, halothane, and nitrous oxide) have little effect on nerve conduction velocity.

2.   **Neuroregulators** play a key role in communication among nerve cells (Table 3-8). They may be subdivided into two groups: small molecule neurotransmitters and neuropeptide modulators.

   a.   **Small molecular neurotransmitters** are synthesized in the cytosol of the presynaptic terminal, absorbed into the transmitter vesicles, and released into the synaptic cleft in response to the arrival of an action potential at the nerve ending. Release of neurotransmitters is voltage dependent and requires calcium influx into the presynaptic terminal.

   b.   **Neuropeptide modulators** are synthesized in the neuronal cell body and are transported to the nerve terminal by axonal streaming. They are released in response to an action potential, but in much smaller quantities than are the small molecule transmitters. The neuropeptides induce prolonged effects to amplify or dampen neuronal activity. In terms of anesthesia, many neuroregulators are known to be of great importance, whereas the significance of others may not be appreciated at this time.

3.   **Cholinergic transmission** occurs when a nerve impulse reaches the synapse and acetylcholine is released. It

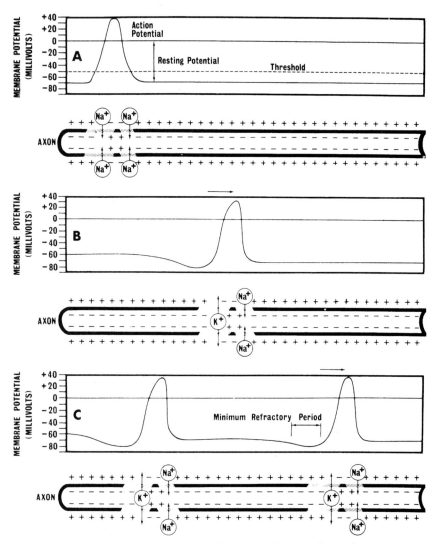

**Figure 3-26.** Nerve impulse. **A,** Depolarizing electrotonic effects result in sodium ions entering the axon. The resting potential is gradually altered until threshold is reached. At this time sodium ions enter the axon in great numbers, creating an action potential. **B and C,** Propagation of the nerve impulse. Sodium ions enter the axon in advance of the nerve impulse, and potassium ions flow out after the impulse has passed. The outflow of potassium ions results in a brief refractory period. Modified from Katz, 1961. Reprinted with permission from Miller ME, Christensen GC, Evans HE. Anatomy of the dog. Philadelphia: Saunders, 1964.

almost instantly crosses the synaptic cleft and unites with receptors on the postjunctional membrane, causing a local increase in ionic permeability of the membrane.

a.  **Acetylcholine esterase** (AChE) is one of two cholinesterases that are present in the body and are capable of hydrolyzing acetylcholine. AChE is a true, specific, e-type cholinesterase that is found principally in neurons and at neuromuscular junctions, but also in erythrocytes, thrombocytes, and placenta. It is responsible for terminating the action of acetylcholine by hydrolysis to acetic acid and choline. Practically all pharmacologic actions of anti-

---

**Table 3-8. Neuroregulators and Modulators**

| | |
|---|---|
| **Small-molecule, rapidly acting neurotransmitters** | α-Melanocyte-stimulating hormone |
| | Prolactin |
| Class I | Luteinizing hormone |
|   Acetylcholine | Thyrotropin |
| Class II (amines) | Growth hormone |
|   Norepinephrine | Vasopressin |
|   Epinephrine | Oxytocin |
|   Dopamine | Peptides that act on gut and brain |
|   Serotonin |   Leucine enkephalin |
|   Histamine |   Methionine enkephalin |
| Class III (amino acids) |   Substance P |
|   GABA |   Gastrin |
|   Glycine |   Cholecystokinin |
|   Glutamate |   Vasoactive intestinal polypeptide |
|   Aspartate |   Neurotensin |
| **Neuropeptide, slow-acting transmitters** |   Insulin |
|   Hypothalamic-releasing hormone |   Glucagon |
|   Thyrotropin-releasing hormone | Peptides that act on other tissues |
|   Luteinizing-releasing hormone |   Angiotensin II |
|   Somatostatin |   Bradykinin |
| Pituitary peptides |   Carnosine |
|   ACTH |   Sleep peptides |
|   β-Endorphin |   Calcitonin |

cholinesterase agents are owing to inhibition of AChE.

b. **Butyrocholinesterase** (BuChE) is a nonspecific, pseudo, plasma, or s-type cholinesterase. It occurs in glial cells of nervous tissue, liver, plasma, and other organs. Its specific physiologic function is unknown; it can hydrolyze ACh but so slowly as to be unimportant physiologically. Inhibition by drugs of pseudocholinesterase produces no functional derangement.

4. **Adrenergic transmission** occurs when catecholamines (dopamine, norepinephrine, and epinephrine) are the neurotransmitters released from the nerve terminal. They are synthesized by a series of enzymes. Generally, enzymatic degradation of catecholamines is not as important as neural membrane uptake in termination of neurotransmitter activity, although in some tissues metabolism of amines does play an important role. The two most important metabolic enzymes are **catechol-*O*-methyltransferase** (COMT) and **monoamine oxidase** (MAO). MAO is associated with mitochondria, whereas COMT is primarily a cytoplasmic enzyme.

## E. Receptors

1. **Cholinergic receptors** are found (in the parasympathetic system, in the brain and the ganglia of the sympathetic system, and at the myoneural junction of voluntary striated skeletal muscle. Pharmacologically, the acetylcholine receptors are classified as muscarinic or nicotinic, based on their selectivity for muscarine or nicotine, and further subtyped based on their affinity for selected antagonist drugs.

2. **Adrenergic receptors** have been divided into $\alpha$ and $\beta$ types based on their pharmacologic properties (i.e., their relative responsiveness to norepinephrine versus isoproterenol). The $\alpha$-receptors have been further subtyped into $\alpha_{1A}$, $\alpha_{1B}$, $\alpha_{1C}$; $\alpha_{2A}$, $\alpha_{2B}$, $\alpha_{2C}$, and $\alpha_{2D}$.

a.  **$\alpha_1$-Receptors** are found in peripheral vascular smooth muscle of the coronary arteries, skin, intestinal mucosa, and splanchnic beds.

b.  **$\alpha_2$-Receptors** occur both presynaptically and postsynaptically in peripheral tissues. $\alpha_2$-Receptors occur on prejunctional sympathetic nerve terminals and decrease the amount of norepinephrine released, thus serving as a negative feedback mechanism. In addition, prejunctional $\alpha_2$-receptors have been identified on cholinergic, serotonergic, and GABA-ergic neurons, where they are thought to be important in neuromodulation. Stimulation of central $\alpha_2$-receptors is associated with sedation, analgesia, decreased sympathoadrenal outflow, anxiolysis, and decreased thermal-induced shivering. $\alpha_2$ Activation indirectly effects cardiac function through centrally mediated decreases in sympathetic tone (CNS postsynaptic receptors), by decreased release of norepinephrine from sympathetic nerve terminals (prejunctional receptors), and by altering coronary blood flow (vascular receptors). In the gastrointestinal tract, $\alpha_2$-receptors act prejunctionally and postjunctionally to regulate motility and secretions. $\alpha_2$ Stimulation decreases gastric secretion and increases net fluid absorption. The uterus is richly supplied with $\alpha_2$-receptors. In the endothelium, $\alpha_2$-receptors have been shown to mediate release of nitric oxide and endothelium-derived relaxing factor. Renal effects of $\alpha_2$ stimulation include diuresis induced by inhibition of release of ADH, blockade of ADH's action at the renal tubule, increased glomerular filtration rate (GFR), and inhibition of renin release. $\alpha_2$-Receptors located on platelets stimulate aggregation.

c.  **$\beta$-Receptors** are characterized as $\beta_1$ (cardiac), $\beta_2$ (noncardiac), and $\beta_3$ (atypical). **$\beta_1$-Receptors** are located in the myocardium, SA node, ventricular conduction system, and adipose tissue. **$\beta_2$-Receptors** are located in the smooth muscle of blood vessels in the skin, muscles, and mesentery and in bronchial smooth muscle. Stimulation of $\beta_2$-receptors results in vasodilation and bronchial relaxation. $\beta_2$-Receptors are much more sensitive to epinephrine than to norepinephrine.

d.   **Dopamine receptors** have been classified as $DA_1$ and $DA_2$. The **$DA_1$** receptor is postsynaptic and mediates splanchnic and renal vasodilation. The **$DA_2$** receptor is presynaptic, and like the $\alpha_2$-receptor, inhibits subsequent release of norepinephrine and induces vasodilation. Centrally, dopamine receptors are found in the basal ganglia, where they coordinate motor function; in the medullary chemoreceptor trigger zone, to stimulate vomiting; and in the hypothalamus associated with prolactin release. A summary of the effects of autonomic stimulation of adrenergic and cholinergic receptors on various organs are presented in Table 3-9.

3.   **Up- and down-regulation** by adrenergic receptors has been shown. The number of receptors is effected by the concentration of agonist to which they are exposed (i.e., there is an inverse relationship between the number of receptors and the ambient concentration of the catecholamines). Extended exposure to the agonist leads to decreased receptor numbers (down-regulation). Up-regulation, the increase in number of receptors, occurs when blood and tissue catecholamine concentrations are low.

## F.   Theories of Anesthesia

Anesthetic agents differ greatly in structure, because they include hydrocarbons, alcohols, ethers, urethanes, sulfones, amides, steroids, and rare gases. Because general anesthesia is produced by a wide range of compounds with no common chemical structure or activity, it is impossible, except in a series of homologous substances, to show any relationship between anesthetic action and chemical constitution. As a result, many of the theories of narcosis have been based on physical properties of the anesthetics. The concept of anesthetic effect has changed from filling of free space to expansion and fluidization of the cell membrane.

Although the majority of investigators favor a lipid anesthetic site, a hydrophobic protein site of action could cause

*Text continued on p. 125.*

**Table 3-9. Responses of Effector Organs to Autonomic Nerve Impulses**

| Effector Organs | Adrenergic Impulses[a] | | Cholinergic Impulses[a] |
| --- | --- | --- | --- |
| | Receptor Type | Responses[b] | Responses[b] |
| *Eye* | | | |
| Radial muscle, iris | α | Contraction (mydriasis) ++ | — |
| Sphincter muscle, iris | | — | Contraction (miosis) +++ |
| Ciliary muscle | β | Relaxation for far vision + | Contraction for near vision +++ |
| *Heart* | | | |
| SA node | β₁ | Increase in heart rate ++ | Decrease in heart rate; vagal arrest +++ |
| Atria | β₁ | Increase in contractility and conduction velocity ++ | Decrease in contractility, and (usually) increase in conduction velocity ++ |
| AV node | β₁ | Increase in automaticity and conduction velocity ++ | Decrease in conduction velocity; AV block +++ |
| His-Purkinje system | β₁ | Increase in automaticity and conduction velocity +++ | Little effect |
| Ventricles | β₁ | Increase in contractility, conduction velocity, automaticity, and rate of idioventricular pacemakers +++ | Slight decrease in contractility claimed by some |
| *Arterioles* | | | |
| Coronary | α, β₂ | Constriction +; dilation[c] ++ | Dilation ± |
| Skin and mucosa | α | Constriction +++ | Dilation[d] |
| Skeletal muscle | α, β₂ | Constriction ++; dilation[c,e] ++ | Dilation[f] + |

Continued

**Table 3-9. (continued)**

| Effector Organs | Adrenergic Impulses[a] | | Cholinergic Impulses[a] |
| --- | --- | --- | --- |
| | Receptor Type | Responses[b] | Responses[b] |
| Cerebral | $\alpha$ | Constriction (slight) | Dilation[d] |
| Pulmonary | $\alpha$, $\beta_2$ | Constriction +; dilation[c] | Dilation[d] |
| Abdominal viscera; renal | $\alpha$, $\beta_2$ | Constriction +++; dilation[e] + | — |
| Salivary glands | $\alpha$ | Constriction +++ | Dilation ++ |
| Veins (Systemic) | $\alpha$, $\beta_2$ | Constriction ++; dilation ++ | — |
| **Lung** | | | |
| Bronchial muscle | $\beta_2$ | Relaxation + | Contraction ++ |
| Bronchial glands | ? | Inhibition (?) | Stimulation +++ |
| **Stomach** | | | |
| Motility and tone | $\alpha_2$, $\beta_2$ | Decrease (usually)[g] + | Increase +++ |
| Sphincters | $\alpha$ | Contraction (usually) + | Relaxation (usually) + |
| Secretion | | Inhibition (?) | Stimulation +++ |
| **Intestine** | | | |
| Motility and tone | $\alpha_2$, $\beta_2$ | Decrease[g] + | Increase +++ |
| Sphincters | $\alpha$ | Contraction (usually) + | Relaxation (usually) + |
| Secretion | | Inhibition (?) | Stimulation ++ |
| *Gallbladder and ducts* | | Relaxation + | Contraction + |
| Kidney | $\beta_2$ | Renin secretion ++ | — |

| | | | |
|---|---|---|---|
| *Urinary bladder* | | | |
| Detrusor | β | Relaxation (usually) + | Contraction +++ |
| Trigone and sphincter | α | Contraction ++ | Relaxation ++ |
| *Ureter* | | | |
| Motility and tone | α | Increase (usually) | Increase (?) |
| *Uterus* | α, β₂ | Pregnant: contraction (α); nonpregnant: relaxation (β) | Variable[h] |
| *Sex organs, male* | α | Ejaculation +++ | Erection +++ |
| *Skin* | | | |
| Pilomotor muscles | α | Contraction ++ | — |
| Sweat glands | α | Localized secretion[i] + | Generalized secretion +++ |
| *Spleen capsule* | α, β₂ | Contraction +++; relaxation + | — |
| *Adrenal medulla* | | — | Secretion of epinephrine and norepinephrine |
| *Liver* | α, β₂ | Glycogenolysis, gluconeogenesis[j] +++ | Glycogen synthesis + |
| *Pancreas* | | | |
| Acini | α | Decreased secretion + | Secretion ++ |
| Islets (β cells) | α | Decreased secretion +++ | — |
| | β₂ | Increased secretion + | — |

*Continued*

**Table 3-9.** (continued)

| Effector Organs | Adrenergic Impulses[a] | | Cholinergic Impulses[a] |
| | Receptor Type | Responses[b] | Responses[b] |
| --- | --- | --- | --- |
| Fat cells | α, β₁ | Lipolysis[j] +++ | — |
| Salivary glands | α | Potassium and water secretion + | Potassium and water secretion |
| | β | Amylase secretion + | +++ |
| Lacrimal glands | | — | Secretion +++ |
| Nasopharyngeal glands | | — | Secretion ++ |
| Pineal gland | β | Melatonin synthesis | — |

Reprinted with permission from Gilman AG, Goodman LS, Gilman A, eds. The pharmacological basis of therapeutics. 6th ed. New York: Macmillan, 1980.

[a] A long dash signifies no known functional innervation.

[b] Responses are designated 1+ to 3+ to provide an approximate indication of the importance of adrenergic and cholinergic nerve activity in the control of the various organs and functions listed.

[c] Dilation predominates in situ owing to metabolic autoregulatory phenomena.

[d] Cholinergic vasodilatation at these sites is of questionable physiologic significance.

[e] Over the usual concentration range of physiologically released, circulating epinephrine, β-receptor response (vasodilation) predominates in blood vessels of skeletal muscle and liver; α-receptor response (vasoconstriction), in blood vessels of other abdominal viscera. The renal and mesenteric vessels also contain specific dopaminergic receptors, activation of which causes dilatation, but their physiologic significance has not been established.

[f] Sympathetic cholinergic system causes vasodilation in skeletal muscle, but this is not involved in most physiologic responses.

[g] It has been proposed that adrenergic fibers terminate at inhibitor β-receptors on smooth muscle fibers and at inhibitory α-receptors on parasympathetic cholinergic (excitatory) ganglion cells of the plexus of Auerbach.

[h] Depends on stage of menstrual cycle, amount of circulating estrogen and progesterone, and other factors.

[i] Palms of hands and some other sites (adrenergic sweating).

[j] There is significant variation among species in the type of receptor that mediates certain metabolic responses.

many of the physical-chemical relationships that point toward the lipid phase. Present evidence supports the assumption that the site of anesthetic action is on the cell membrane. It is believed that anesthetics act chiefly by depressing synaptic transmission. It has also been shown that several general anesthetics hyperpolarize CNS neurons, apparently because of an increase in potassium permeability. This is a nonsynaptic activity that, combined with synaptic depression, can result in decreased neuronal excitability and CNS unresponsiveness. The concepts of membrane volume expansion on critical hydrophobic sites, altered fluidity of the lipid matrix of cell membranes, and altered binding to protein sites that interfere with signal transduction are reasonable explanations for the mechanism of generalized altered CNS activity that is defined as general anesthesia.

## G.    Effects of Anesthetics on Central Nervous System Homeostasis

Physiologic mechanisms that protect brain function can be altered by sedatives, analgesics, and anesthetics. Within reasonable limits, autoregulation and coupling of EEG, cerebral blood flow (CBF), and cerebral metabolic rate of oxygen consumption ($CMRO_2$) protect brain cells against irreversible damage. Some parameters are well established at normal body temperatures. It is known that 60% of metabolism as measured by $CMRO_2$ supports cell function, whereas 40% supports cell integrity. CBFs < 20 mL/100 g/min are detrimental to all function and possible integrity. CNS stimulants increase cell requirements, metabolism, and blood flow, just as depressants do the opposite.

As considerations are made for selection of anesthetics, the primary objectives of providing analgesia and avoiding distress should be coupled to the necessity of adequate cerebral perfusion and metabolism. It should be appreciated that prolonged recovery is not always the result of lingering anesthetic action but may, in a small percentage of patients, result from cerebral dysfunction. Reports of postanesthetic seizures in dogs and horses after ketamine, prolonged CNS depression in animals after low oxygen availability or low cardiac output, postanesthetic blindness or deafness, and other possible CNS dysfunction manifested as incoordination or ataxia suggest adverse CNS sequela. Proper selection of anesthetics and maintenance of needed ventilation and perfusion undoubtedly improves anesthetic outcome.

# Chapter 4

---

## Pharmacology

### Introductory Comments

*Preanesthetic drugs are used to prepare the patient for induction and contribute to maintenance and smooth recovery from anesthesia. Injectable anesthetics can be used to induce unconsciousness and maintain anesthesia (e.g., propofol). Total intravenous anesthesia refers to the production of general anesthesia with injectable drugs only. The advantage of total intravenous anesthesia is its ability to provide each component of anesthesia (CNS depression, analgesia, muscle relaxation) with specific drugs that minimize overall CNS depression. In contrast, inhalation anesthetics increase or decrease the intensity of all components of anesthesia at the same time. Dissociative anesthesia interrupts ascending transmission from the unconscious to conscious parts of the brain, rather than by generalized depression of all brain centers. Muscle relaxants do not affect CNS function but limit their actions to peripheral neuromuscular blockade causing paralysis.*

**Preanesthetics and Anesthetic Adjuncts**
**Injectable Anesthetics**
**Inhalant Anesthetics**
**Muscle Relaxants and Neuromuscular Block**

---

## I.   PREANESTHETICS AND ANESTHETIC ADJUNCTS
*Kip Lemke*

Preanesthetic drugs are used to calm the patient, induce sedation, provide analgesia and muscle relaxation, decrease salivation and airway secretions, obtund autonomic reflex responses, decrease gastric fluid volume and acidity, suppress or prevent vomiting or re-gurgitation, decrease anesthetic requirements, and promote smooth induction and recovery from anesthesia. Preanesthetic drugs should be selected according to patient needs rather than clinical routine. When selecting preanesthetic drugs, the following factors should be considered: age, physical status, disposition, species, surgical procedure and duration, inpatient or outpatient surgery, elective or emergency surgery, and personal experience with different drugs. Commonly used preanesthetic drugs include anticholinergics, phenothiazines, benzodiazepines, opioids, and $\alpha_2$-agonists.

### A.  Anticholinergics

1.  **Atropine** blocks acetylcholine at postganglionic terminations of muscarinic, cholinergic fibers in the autonomic (parasympathetic) nervous system. Oral, pharyngeal, and respiratory tract secretions are decreased, and bronchi are dilated. Atropine increases both anatomic and physiologic respiratory dead space and can accentuate postoperative hypoxemia caused by ventilation-perfusion impairment. Motor and secretory activity in the gastrointestinal tract are decreased, and vagal influence on the heart is suppressed. In therapeutic doses, atropine has little effect on arterial blood pressure. Atropine blocks cholinergic fibers of the short ciliary nerves and relaxes the sphincter muscle of the iris, dilating the pupil. Tear formation is decreased in awake and anesthetized dogs. It also suppresses the muscarinic effects of anticholinesterase drugs used to reverse nondepolarizing muscle relaxants.

    a.  Atropine can be given **subcutaneously, intramuscularly,** or **intravenously** to healthy dogs and cats at a dosage of 0.02 to 0.04 mg/kg. When given intravenously, atropine may increase vagal tone transiently, causing a slowing of heart rate and occasionally 1st- and 2nd-degree atrioventricular blockade. Subsequently, vagal tone decreases and heart rate increases. Atropine is contraindicated in patients with pre-existing tachycardia (e.g., fever, pain, or thyrotoxicosis). Indiscriminate preoperative use is not recommended.

b.   **Metabolism and elimination** of atropine vary among species. Cats, rats, and rabbits can destroy large quantities of atropine, because they have atropine esterase in the liver. Dogs clear atropine quickly from the blood and excrete it in the urine.

2.   **Glycopyrrolate** is a synthetic, quaternary ammonium, compound. Like atropine, it inhibits the action of acetylcholine on structures innervated by postganglionic, cholinergic (muscarinic) nerves. Glycopyrrolate decreases the volume and acidity of gastric secretions, intestinal motility, and pharyngeal, tracheal, and bronchial secretions. Because it is a large polar molecule, diffusion across lipid membranes such as the blood–brain barrier and placenta is limited.

Glycopyrrolate can be given **subcutaneously, intramuscularly,** or **intravenously** to healthy dogs and cats at a dosage of 0.005 to 0.01 mg/kg. After subcutaneous or intramuscular administration of glycopyrrolate, peak effect occurs in 30 to 45 min. Its cardiovascular effect is evident within 1 min of intravenous injection. Vagal inhibition lasts for 2 to 3 h, and the antisialagogue effect may persist for up to 7 h.

## B.   Phenothiazines

**Phenothiazine tranquilizers** are used to induce sedation and relieve anxiety before induction of anesthesia. In addition, they can be used to quiet patients for physical examination, diagnostic procedures, or transport and to prevent animals from licking wounds or chewing bandages and splints. When used as preanesthetics, phenothiazine tranquilizers can be given orally or parenterally. Response to oral administration is slow and unpredictable, and these drugs are usually given intramuscularly 20 to 30 min before induction of anesthesia. Shortly after administration of a phenothiazine tranquilizer, animals relax with their heads hanging and ears drooping. Some animals lie down; eyes can appear glazed, and the nictitating membrane often protrudes. Phenothiazines are also effective antiemetics and reduce the incidence of perioperative vomiting. These drugs can cause hypotension and hypothermia and can reduce the seizure threshold. Occasionally, acute adverse reactions occur. Among these are extreme depression, hypotension, dyspnea, and death.

Phenothiazine tranquilizers can also potentiate the toxic effects of organophosphates and procaine hydrochloride. **A decrease in arterial blood pressure** results from the depression of vasomotor reflexes mediated by the hypothalamus and brainstem, peripheral α-adrenergic blockade, a direct relaxing effect on vascular smooth muscle, and direct cardiac depression. Aggressive intravenous fluid therapy with a balanced electrolyte solution is the primary treatment of phenothiazine-induced hypotension. Epinephrine is contraindicated. Norepinephrine, phenylephrine, and ephedrine are indicated, because they have little β-2 activity, and act primarily at $\alpha_1$-receptor sites.

1. **Acepromazine,** a phenothiazine tranquilizer, is a relatively safe, effective sedative in dogs and cats. The recommended oral dosage for healthy dogs and cats is 0.5 to 1 mg/kg. In healthy dogs, the recommended parenteral dosage is 0.05 to 0.1 mg/kg IM or SC, not to exceed a total dose of 3 mg. In healthy cats, the recommended parenteral dosage is 0.1 to 0.2 mg/kg IM or SC. Acepromazine reportedly lowers the convulsive seizure threshold and is contraindicated in epileptic patients and in animals with drug-induced seizures. In dogs, high dosages (0.4 to 1.0 mg/kg) of acepromazine effectively prevent epinephrine-induced cardiac arrhythmias and ventricular fibrillation during barbiturate, methoxyflurane, and halothane anesthesia.

## C. Benzodiazepines

1. **Diazepam** is a safe, effective sedative in dogs but is not a reliable sedative in cats. Diazepam has calming, muscle relaxant, and anticonvulsant effects. It is used as a tranquilizer, a muscle relaxant, an anticonvulsant, and a preanesthetic in dogs with a history of seizure disorders. It is frequently given before ketamine to prevent muscle tremors and seizures. It can, however, also be given before propofol or thiopental to reduce the amount of drug required to induce anesthesia.

    a. Diazepam acts on specific **benzodiazepine receptor sites** located on postsynaptic nerve endings within the CNS. The greatest concentration of these receptors is found in the cerebral cortex. The anxiolytic and muscle relaxant effects are a result of increased availability of the inhibitory neurotransmitter glycine. Diazepam enhances blockade induced by myoneural-blocking agents and other central-acting muscle relaxants. Sedation and anticonvulsant activity are mediated by γ-aminobutyric acid (GABA) in the cerebral cortex and motor centers, respectively. Pentobarbital appears to increase the affinity of diazepam for the benzodiazepine receptor.

b. **The recommended intravenous dosage** of diazepam for healthy dogs is 0.1 to 0.5 mg/kg. Diazepam solution should be injected slowly to decrease the incidence of venous thrombosis. Clinical doses cause only minimal respiratory and cardiac depression.

2. **Midazolam** is a water-soluble benzodiazepine with a pH of 3.5. At pH values above 4.0, the chemical configuration of midazolam changes, and it becomes lipid soluble. It has a rapid elimination half-life and total body clearance.

a. Midazolam induces mild sedation in some dogs but is not a reliable sedative in cats. In dogs, midazolam is often given with ketamine to prevent muscle tremors and seizures.

b. Midazolam, unlike diazepam, can be given either intramuscularly or intravenously. In older dogs, midazolam is often given intramuscularly, alone or in combination with an opioid, 20 to 30 min before induction of anesthesia with ketamine or thiopental. An **intramuscular dosage** of 0.1 to 0.2 mg/kg of midazolam has been recommended for premedication of dogs before induction of anesthesia with ketamine or thiopental. Midazolam is nonirritating and well absorbed after intramuscular injection.

c. Midazolam can induce **aberrant behavior in cats.** Some animals become irritable, restless, and difficult to approach after drug administration.

d. Midazolam has been used as an **appetite stimulant** in dogs and cats.

### D. Benzodiazepine Antagonist

1. **Flumazenil** effectively antagonizes CNS action of the benzodiazepines. This drug has a high affinity for benzodiazepine receptors. It reverses all agonist, as well as inverse agonist, effects of benzodiazepines. Flumazenil's action is rapid, occurring in 2 to 4 min. Reversal is not accompanied by anxiety, tachycardia, or hypertension. Flumazenil dosage calculation is based on the amount of benzodiazepine given initially and the interval since drug administration. In dogs, the recommended agonist to antagonist ratio for reversal of diazepam-induced sedation is 26:1 (diazepam to flumazenil). Similarly, the recommended agonist to antagonist ratio for reversal of midazolam-induced sedation is 13:1 (midazolam to flumazenil). Flumazenil's duration of action is relatively short (approximately 60 min), and redosing may be required when attempting to antagonize a large dose of benzodiazepine.

### E. Opioids

The term *opioid* is used to refer to all exogenous and synthetic compounds that bind to specific subpopulations of opioid receptors. Three sites of action appear to be involved: (1) inhibition of pain transmission in the dorsal horn, (2) inhibition of somatosensory afferents at supraspinal levels, and (3) activation of descending inhibitory pathways. The opioids are conveniently classified as agonists, agonist–antagonists, and antagonists (Table 4-1). There are three major opioid receptors:

**Table 4-1. Opioid Agonists, Agonist–Antagonists, and Antagonists**

I. Agonists
  A. Meperidine
  B. Morphine
  C. Hydromorphone
  D. Oxymorphone
  E. Alfentanil
  F. Fentanyl
  G. Sufentanil

II. Agonist–antagonists
  A. Butorphanol
  B. Buprenorphine
III. Antagonist
  A. Naloxone

| Class | μ | δ | κ |
|-------|---|---|---|
| **Table 4-2. Opioid Receptor Selectivity and Activity** | | | |
| **AGONISTS** | | | |
| Morphine | + + + | | + |
| Fentanyl | + + + | | |
| Sufentanil | + + + | + | + |
| **AGONIST–ANTAGONISTS** | | | |
| Butorphanol | P | NA | + + + |
| Buprenorphine | P | NA | – – |
| **ANTAGONIST** | | | |
| Naloxone | – – – | – | – – |

Modified from Reisine T, Pasternak G. Opioid analgesics and antagonists. In: A Goodman Gillman, LS Goodman, A Gillman, eds. Goodman and Gillman's the pharmacological basis of therapeutics. 9th ed. New York: McGraw-Hill, 1996.
*P,* partial agonist; *NA,* not available.

**mu** (μ), **kappa** (κ), and **delta** (δ) (Table 4-2). Activation of μ and κ receptors is associated with sedation and reduced gastrointestinal motility in most species. Respiratory depression appears to be mediated primarily by μ receptors.

1. **Morphine** is the prototypical opioid agonist. Its major pharmacologic effect is analgesia. Morphine induces a rapid, marked increase in serotonin (5-hydroxytryptamine; 5-HT) synthesis, which correlates with its analgesic effect. The supraspinal site of action is probably the nucleus raphe magnus and the spinal system. With therapeutic doses, there is a decrease in the basal metabolic rate, resulting in a decrease in body temperature of 1 to 3°F.

    a. **Depression of the respiratory centers** results in decreased respiratory minute volume and increased alveolar carbon dioxide tension. Morphine can cause histamine release, peripheral vasodilation, bradycardia, and increases in antidiuretic hormone.

    b. Morphine directly **stimulates the vomiting center.** The sphincters of the gastrointestinal tract are stimulated and the amplitude of nonpropulsive segmental contractions in the small and large intestines are increased, resulting in constipation.

c. Morphine **induces sedation in dogs,** but may cause excitement in other species. In cats, morphine given subcutaneously at a dosage of 0.1 mg/kg causes no excitement, and analgesia lasts for > 4 h. When morphine is given to cats at dosage of 1.0 mg/kg, however, mydriasis, salivation, and anxiety typically occur.

d. **In dogs,** low intramuscular dosages of morphine (0.1 to 0.5 mg/kg) can be used preoperatively, but vomiting is relatively common. Concurrent administration of acepromazine may reduce the incidence of vomiting. Epidural administration of preservative-free morphine (0.1 mg/kg) provides analgesia for 12 to 24 h.

2. **Meperidine** potency is one-tenth that of morphine. It has a spasmolytic effect similar to atropine and reduces salivary and respiratory secretions. When meperidine is used as a preanesthetic, it reduces the amount of general anesthetic needed. Rapid intravenous injection can cause histamine release, hypotension, excitement, and convulsions; thus this route of administration is not recommended. The intramuscular preanesthetic dosage of meperidine for dogs and cats is 4 to 6 mg/kg. Although sedation is not marked, cats given meperidine are tractable and easier to handle. Duration of effect is relatively short (30 to 60 min).

3. **Methadone** is a synthetic µ agonist unrelated to morphine. Its pharmacologic effects are qualitatively similar to those of morphine, and the drug is active both orally and parenterally. Large intravenous doses of methadone cause generalized depression, loss of postural control, copious salivation, and defecation. Methadone can be used as a preanesthetic or a postoperative analgesic. The intramuscular dose of methadone for dogs is 0.1 to 0.5 mg/kg. The drug should be given 20 to 30 min before induction of anesthesia. In cats, methadone may cause excitation and seizures, and its use in this species is not recommended.

4. **Hydromorphone** is a semisynthetic μ agonist with an analgesic potency approximately 5 times that of morphine. The respiratory and cardiovascular effects of the drug are comparable to other μ agonists. In dogs, it appears to cause less vomiting than does morphine. Hydromorphone can be used as a preanesthetic or analgesic and is given intramuscularly to dogs and cats at a dosage of 0.1 to 0.2 mg/kg.

5. **Oxymorphone** is a semisynthetic μ agonist with an analgesic potency approximately 10 times that of morphine. In dogs, oxymorphone appears to induce more sedation and less hypnosis than does morphine. Bradycardia may occur, but other alterations in cardiovascular function are minimal.

   a.  Oxymorphone is used as a **preanesthetic** and an analgesic for dogs and cats. The recommended dosage of oxymorphone for healthy animals is 0.05 to 0.1 mg/kg given intramuscularly or intravenously. Oxymorphone can also be given intraoperatively at a reduced dosage to enhance analgesia during surgery and the postoperative period.

   b.  **Neuroleptanalgesia** is induced when oxymorphone is given in combination with a tranquilizer (e.g., acepromazine). The degree of sedation and analgesia obtained depends on the tranquilizer and dosages selected. When combined with acepromazine (0.05 to 0.1 mg/kg IM), oxymorphone (0.05 to 0.1 mg/kg IM) safely induces neuroleptanalgesia in healthy dogs and cats.

6. **Fentanyl** is a synthetic μ agonist structurally related to meperidine and is approximately 80 to 100 times more potent than morphine. It has a rapid onset and a short duration of action.

   a.  **Respiratory depression,** analgesia, sedation, and ataxia develop 3 to 8 min after intravenous or intramuscular injection; peak effects are observed in < 30 min, and duration of action is 1 to 2 h. Respiratory effects range from panting to a reduction in minute ventilation with occasional apnea. Although fentanyl is short acting, respiratory depression may persist for several hours after drug administration.

b. Fentanyl is a **highly lipophilic drug**, and equilibration of plasma and cerebrospinal fluid (CSF) concentrations occurs rapidly. Plasma and CSF concentrations correlate closely with the degree of drug-induced respiratory depression.

c. **Changes in acid–base status** on fentanyl pharmacokinetics is complex and difficult to predict. Decreases in plasma pH associated with respiratory depression, however, tend to increase the amount of active, ionized fentanyl available to extracellular receptors and produce an enhanced opioid effect.

d. Fentanyl can be used as a **preanesthetic** or intraoperatively as part of a balanced anesthetic technique. Intravenous or intramuscular injection of fentanyl can cause vagally mediated bradycardia. Prior administration of atropine or glycopyrrolate prevents bradycardia but can cause severe tachycardia. There is little effect on cardiac output or blood pressure with normal clinical dosages (5 to 10 µg/kg) of fentanyl. Unlike morphine and meperidine, fentanyl does not cause histamine release. Low intravenous dosages (2.5 to 5 µg/kg) of fentanyl can be used to enhance analgesia during inhalation anesthesia.

e. Fentanyl **transdermal patches** have been used to manage postoperative pain in dogs and cats. Patches are applied to the skin following clipping, and the area is bandaged to keep the animal from removing, and possibly ingesting, the patch. Fentanyl uptake through skin is highly variable. Patches are available in four sizes and are designed to deliver fentanyl at rates of 25, 50, 75, and 100 µg/kg/h. A 25-mg/kg/h patch is used for cats and small dogs. Patches delivering 50, 75, and 100 µg/kg/h are used for dogs weighing 10 to 20, 20 to 30, and 40 to 50 kg, respectively. After patch application, steady-state plasma fentanyl concentrations may not be reached for 24 h, and supplemental opioids should be given parenterally for the first 12 to 24 h. The use of fentanyl transdermal patches in animals is off label, and there is a potential for human injury and abuse.

**F.    Agonist–Antagonists**

The term **agonist–antagonist** was originally used to describe nalorphine and similar drugs. Perhaps a practical and broadly applicable definition of an agonist–antagonist drug is one that has agonist or partial agonist activity at one or more types of opioid receptors and the ability to antagonize the effects of a full agonist at one or more types of opioid receptors. Many of the opioid agonist–antagonists appear to be partial agonists at more than one type of receptor.

1.   **Butorphanol** is a synthetic opioid that has both agonist and antagonist properties. Its analgesic potency is 3 to 5 times that of morphine. As an antagonist, it is comparable to nalorphine and about 50 times less potent than naloxone. Because butorphanol has greater receptor affinity, the dose of naloxone required to reverse butorphanol is higher than that required to antagonize opioid agonists such as morphine.

   a.   **The depressant effects** of butorphanol on ventilation are less than those of morphine. Respiratory depression appears to reach a ceiling beyond which higher doses do not cause appreciable changes in minute ventilation.

   b.   **Mild sedation** in dogs is induced by intravenous butorphanol (0.5 mg/kg); but the drug does not cause histamine release.

   c.   Butorphanol **will antagonize** the sedative and respiratory depressant effects of some opioid agonists (e.g., morphine and oxymorphone).

   d.   Butorphanol is given intramuscularly to dogs and cats at a dosage of 0.1 to 0.4 mg/kg and can be given intravenously at lower dosages. As a **preanesthetic,** it can be used alone or in combination with phenothiazines, benzodiazepines, or $\alpha_2$-agonists. Limited respiratory depression, minimal cardiovascular effects, and a lack of gastrointestinal side effects (i.e., vomiting and defecation) are significant advantages over other opioids.

2. **Buprenorphine** is a partial agonist at the μ receptor and an antagonist at the κ receptor. Its agonist effects are approximately 30 times that of morphine. Buprenorphine's onset of action is relatively slow, requiring 20 to 30 min to reach full effect. Its analgesic action may last as long as 8 to 12 h. In dogs and cats, buprenorphine is given intramuscularly at a dosage of 5 to 10 μg/kg and can be given intravenously at lower dosages. Buprenorphine is commonly used to provide **postoperative analgesia** because of its long duration of action.

### G. α₂-Receptor Agonists

The **α₂-receptor** is a distinct subclassification of the α-adrenergic receptor family. These receptors hold promise because, when activated, they induce sedation, analgesia, anxiolysis, and sympatholysis in most mammalian species. They serve as prejunctional inhibitory receptors (autoreceptors) within the sympathetic nervous system, and induce **vasoconstriction** and endothelial-dependent vasodilation. They are also found in the gastrointestinal tract, uterus, kidney, and platelets. Within the CNS, α₂-receptor activation induces both sedation and analgesia. α₂-Receptors and opioid receptors are found in similar regions of the brain and even on some of the same neurons.

1. **Xylazine** was the first α₂-agonist to be used as a sedative analgesic and in combination to prevent muscular hypertonicity in dogs and cats given ketamine.

   a. Xylazine is currently **approved for use in dogs and cats** in Canada and the United States. Xylazine is given intramuscularly to healthy dogs at a dosage of 0.25 to 0.5 mg/kg and to healthy cats at a dosage of 0.5 to 1.0 mg/kg. In both species, xylazine can be given intravenously at lower dosages.

   b. **Sedation and muscle relaxation** are evident 10 to 15 min after intramuscular administration and 3 to 5 min after intravenous administration. In dogs, peak plasma concentrations are reached 12 to 14 min after intramuscular injection. A sleep-like state is usually maintained for approximately 1 h. Duration of analgesia is much shorter.

c.  Xylazine-induced **decreases in heart rate and cardiac output** are attenuated somewhat by ketamine's sympathomimetic effect. When xylazine and ketamine are given intravenously, blood pressure, systemic vascular resistance, and presumably myocardial oxygen consumption are increased. These acute hemodynamic changes, coupled with moderate decreases in venous $Po_2$ and oxygen content, caution against its use in patients with myocardial disease or reduced cardiopulmonary reserve.

d.  The most commonly encountered **arrhythmogenic effects** of xylazine include bradycardia, atrioventricular block, atrioventricular dissociation, and sinoatrial block.

e.  Although **respiratory rate decreases** with the administration of clinically recommended doses of xylazine, arterial pH, $Pao_2$, and $Paco_2$ values remain virtually unchanged in dogs and cats. Decreases in respiratory rate are accompanied by increases in tidal volume to maintain alveolar minute ventilation. When xylazine is given intravenously to healthy dogs at a relatively large dosage (1.0 mg/kg), however, minute ventilation, physiologic dead space, oxygen transport, venous $Pao_2$ and oxygen content, and oxygen consumption decrease and tidal volume increases.

f.  Xylazine alters **gastrointestinal function.** In dogs, xylazine decreases gastroesophageal sphincter pressure, prolongs gastrointestinal transit time, and may increase the likelihood of gastric reflux. Subcutaneous and intramuscular administration of xylazine induces vomiting during the early onset of sedation in some dogs and cats.

g.  **Increased urine** production is common in dogs and cats. Although decreased urethral closure pressure has been noted in both female and male dogs, normal micturition reflexes are maintained. Xylazine administration does not appear to alter the detrusor reflex in dogs.

h. **Transient hypoinsulinemia and hyperglycemia** have been observed in dogs. The magnitude and duration of these effects appear to be dose dependent.

i. **Increased myometrial tone and intrauterine pressure** have been observed.

j. **Mydriasis** is commonly observed. This effect is caused by central inhibition of parasympathetic innervation to the iris or direct sympathetic stimulation of $\alpha_2$-receptors located in the iris and CNS.

k. Failure to achieve **optimum sedation** with $\alpha_2$-agonists may be the result of pre-existing stress, fear, excitement, or pain that increases endogenous catecholamine levels.

2. **Medetomidine** is lipophilic, is rapidly eliminated, and possesses more potency and efficacy than other $\alpha_2$-agonists. Its $\alpha_2$- to $\alpha_1$-receptor selectivity binding ratio is 1620 compared to 220 and 160 for clonidine and xylazine, respectively.

a. Medetomidine induces dose-dependent **sedation and analgesia** in dogs and cats within the recommended dose range. Higher doses do not result in more sedation but increase the duration of effect. Atropine or glycopyrrolate premedication prevents bradycardia but may increase medetomidine's initial hypertensive effects. After subcutaneous or intramuscular administration, vomiting may occur with the onset of sedation. Diuresis is observed with doses as low as 10 µg/kg.

b. The optimal intramuscular **preanesthetic dose** in dogs is between 5 and 10 µg/kg. After a 10-µg/kg dose, bradycardia and sedation consistently occur.

c. **In cats,** as in other species, when ketamine is combined with medetomidine, the sympathomimetic properties of ketamine offset the bradycardic effects of medetomidine to some degree. Medetomidine–ketamine combinations effectively induce immobilization and short periods of anesthesia. The coadministration of an opioid or benzodiazepine with medetomidine enhance both sedation and analgesia.

3. **Romifidine** is the newest $\alpha_2$-agonist to be evaluated for use as a sedative analgesic in animals. Romifidine is an effective sedative in dogs when given intramuscularly at dosages of 20 to 40 µg/kg. Compared to xylazine, its sedative effects are longer in duration.

## H. $\alpha_2$-Receptor Antagonists

1. **Yohimbine** has proven to be an effective antagonist for the sedative-immobilizing effects of anesthetic regimens incorporating xylazine. Reversal can be achieved by combining yohimbine with 4-aminopyridine to antagonize the sedative actions of xylazine, xylazine–ketamine, and xylazine–pentobarbital in dogs, cats, and several other species.

2. **Tolazoline** has been used in a number of species to reverse xylazine sedation or partially reverse the depressant effects achieved with anesthetic combinations incorporating $\alpha_2$-agonists. Tolazoline induces potent $H_2$ receptor–mediated effects and has been associated with gastrointestinal bleeding, abdominal pain, nausea, diarrhea, and exacerbation of peptic ulcer.

3. **Atipamezole** is the newest $\alpha_2$-antagonist available for use in dogs. The $\alpha_2$- to $\alpha_1$-selectivity ratio of atipamezole is 200 to 300 times higher than that of yohimbine. Atipamezole is devoid of activity at $\beta$-, histaminergic, serotonergic, muscarinic, dopaminergic, GABA, opioid, and benzodiazepine receptors. Dosage recommendations for atipamezole vary according to species, dosage, and agonist.

   a. **Reversal** of medetomidine (1 mg/mL) in dogs is accomplished with an equal volume of atipamezole (5 mg/mL). Cats can be given half of the medetomidine dose injected. In the United States, atipamezole is approved for intramuscular use only in dogs.

4. **Severe hypotension and tachycardia** can occur following the rapid intravenous injection of $\alpha_2$-antagonists. Nevertheless, the incidence of unfavorable reactions to $\alpha_2$-antagonists when given appropriately is extremely rare.

The use of more selective $\alpha_2$-antagonists, such as atipamezole, lessens the likelihood of untoward reactions.

## II. INJECTABLE ANESTHETICS
*Kip Lemke*

There is no injectable anesthetic that produces all of the components of anesthesia without depressing some vital organ function. Because available drugs have rather selective actions within the CNS, combinations of drugs are necessary to provide surgical anesthesia without depressing vital functions. Injectable anesthetics induce unconsciousness, but do not necessarily obtund nociception or provide muscle relaxation. Additional analgesics and muscle relaxants are usually required to safely provide all of the components of balanced anesthesia. Characteristics of the ideal injectable anesthetic are given in Table 4-3.

### A. Mechanisms of Action

The complexity of the CNS has contributed to a lack of understanding of the mechanisms of action of injectable

---

**Table 4-3. Characteristics of an Ideal Injectable Anesthetic**

I. Physiochemical and pharmacokinetic
  A. Water soluble
  B. Long shelf life
  C. Stable when exposed to light
  D. Small volume required for induction of anesthesia
II. Pharmacodynamics
  A. Minimal individual variation
  B. Safe therapeutic ratio
  C. Onset, one vein to brain circulation time
  D. Short duration of action
  E. Inactivated to nontoxic metabolites
  F. Smooth emergence
  G. Absence of anaphylaxis
  H. Absence of histamine release
III. Side effects
  A. Absence of local toxicity
  B. No effect on vital organ function, except anesthetically desirable CNS effects

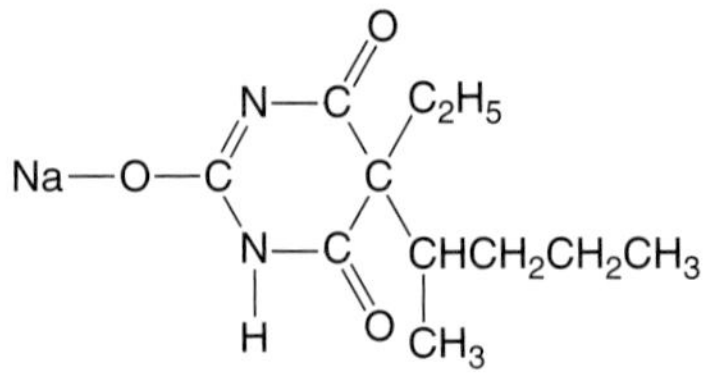

**Figure 4-1.** Pentobarbital sodium.

anesthetics. No drug has a single action. Some theories suggest that anesthetics alter cell membranes, whereas others emphasize receptor-specific interactions. Considerable evidence suggests that most injectable anesthetics alter **GABA**-mediated neurotransmission. GABA activates postsynaptic receptors that in turn increase chloride conductance, thus hyperpolarizing and inhibiting the neuron. At high concentrations, barbiturates directly activate chloride channels. Propofol and etomidate may also induce CNS depression by modulation of GABA-mediated neurotransmission.

**B.    Barbiturate Anesthetics**

1.    **Pentobarbital sodium** came into general use as an anesthetic agent for dogs and cats in the early 1930s and slowly supplanted ether administration by open mask as the anesthetic of choice (Fig. 4-1). By 1940 its use was widespread. Today, it has largely been replaced by inhalation and balanced anesthetic techniques. The estimated **intravenous dose** for healthy, unpremedicated dogs and cats is 20 to 30 mg/kg. It should be emphasized, however, that pentobarbital is given to effect. The use of pentobarbital in dogs and cats is approved by the FDA.

    a.    **Cardiovascular responses** after an intravenous anesthetic dose of pentobarbital typically include a decrease in arterial blood pressure and an initial increase in heart rate (for 10 to 20 min), which then stabilizes or decreases. Cardiac output is variable, and peripheral vascular resistance increases. Intravenous pentobarbital administration alters myocardial function and distribution of blood flow. Pentobarbital causes enlargement of the spleen, which presumably accounts for the decrease in erythrocytes. Maximum enlargement usually occurs 20 to 30 min after barbiturate administration.

b. **Method of administration** can significantly alter the cardiovascular response to pentobarbital administration. About 25% of animals rapidly given pentobarbital intravenously at a dosage of 30 mg/kg develop side effects that mimic shock.

c. Pentobarbital is **metabolized** primarily by hepatic microsomal enzymes. The sensitivity of an animal to the action of barbiturates may be increased by uremia. This phenomenon is probably caused by the decreased capacity of plasma protein to bind acidic drugs.

d. Pentobarbital freely crosses the **placental barrier** and enters the fetal circulation. Neonatal survival is very low when pentobarbital is used at high dosages as a monoanesthetic for cesarean section.

e. **During recovery** from pentobarbital anesthesia, animals tend to exhibit the same signs as they do during induction of anesthesia, except in reverse order. These signs include crying, shivering, involuntary running movements, thrashing, and increased respiratory movements followed by recovery of the righting reflex and, later, the ability to stand with a staggering gait.

2. **Thiopental** is the 2-thio analogue of pentobarbital and was the first thiobarbiturate to gain popularity as an injectable anesthetic for animals (Fig. 4-2). Thiopental sodium is a yellow crystalline powder that is unstable when exposed to air and in aqueous solution. For this reason, it is dispensed in sealed containers as a powder buffered with sodium carbonate. It is usually mixed with sterile water or saline to

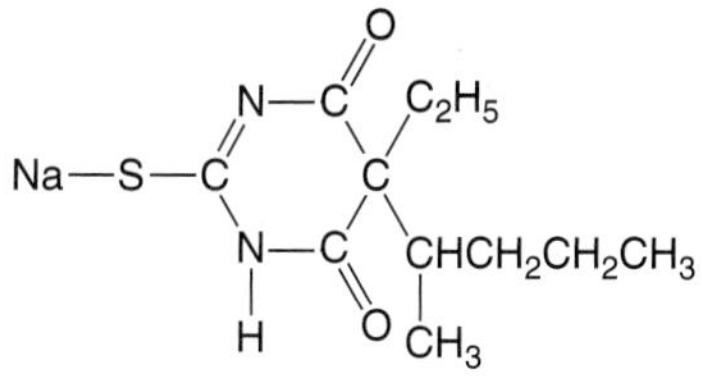

**Figure 4-2.** Thiopental sodium.

form 2.5 or 5.0% solutions. Once prepared, thiopental solutions should be stored in a refrigerator at 5 to 6°C (41 to 42°F) to retard deterioration. As solutions age, there is a progressive loss of activity.

a.  **The lethal dose (LD$_{50}$)** of thiopental is approximately twice the anesthetic dose (AD$_{50}$), and animals die because of respiratory failure.

b.  Thiopental administration **depresses pulmonary and cardiovascular function.** Initially, there is a reduction in respiratory rate and tidal volume. Thiopental administration may induce the development of ventricular arrhythmias (e.g., premature ventricular depolarizations and bigeminy). Concurrent administration of lidocaine reduces the incidence of ventricular arrhythmias and has been advocated for use in animals with cardiovascular disease. Premedication with acepromazine may reduce the incidence of epinephrine-induced ventricular arrhythmias.

c.  Thiopental is used as **a sole anesthetic** for brief procedures and for induction of anesthesia before administration of inhalation anesthetics. Thiopental should always be given intravenously. Accidental perivascular injection can cause severe tissue damage, and the use of properly placed intravenous catheters is strongly advised. Dilute solutions ($\leq 2.5\%$) of thiopental should be used whenever possible. For induction of anesthesia in healthy, unpremedicated dogs and cats, the estimated dosage is 15 to 20 mg/kg. One-third of the estimated dose is injected rapidly, and the remainder is administered slowly to effect. Thiopental should not be used to maintain anesthesia for extended periods of time.

d.  **Recovery** from anesthesia occurs as thiopental redistributes from the CNS to muscle and fat (Fig. 4-3). If repeated doses of thiopental are given, muscle and fat become saturated, and redistribution cannot occur. Apnea is common if too much thiopental is given, and animals should be intubated and manually ventilated until the drug redistributes and spontaneous breathing returns. Recovery from thiopental anesthesia may be prolonged in sighthounds and other thin, athletic breeds.

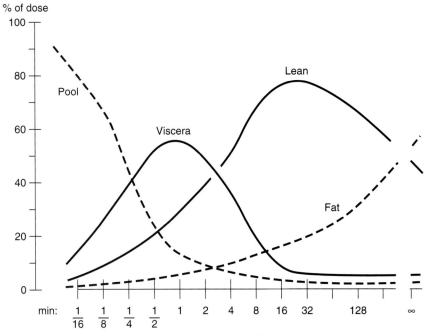

**Figure 4-3.** Percentage of thiopental dose in the central blood pool, viscera, lean tissue, and fat after rapid intravenous administration.

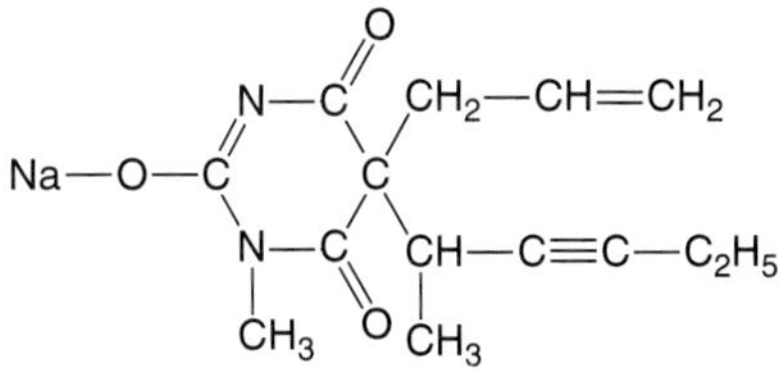

**Figure 4-4.** Methohexital sodium.

3. **Methohexital sodium** is a rapid onset, ultra-short-acting oxybarbiturate (Fig. 4-4). The drug's short duration of action is primarily the result of rapid metabolism and redistribution from the CNS to other body tissues. Methohexital is at least twice as potent as thiopental, and its duration of action is half as long. Methohexital is approved for use in dogs and cats.

   a.    Methohexital is used primarily for **induction of anesthesia,** but can also be used to maintain anesthesia. The drug is given intravenously, and perivascular injection does not cause tissue irritation. The estimated dosage for healthy, unpremedicated dogs and cats is 8 to 10 mg/kg. For healthy, premedicated dogs and cats, the estimated dosage is 5 mg/kg. Half the estimated dose is injected rapidly, and the rest is given slowly to effect. Anesthesia is rapidly induced, lasts for 5 to 10 min, and can be maintained by intermittent bolus administration or by continuous infusion.

   b.    **Emergence from anesthesia is quick,** and animals are usually alert within 30 min. Excitement, muscle tremors, and convulsions can occur during induction or recovery, and these side effects limit the usefulness of the drug. Premedication with phenothiazines or benzodiazepines may reduce the incidence and severity of CNS excitation upon recovery.

   c.    **In brachycephalic animals and sighthounds,** methohexital may be a better choice than thiopental for induction of anesthesia because of its quick onset and rapid metabolism. Methohexital should not be used in animals predisposed to seizure activity.

## C.    Nonbarbiturate Anesthetics

   1.    **Propofol (2,6-diisopropylphenol)** is a rapid-onset, ultra-short-acting injectable anesthetic formulated in an aqueous emulsion that contains propofol (10 mg/mL), soybean oil (100 mg/mL), glycerol (2.5 mg/mL), egg lecithin (12 mg/mL), and sodium hydroxide to adjust the pH (Fig. 4-5). The emulsion is capable of supporting microbial

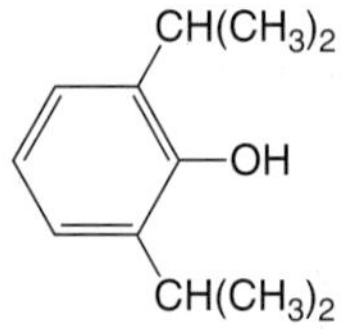

**Figure 4-5.** The structure of propofol, an alkylphenol derivative.

growth and endotoxin production. Strict aseptic technique should be used when administering propofol, and any unused drug should be discarded at the end of the day. Propofol is currently approved for use in dogs.

a.  **The pharmacokinetic profile** of propofol in dogs fits a two-compartment open model. Rapid uptake by the CNS results in a quick onset of action. Termination of the drug's anesthetic effect is the result of extensive redistribution from the CNS to other tissues and rapid metabolic clearance. Propofol is metabolized primarily by the liver; however, the drug's clearance exceeds hepatic blood flow, suggesting extrahepatic sites of metabolism. Propofol is excreted primarily in the urine.

b.  Propofol is used to **induce and maintain anesthesia.** Induction of anesthesia is usually rapid and smooth. The estimated dosage for healthy, unpremedicated dogs and cats is 8 to 10 mg/kg. For healthy, premedicated dogs and cats, the estimated dosage is 4 to 6 mg/kg. The estimated dose is injected over a 60- to 90-s period to effect. A more rapid injection will often result in apnea.

c.  **Recovery** from propofol anesthesia is usually rapid and smooth. Dogs recover completely in about 20 min. Cats given propofol at a similar dosage recover in about 30 min. Anesthesia can be maintained with propofol by either intermittent bolus administration or continuous infusion. The rate of administration depends on the adjunctive drugs administered and the degree of surgical stimulation. Intermittent boluses are given at a dosage of 0.5 of 2.0 mg/kg, and continual infusion rates range from 0.2 to 0.4 mg/kg/min.

d.  **Blood pressure and cardiac output** decrease after propofol administration. Heart rate usually does not change. Propofol increases myocardial sensitivity to catecholamines but is not inherently arrhythmogenic. Short periods of apnea are common after induction of anesthesia with propofol. Mild hypercapnia and respiratory acidosis are common when anesthesia is maintained with propofol. Intracranial

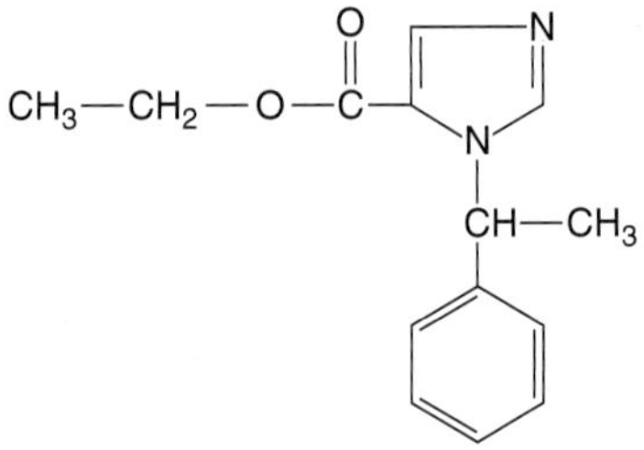

**Figure 4-6.** The structure of etomidate, an imidazole derivative.

pressure (ICP) and intraocular pressure (IOP) decrease after propofol administration.

e.   Propofol may cause **pain** when injected intravenously but does not cause tissue irritation when given perivascularly. In dogs, muscle tremors and seizure activity have been reported. In cats, propofol can cause oxidative injury to red blood cells. Heinz body formation, anorexia, malaise and diarrhea can occur in cats given propofol repeatedly over several days.

2.   **Etomidate** is an imidazole derivative first used for induction of anesthesia in people in 1975 (Fig. 4-6). It is a congener of metomidate and contains 2 mg/mL of the drug in 35% ethylene glycol. It should be refrigerated at 2 to 8°C (36 to 46°F) and not frozen or exposed to extreme heat.

a.   **Intravenous administration** of etomidate in dogs at dosages of 1.5 and 3.0 mg/kg induces unconsciousness for 8 and 21 min, respectively. In cats, the pharmacokinetics of a 3-mg/kg intravenous dose of etomidate is best described as a three-compartment open model. Induction and recovery are rapid, with brief periods of myoclonus occurring early in the recovery period. Etomidate is rapidly hydrolyzed in the liver and excreted in the urine.

b.   Etomidate is a safe **induction agent** because it does not depress the cardiovascular and respiratory systems or cause histamine release.

c.   **Heart rate, blood pressure,** and myocardial performance do not change after etomidate administration. It decreases the cerebral metabolic rate of oxygen consumption ($CMRO_2$) and intracranial pressure and may have brain-protective properties after episodes of global ischemia associated with cardiac arrest. Muscle tremors and seizures, however, may occur after etomidate administration. Neonates born to mothers anesthetized with etomidate have minimal respiratory depression.

d.    Etomidate inhibits **steroid production** by the adrenal glands, suppressing the usual increase in plasma cortisol observed during surgery. A single induction dose of etomidate may depress adrenal function for up to 3 h. Lack of a normal stress response to surgery may not have deleterious effects, and attenuation of metabolic and endocrine responses to surgery may actually reduce morbidity. Prolonged administration of etomidate to maintain sedation in intensive care patients may lead to adrenocortical suppression and the development of an Addisonian crisis. Consequently, long-term infusion in critically ill patients is not recommended.

e.    Etomidate (2 mg/kg) can cause **acute hemolysis.** The mechanism of hemolysis appears to be owing to propylene glycol, which causes a rapid increase in osmolality, resulting in red cell rupture.

f.    Etomidate may cause **pain** when injected intravenously. Vomiting may occur during induction or recovery. Myoclonus may also occur in dogs and cats. For the most part, these side effects can be prevented by administration of appropriate preanesthetic drugs. In summary, etomidate may be a useful induction drug for animals with severe trauma, advanced cardiovascular or hepatic disease, or intracranial lesions, and for compromised animals requiring cesarean section.

3.    **Althesin** is a combination of two steroids: alphaxalone (9 mg/mL) and alphadolone acetate (3 mg/mL) (Fig. 4-7). Alphaxalone is insoluble in water, but can be dissolved in Cremophor EL (polyhydroxylated castor oil). Addition of alphadolone further increases the solubility of alphaxalone. The solution is clear and viscous and has a neutral pH. Althesin has a higher therapeutic index than

do barbiturate anesthetics, and repeated administration has little cumulative effect. The use of althesin in animals has not been approved by the FDA.

a.   Althesin is used primarily for **induction of anesthesia** but can also be used to maintain anesthesia. The drug is usually given intravenously, and perivascular injection does not cause tissue irritation. Dosage calculations for althesin are based on the total steroid content (12 mg/mL). The estimated dosage for healthy, unpremedicated cats is 8 to 10 mg/kg. For healthy, premedicated cats, the estimated dosage is 5 mg/kg. Half of the calculated dose is injected rapidly, and the rest is given slowly to effect. Anesthesia is rapidly induced, lasts for 5 to 10 min, and can be maintained by intermittent administration or by continuous infusion.

b.   **Emergence is rapid** once althesin administration is discontinued, and animals are usually alert in 30-45 min. Excitement, muscle tremors, and convulsions can occur during recovery. Premedication with acepromazine may reduce the incidence and severity of CNS excitation during the recovery period.

c.   Althesin causes **histamine release** in cats and dogs. Scratching, hyperemia of the ears, and swelling of the face and paws occur commonly in cats. Cardiovascular collapse may occur in dogs, and althesin is not recommended for use in this species.

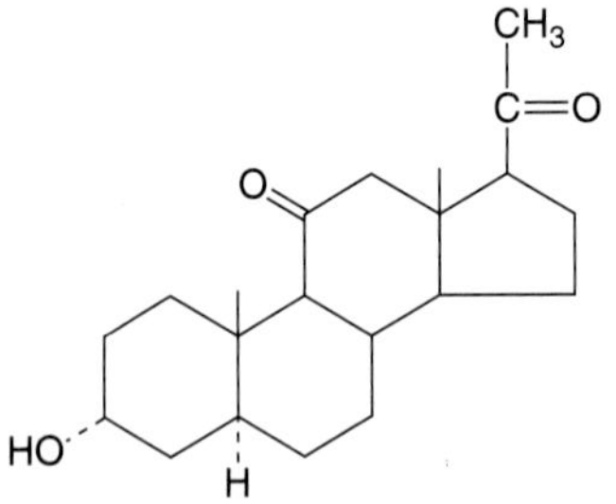

Steroid I (alphaxalone;
3α-hydroxy-5α-pregnane-
11,20, dione)

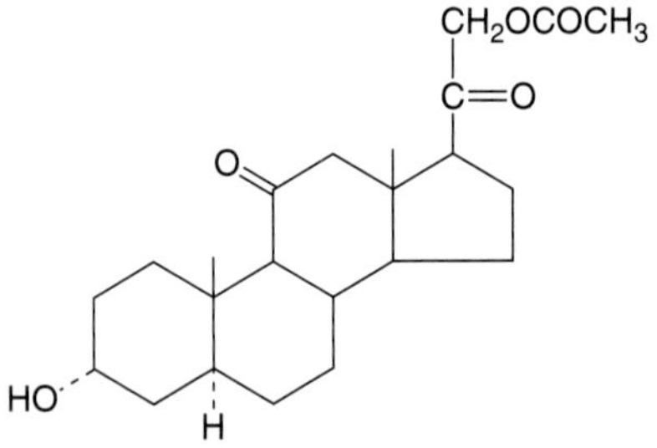

Steroid II (alphadolone;
21-acetoxy-3α-hydroxy-
5α-pregnane-11,20, dione)

**Figure 4-7.** Steroids I and II.

### D.  Dissociative Anesthetics
*Hui Chu Lin*

Dissociative anesthetics include phencyclidine, tiletamine, ketamine (in order of greater to less potency). Phencyclidine is no
longer available to the practicing veterinarian. Ketamine is the
most commonly used dissociative for animal anesthesia. Tiletamine is approved for use only in combination with the
benzodiazepine derivative zolazepam in a 1 : 1 ratio, marketed as
Telazol. These drugs are used to induce taming and immobilization as well as general anesthesia. Characteristic responses of
dissociation include the development of a cataleptoid state.
Varying degrees of hypertonus, purposeful, and reflexive
skeletal muscle movements unrelated to surgical stimulation
commonly occur.

1. **Ketamine** has a **rapid onset of action,** with maximal effect
   occurring in approximately 1 min. It produces dose-
   related unconsciousness and analgesia. Recovery from
   anesthesia is caused by rapid redistribution of the drug
   from the brain to other tissues. Duration of anesthesia
   usually lasts 10 to 20 min after intravenous administration.
   Ketamine-induced seizure has been reported in some
   dogs and cats known to be epileptic. In general, its use in
   animals with a history of epilepsy, should be avoided.

   a. **Analgesia** produced by ketamine occurs at subanes-
      thetic doses, and elevated pain thresholds are corre-
      lated with plasma levels of $\geq 0.1$ mg/mL. The degree
      of analgesia appears to be greater for somatic pain
      than for visceral pain. In cats, visceral analgesia
      induced by ketamine (2, 4, and 8 mg/kg IV) is
      similar to that produced by butorphanol (0.1 mg/kg
      IV). Ketamine alone is not recommended for reliev-
      ing visceral pain associated with abdominal or tho-
      racic procedures.

   b. Ketamine induces significant increase in **cerebral
      blood flow** (CBF), ICP, and CSF pressure as a result
      of cerebral vasodilation and elevated systemic blood
      pressure. Regardless of the mechanism, if controlled
      ventilation is used to maintain $Paco_2$ between 25 and
      30 mm Hg, further increases in ICP can be pre-

vented. Ketamine should be avoided in spontaneously breathing patients with increased CSF pressure or head injury.

c. **Hallucinatory behavior,** which may progress to delirium, may occur during emergence from ketamine anesthesia. In cats, emergence reactions are characterized by ataxia, increased motor activity, hyperreflexia, sensitivity to touch, avoidance behavior of an invisible object, and sometimes violent recovery. Premedication or concurrent administration of $\alpha_2$-agonists, acetylpromazine, or a benzodiazepine (e.g., diazepam) decreases the incidence of adverse emergence reactions.

d. **Cardiovascular effects** on target organs include sympathomimetic effects mediated within the CNS, inhibition of neuronal uptake of catecholamines by sympathetic nerve endings, direct vasodilation of vascular smooth muscle, and an inotropic effect on the myocardium. Increased myocardial stimulation is associated with increased cardiac work and myocardial oxygen consumption. A positive inotropic effect as a result of the inhibition of catecholamine uptake at the neuro-effector junction, leading to activation of $\beta$-adrenoceptors, requires an intact and normally functioning CNS.

e. Ketamine has been recommended for anesthesia of **critically ill patients,** for which there is a risk of cardiac depression and hypotension. Although blood pressure may be better maintained in animals anesthetized with ketamine as a result of its vasoconstricting effect, arterial lactate concentrations increase more than in animals with lower blood pressure anesthetized with a volatile anesthetic.

f. Ketamine does not depress **ventilatory responses** to hypoxia, and pulmonary gas exchange is only minimally affected. The transient apnea induced by ketamine appears to be dose dependent. At higher doses, respiration is characterized by an apneustic, shallow, and irregular pattern.

g. Ketamine often causes **increased salivation** and secretion of respiratory tract mucus, which can easily be controlled by administration of an anticholinergic. Laryngeal and pharyngeal reflexes are usually well maintained during ketamine anesthesia.

h. **Increases in extraocular muscle tone** induced by ketamine may be responsible for the increase in IOP. Therefore, ketamine should be used with caution in patients with corneal injuries, for which increased IOP may result in expulsion of intraocular contents.

i. Ketamine undergoes extensive **hepatic metabolism** in dogs. Very little hepatic metabolism occurs in cats, and the majority of the injected ketamine is eliminated unchanged via the kidney. Rapid recovery following ketamine administration is caused by rapid redistribution of ketamine from the CNS to all body tissues, primarily body fat, lung, liver, and kidney. Ketamine should be given in low doses only to animals with hepatic or renal dysfunction.

j. Ketamine alone can induce **extreme catatonia,** exuberant spontaneous movement, violent recovery, and occasional convulsions in dogs. Clinically, ketamine is used in combinations with or after a tranquilizer or sedative to eliminate many of these side effects (Table 4-4).

k. In cats, ketamine produces **profound anesthesia** with doses ranging from 11 to 44 mg/kg IM (Table 4-5). Rapid induction and short duration of anesthesia (10 to 15 min) occur when ketamine (2 to 6 mg/kg) is administered intravenously. Cardiac arrest or apnea may occur when a large intravenous dose is rapidly injected. Intravenous ketamine should be administered slowly to effect.

2. **Telazol** (CI-744), is a nonopioid, nonbarbiturate injectable anesthetic that is a 1:1 (wt/wt) combination of tiletamine and zolazepam. **Tiletamine** (CI-634), a dissociative anesthetic agent, has a longer duration of action and greater analgesic effect than does ketamine. **Zolazepam** (CI-716), a benzodiazepine tranquilizer, is combined with tiletamine because of its effectiveness as an anticonvulsant and muscle relaxant. Anesthesia is characterized by excellent muscle relaxation, no nystagmus or athetoid movement, and smooth recovery. Telazol has a wide margin of safety, and reactions to intramuscular injection are minimal.

Induction of anesthesia is rapid and smooth, as is recovery in most species. It is supplied in a sterile vial as a lyophilized powder containing 250 mg tiletamine and 250 mg zolazepam. It is recommended that the drug be reconstituted with 5 mL sterile water, resulting in a combination of 50 mg tiletamine and 50 mg zolazepam per milliliter.

**Table 4-4. Ketamine Use in Canines**

| Drugs | Dose, mg/kg, and Route | Duration, min | Comments |
|---|---|---|---|
| Acetylpromazine Ketamine Thiamylal | 0.22–0.55 IM 11–22 IM To effect IV | 20–90 | Occasional seizures; restraint for aggressive dogs; spastic movements; prolonged recovery |
| Acetylpromazine Ketamine Butorphanol | 0.1–0.2 IV or IM 10 IV or IM 0.2–0.4 IM | 39 | Good restraint; less muscle rigidity than ketamine alone; useful for clinical anesthesia |
| Romifidine Ketamine | 0.08 IV 7–14 IV | | Good muscle relaxation; smooth recovery |
| Medetomidine Ketamine | 0.04 IM 2.5–5 IM | 7±0.9 30–75 | Longer duration of muscle relaxation and recovery than xylazine–ketamine; prolonged recovery; significant cardiovascular changes |
| Diazepam Ketamine | 0.28 IV 5.5 IV | | Suitable induction combination for dogs |
| Midazolam Ketamine | 0.28–0.5, IV 5.5–10, IV | 13.3±3.1 | More myoclonic movements; shorter time to intubation; suitable induction combination; increased heart rate; mild respiratory depression |

| Table 4-5. Ketamine Use in Felines | | | |
| --- | --- | --- | --- |
| **Drug(s)** | **Dose, mg/kg, and Route** | **Duration, min** | **Comments** |
| Ketamine | < 22 IM | 20–40 | Chemical restraint |
| Ketamine | 11–44 IM | 20–77 | Cataleptoid anesthesia; lack of muscle relaxation; little analgesia; respiratory depression, occasional apnea |
| Xylazine<br>Ketamine | 0.23–2.2 IM<br>4.6–22 IM | 25–120 | Vomiting; longer duration of anesthesia than acepromazine–ketamine |
| Diazepam<br>Ketamine | 0.2 IV<br>2–8 IV | 20–100 | Visceral analgesia of short duration |
| Medetomidine<br>Ketamine | 0.08 IM<br>2.5–7.5 IM | 36–65 | Better muscle relaxation; satisfactory anesthesia; vomiting |
| Butorphanol<br>Ketamine | 0.1 IV<br>2–8 IV | 280–360 | Visceral analgesia |
| Midazolam<br>Ketamine | 0.05–2 IV<br>3 IV | | Dose-related behavioral signs; dose-dependent muscle relaxation; suitable for clinical use |

a. Telazol induces **analgesia** by interruption of sensory input into the brain, which usually persists after the anesthetic effect has subsided. The patient's eyes remain open, even during surgical anesthesia. Protective reflexes, such as coughing, swallowing, and corneal and pedal reflexes, are maintained. Most animals given Telazol salivate. This can be easily prevented by administration of atropine or glycopyrrolate.

    b.     In cats and dogs, Telazol produces generalized **cardiovascular stimulation.** Tiletamine may play a major role in the biphasic hemodynamic changes occurring after Telazol injection.

    c.     **Breathing rate** increases in most species after Telazol injection. When 2 to 4 mg/kg is given intravenously to dogs without premedication, the ventilatory pattern is characterized by a short period of apnea (1 min) followed by irregular, slow, shallow breathing. The rate of breathing in cats generally decreases and is characterized by an apneustic breathing pattern after intramuscular or intravenous injection.

    d.     Telazol can be used concurrently with other anesthetics (e.g., ultra-short-acting barbiturates and inhalation anesthetics). In dogs, **onset of surgical anesthesia** occurs within 7 to 8 min following the recommended intramuscular dose of Telazol and within 30 to 60 s after low-dose intravenous injection. Recommended doses and duration of surgical anesthesia for dogs are given in Table 4-6. Dogs are usually fully recovered within 4 h after a single intramuscular injection. When dogs emerge, the tranquilizing effects of zolazepam appear to wane first. Therefore, the characteristic rough recovery seen with dissociatives alone is often seen in dogs.

| Table 4-6. Telazol Use in Canines | | | |
|---|---|---|---|
| **Drug(s)** | **Dose, mg/kg, and Route** | **Duration, min** | **Comments** |
| Telazol | 4–5 IV | 20–40 | Satisfactory anesthesia; good muscle |
| | 4–12 IM | 40–90 | relaxation; occasional rough recovery |
| Telazol | 8.8 IM | 100 | Anesthesia; good muscle relaxation; |
| Xylazine | 1.1 IM | | good analgesia |
| Butorphanol | 0.22 IM | | |

| Drug(s) | Dose, mg/kg, and Route | Duration, min | Comments |
|---------|------------------------|---------------|----------|
| **Table 4-7. Telazol Use in Felines** | | | |
| Telazol | 6–12.8 IM or IV | 20–60 | Recommend low doses for intravenous use; salivation and apneustic breathing common; manufacturer-recommended doses can result in prolonged recoveries |
| Acepromazine Telazol | 0.1 IM 2.7 ± 0.97 IV or 3.0 ± 1.0 IM | | Adequate anesthesia for castration |
| Telazol[a] Ketamine Xylazine | 3.3 IM 2.64 IM 0.66 IM | 43.4 ± 9.1 | Smooth induction and recovery; excellent muscle relaxation; good analgesia |

[a]Reconstitute with 4 mL ketamine and 1 mL of 10% xylazine (TKX). Dose at 0.1 mL/10 lbs.

    e.    **Recommended doses** and duration of surgical anesthesia for cats are given in Table 4-7. Cats react painfully to intramuscular injection of Telazol. The margin of safety of Telazol in cats is 4.5 times the recommended dose. The **plasma** half-lives of tiletamine and zolazepam in cats are 2.5 and 4.5 h, respectively. Cats usually emerge from anesthesia quietly. Typically, the recovery time for cats is twice that of dogs.

## III. INHALANT ANESTHETICS
*Eugene P. Steffey*

Inhalant anesthetics are used widely for the anesthetic management of animals. They are unique among the anesthetic drugs because they are administered, and in large part removed from the body, via the lungs. Over the nearly 150 years that inhalation anesthesia has been used in clinical practice, < 20 agents have actually been introduced and approved for use in patients, and only 6 are in current clinical use in North America (Fig. 4-8).

## A.    Characteristics of Inhalant Agents

The chemical structure of inhalant anesthetics and their physical properties are important determinants of their actions and safety of administration. A knowledge and understanding

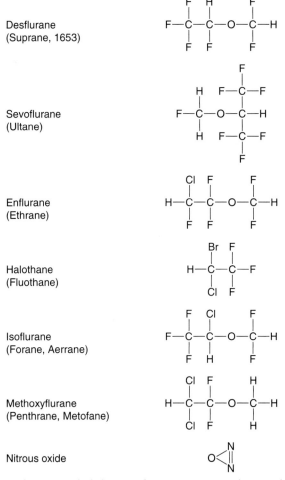

**Figure 4-8.** Chemical structure of inhalant anesthetics in current use for animals. Trade names are given in parentheses.

of fundamental properties permits intelligent use of contemporary anesthetics (Table 4-8).

1.  *Chemical Characteristics*

All contemporary inhalation anesthetics are organic compounds except nitrous oxide ($N_2O$). Agents of current interest are further classified as either **aliphatic hydrocarbons** or **ethers.** In the continued search for a less-reactive, more potent, nonflammable inhalation anesthetic, focus on halogenation of these compounds has predominated. Chlorine and bromine can convert compounds of low anesthetic potency into more potent drugs. Fluorine can be substituted for chlorine or bromine to improve stability, but at the expense of reduced anesthetic potency and solubility.

a.  **Halothane** is an example of a halogenated, aliphatic-saturated hydrocarbon (Fig. 4-8). Soon after clinical introduction, it was observed that the concurrent presence of halothane and catecholamines increased the incidence of cardiac arrhythmias. An ether linkage in the molecule favors a reduced incidence of cardiac arrhythmias. Consequently, this chemical structure is a predominant characteristic of all agents developed or proposed for clinical use since the introduction of halothane. Halothane is susceptible to decomposition. Accordingly, halothane is stored in dark bottles and a very small amount of a preservative, thymol, is added to it to retard breakdown. Thymol is much less volatile than halothane and over time collects within the vaporizer, causing them to malfunction.

2.  *Physical Characteristics*

The important **physical characteristics** can be divided into two general categories: those that determine the means by which the agents are administered and those that help determine their kinetics in the body.

a.  A variety of physical and chemical properties determine the means by which inhalant anesthetics are administered, including molecular weight, boiling

**Table 4-8. Some Physical and Chemical Properties of Inhalant Anesthetics in Current Clinical Use for Animals**

| Property | Enflurane | Halothane | Isoflurane | Methoxyflurane | Nitrous Oxide |
|---|---|---|---|---|---|
| Molecular weight | 185 | 197 | 185 | 165 | 44 |
| Liquid specific gravity (20° C), g/mL | 1.52 | 1.86 | 1.49 | 1.42 | |
| Boiling point, °C | 57 | 50 | 49 | 105 | −89 |
| Vapor pressure, mm Hg | | | | | |
|   20°C (68°F) | 172 | 243 | 240 | 23 | |
|   24°C (75°F) | 207 | 288 | 286 | 28 | |
| Milliliter vapor/milliliter liquid (20°C) | 197.5 | 227 | 194.7 | 206.9 | |
| Preservative | None | Required | None | Required | None |
| Stability in | | | | | |
|   Soda lime | Stable | Decomposes | Stable | Decomposes | Stable |
|   UV light | Stable | Decomposes | Stable | Decomposes | Stable |

Modified from Lowe HJ, Ernst EA. The quantitative practice of anesthesia: Use of closed circuit. Baltimore: Williams & Wilkins, 1981; and Eger EJ, II. Isoflurane (forane). A compendium and reference. Madison WI: Ohio Medical Products, 1982.

point, liquid density (specific gravity), and vapor pressure. Whether inhalation agents are supplied as a gas or volatile liquid under ambient conditions, the same physical principles apply to each agent when it is in the gaseous state. The behavior of gases is predictably described by various gas laws. Relationships such as those described by **Boyle's law** (volume versus pressure), **Charles's law** (volume versus temperature), **Gay-Lussac's law** (temperature versus pressure), **Dalton's law of partial pressure** (the total pressure of a mixture of gases is equal to the sum of the partial pressures of all of the gaseous substances present), and others are important to our understanding of anesthetic gases and vapors. The **saturated vapor pressure** of most volatile anesthetics is of such magnitude that the maximum concentration of anesthetic attainable at the usual operating room conditions is above the range of concentrations that are commonly necessary for safe clinical anesthetic management. Therefore, some control of the delivered concentration is necessary and is usually provided by a device known as a **vaporizer.** The purpose of the vaporizer is to dilute the vapor generated from the liquid anesthetic with oxygen (or an oxygen and $N_2O$ mixture) to produce a more satisfactory inspired anesthetic concentration.

b.  **Solubility** is one of the properties influencing drug kinetics. Anesthetic gases and vapors dissolve in liquids and solids. The solubility of an anesthetic is a major characteristic of the agent and has important clinical ramifications. For example, anesthetic solubility in blood and body tissues is a primary factor in the rate of uptake and its distribution within the body. It is, therefore, a primary determinant of the speed of anesthetic induction and recovery. Solubility in lipid bears a strong relationship to anesthetic potency, and its tendency to dissolve in anesthetic delivery components, such as rubber goods, influences equipment selection and other aspects of anesthetic management. The total number of molecules of a given gas dissolving in a solvent depends on the chemical nature of the gas itself, the partial pressure of the gas, the nature of the solvent, and the temperature. This relationship is described by **Henry's law:**

$$V = S \times P$$

where $V$ is the volume of gas, $S$ is the solubility coefficient for the gas in the solvent at a given temperature, and $P$ is the partial pressure of the gas.

i.   Within the body there is a **partition of anesthetic gases** between blood and body tissues in accordance with Henry's law. This process can perhaps be better understood by visualizing a system composed of three compartments (e.g., gas, water, and oil) contained in a closed container (Fig. 4-9). In such a system, the gas overlies the oil, which in turn overlies the water.

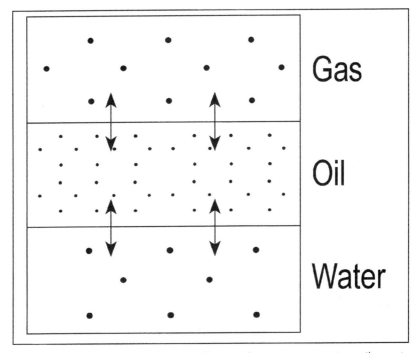

**Figure 4-9.** An anesthetic gas distributing itself among three compartments (gas, oil, water). At equilibrium, the number of anesthetic molecules in the three compartments differ but the pressure exerted by the anesthetic molecules is the same in each compartment.

Because there is a passive gradient from the gas phase to the oil, gas molecules move into the oil compartment. This movement in turn develops a gradient for the gas molecules in oil relative to water. If gas is continually added above the oil, there will be a continual net movement of the gas molecules from the gas phase into both the oil and, in turn, the water. At a given temperature, when no more gas dissolves in the solvent, the solvent is said to be fully saturated. At this point, the pressure of the gas molecules within the three compartments will be equal, but the amount (i.e., concentration) partitioned between the two liquids will vary with the nature of the liquid and gas. The extent to which a gas will dissolve in a given solvent is usually expressed in terms of its **solubility coefficient.** For inhalation anesthetics, solubility is most commonly measured and expressed as a **partition coefficient** (PC).

## B. Pharmacokinetics

The **pharmacokinetics** of inhaled anesthetics describes the rate of their uptake by the blood from the lungs, distribution in the body, and eventual elimination by the lungs and other routes. Inhalation anesthetics, similar to oxygen and carbon dioxide, move down a series of partial pressure gradients from regions of higher tension to those of lower tension until equilibrium is established.

1. *Anesthetic Uptake: Factors That Determine the Alveolar Partial Pressure of Anesthetic*
   The alveolar partial pressure ($P_A$) of anesthetic is a balance between anesthetic input (i.e., delivery to the alveoli) and loss (uptake by blood and body tissues) from the lungs. A rapid rise in the $P_A$ of anesthetic is associated with a rapid anesthetic induction or change in anesthetic depth.

   a. **Delivery of anesthetic to the alveoli** and, therefore, the rate of rise of the alveolar concentration or fraction (F$_A$) toward the inspired concentration or fraction (F$_I$) depends on the **inspired anesthetic concentration** itself and the magnitude of alveolar ventilation. Increasing either one or both of these increases the rate of rise of the P$_A$ of anesthetic.

b.    **The inspired concentration** has a number of variables controlling it. The upper limit of inspired concentration is dictated by the agent vapor pressure, which in turn depends on temperature. Characteristics of the patient breathing system can also be major factors in generating a suitable inspired concentration under usual operating room conditions. Characteristics of special importance include the volume of the system, the amount of rubber or plastic components in the system, the position of the vaporizer relative to the breathing circuit (i.e., within or outside of the circuit), and the fresh gas inflow to the patient breathing circuit. The patient breathing circuit contains a gas volume that must be replaced with gas containing the desired anesthetic concentration. Thus the volume of the breathing circuit is a buffer, delaying the rise of anesthetic concentration. In the management of small animals (i.e., animals < 5 kg), a **nonrebreathing patient circuit** and/or a relatively high fresh gas inflow into the patient breathing circuit is usually used, so there should be no clinically important difference between the delivered (e.g., vaporizer dial setting) and the inspired concentration. For animals > 5 kg, however, a **circle patient breathing circuit** is most commonly used for inhalation anesthesia. The volume of this breathing circuit may be very large compared to the fresh gas inflow. This volume markedly delays the rate of rise of inspired anesthetic concentration, because the residual gas volume must be washed out and replaced by fresh gas containing anesthetic so the inspired concentration can increase to that delivered from the vaporizer.

c.    **Positioning the vaporizer** in relation to the patient breathing circuit will influence the inspired anesthetic concentration. For example, when the vaporizer is positioned within a circle rebreathing circuit (**VIC**), a decrease in inspired concentration will

| Table 4-9. Influence of Vaporizer Positioning on the Inspired Anesthetic Concentration | | |
| --- | --- | --- |
| Factor | VOC | VIC |
| Increase ventilation | Decrease | Increase |
| Increase fresh gas oxygen inflow to circuit | Increase | Decrease |

Modified from Mapleson WW. The concentration of anaesthetics in closed circuits, with special reference to halothane. I. Theoretical studies. Br J Anaesth 1960;32:298–309.

follow an increase in fresh gas inflow to the circuit; when the vaporizer is positioned outside the circuit (**VOC**), there will be an increase in the inspired concentration (Table 4-9).

d.  **An increase in alveolar ventilation** increases the rate of delivery of inhalation anesthetic to the alveolus (Fig. 4-10). If unopposed by anesthetic tissue uptake, alveolar ventilation would rapidly increase the alveolar concentration of anesthetic so that within minutes the alveolar concentration would equal the inspired concentration. In reality, however, the input created by alveolar ventilation is countered by absorption of anesthetic into blood. Predictably, hypoventilation decreases the rate at which the alveolar concentration increases over time compared to the inspired concentration (i.e., anesthetic induction is slowed).

2.  *Removal from Alveoli: Uptake by Blood*
    Anesthetic uptake is the product of three factors: **solubility** (*S*, the blood/gas solubility), **cardiac output** (CO), and the **difference** in the anesthetic partial pressure between the alveolus and the venous blood returning to the lungs ($P_A - P_V$; expressed in millimeters of mercury):

$$\textbf{Uptake} = \textbf{S} \times \textbf{CO}(\textbf{P}_A - \textbf{P}_V/\textbf{P}_{bar})$$

    where $P_{bar}$ is the barometric pressure in millimeters of mercury. Note that if any of these three factors equals zero, there is no further uptake of anesthetic by the blood.

3. *Anesthetic Elimination*

Recovery from inhalation anesthesia results from the elimination of anesthetic from the brain. This requires a decrease in alveolar anesthetic partial pressure, which in turn fosters a decrease in arterial and then brain anesthetic partial pressure. The prominent factors accounting for recovery are the same as those for anesthetic induction. Alveolar ventilation, cardiac output, and especially agent solubility greatly influence recovery from inhalation anesthesia. Indeed, the graphic curves representing the wash out of anesthetic from the alveoli versus time are essentially inverses of the wash-in curves (Fig. 4-11). If a patient rebreathing anesthetic circuit (e.g., circle system) is in use, and the patient is not disconnected from the circuit at the

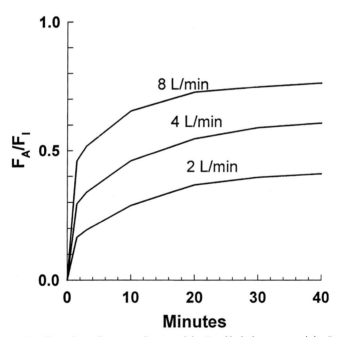

**Figure 4-10.** The effect of ventilation on the rise of the $F_A$ of halothane toward the $F_I$ concentration. As noted, the $F_A:F_I$ ratio increases more rapidly as ventilation is increased from 2 to 8 L/min. Redrawn from Eger EI, II. Anesthetic uptake and action. Baltimore: Williams & Wilkins, 1974.

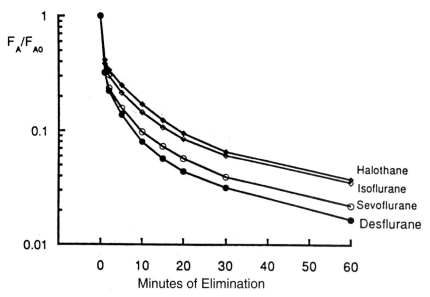

**Figure 4-11.** The fall in $F_A$ relative to the alveolar concentration at the end of anesthesia $F_{AO}$. Note that the newest, most insoluble volatile anesthetic, desflurane, is eliminated in humans more rapidly than the other contemporary potent anesthetics. Not shown is information for methoxyflurane; the curve for this drug would appear above the one for halothane. Reprinted with permission from Eger EI, II. Anesthetic uptake and action. Baltimore: Williams & Wilkins, 1974.

end of anesthesia, the circuit itself may also reduce the rate of recovery. This influence of rebreathing circuits can be reduced by directing high flow rates of anesthetic-free oxygen into the anesthetic circuit.

a.  **Diffusion hypoxia** is a possibility at the end of $N_2O$ administration if the patient immediately breathes air rather than oxygen. In this case, a large volume of $N_2O$ enters the lungs from the blood, displacing other gases. If at this time the patient is breathing air (only about 21% oxygen) rather than 100% oxygen, the $N_2O$ dilutes the alveolar oxygen, further reducing oxygen tension from levels found in ambient air. This action may cause life-threatening reductions in arterial oxygenation. Because the major effect is in the first few minutes after discontinuing $N_2O$, the condition can be prevented by administering pure oxygen at the conclusion of $N_2O$ administration, rather than allowing the patient to immediately breathe ambient air.

4. *Biotransformation*

Inhalation anesthetics undergo varying degrees of metabolism, primarily in the liver but also in lesser degrees in the lung, kidney, and intestinal tract (Table 4-10). The importance of this is twofold. First, metabolism may facilitate anesthetic recovery in a limited way. Second is the potential for acute and chronic toxicities by intermediary or end metabolites of inhalation agents, especially on the kidneys, liver, and reproductive organs.

## C.   Anesthetic Dose: The Minimum Alveolar Concentration

The term **potency** refers to the quantity of an inhalant anesthetic that must be administered to cause a desired effect (e.g., general anesthesia), and the standard index of anesthetic potency for inhalation anesthetics is the minimum alveolar concentration (MAC). The anesthetic potency of an inhaled agent is inversely related to MAC (i.e., potency = 1/MAC). MAC is inversely related to the oil/gas PC. Thus a very potent anesthetic (e.g., methoxyflurane) has a low MAC value and a high oil/gas PC, whereas a low potency agent (e.g., $N_2O$) has a high MAC and low oil/gas PC.

| Table 4-10. Biotransformation of Inhalation Anesthetics in Humans | |
|---|---|
| **Anesthetic** | **Anesthetic Recovered as Metabolites, %** |
| Methoxyflurane | 50 |
| Halothane | 20–25 |
| Sevoflurane | 3.0 |
| Enflurane | 2.4 |
| Isoflurane | 0.17 |

1. **MAC** is defined as the **minimum alveolar concentration** of an anesthetic at one atmosphere that produces immobility in 50% of subjects exposed to a supramaximal noxious stimulus. Thus MAC corresponds to the medium effective dose ($ED_{50}$). The dose that corresponds to $ED_{95}$ (95% of the individuals are anesthetized), at least in humans, is 20 to 40% greater than MAC.

2. In a single species the **variability in MAC** is generally small. Even between species, the variability in MAC for a given agent is usually not large. There is at least one notable exception. In humans, the MAC for $N_2O$ is 104%, making it the least potent of the inhalation anesthetics currently used. Its potency in other species is less than half that in humans (i.e., around 200%).

3. **The anesthetic dose** is commonly defined in terms of multiples of MAC (i.e., 1.5 or 2.0 times MAC or, simply, 1.5 MAC or 2.0 MAC). The $ED_{50}$ equals MAC or 1.0 MAC and represents a light level of anesthesia (clearly inadequate in 50% of otherwise unmedicated healthy animals).

## D. Pharmacodynamics

All contemporary inhalation anesthetic agents in one way or another influence vital organ function. Some actions are inevitable and accompany the use of all agents, whereas other actions are a special or prominent feature of one or a number of the agents. Differences in action, and especially undesirable action, of specific anesthetic agents form the basis for selecting one agent over another for a particular patient and/or procedure.

1. *CNS*

   Inhalation anesthetics induce a reversible generalized CNS depression. **Cerebral electric activity** varies with anesthetic dose. In general, as the depth of anesthesia is increased from awake states, the electric activity of the cerebral cortex becomes desynchronized. There is initially an increased frequency of EEG activity. With further increases in anesthetic concentration, a decrease in frequency and increased amplitude of EEG waves occur.

2. *Respiratory System*

   Inhalation anesthetics depress respiratory system function. The volatile agents affect ventilation in a drug- and species-specific manner. In general, spontaneous ventilation progressively decreases as inhalation anesthetic dose is increased. In otherwise unmedicated animals **respiratory arrest** occurs at 2 to 3 MAC. Decreases in alveolar ventilation are out of proportion to decreases in carbon dioxide ($CO_2$) production, so that $Paco_2$ increases. In addition, the normal stimulation to ventilation caused by an increased $Paco_2$ (or decreased $Pao_2$) is depressed by the inhalation anesthetics.

3. *Cardiovascular System*

   All of the volatile inhalation anesthetics cause dose-dependent and drug-specific changes in cardiovascular performance. The mechanisms of cardiovascular effects are diverse but often include direct myocardial depression and a decrease in sympathoadrenal activity.

   a. All of the volatile anesthetics **decrease cardiac output.** The magnitude of change is related to the dose and depends on the agent. The decrease in cardiac output (CO) is largely caused by a decrease in stroke volume as a result of dose-related depression in myocardial contractility.

   b. The effect of inhalation anesthetics on **heart rate** (HR) is variable and depends on the agent and species. The HR usually remains constant over a range of clinically useful alveolar concentrations in the absence of other modifying factors (e.g., noxious stimulation).

   c. Volatile anesthetics cause a dose-dependent decrease in **arterial blood pressure** (Fig. 4-12). In general, the dose-related decrease in arterial blood pressure is similar regardless of the species. The decrease in blood pressure is usually related at least to a decrease in stroke volume, regardless of the agent or species. In some cases (agent and/or species), a decrease in peripheral vascular resistance may also play an important but lesser role.

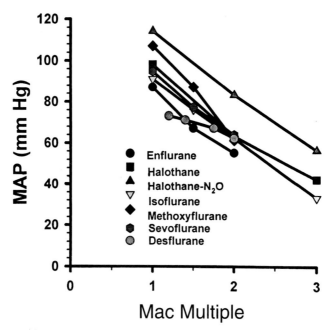

**Figure 4-12.** Inhalant anesthetics cause a dose-dependent decrease in mean arterial blood pressure (MAP) in dogs undergoing mechanically controlled ventilation to produce eucapnia. Dose is expressed as multiples of MAC.

d. Inhalation anesthetics may sensitize the heart to **arrhythmogenic effects of catecholamines.** Halothane is most notable in this regard, as it markedly reduces the amount of epinephrine necessary to cause ventricular premature contractions.

e. Cardiovascular function is usually depressed during **intermittent positive-pressure ventilation** (IPPV) relative to actions during spontaneous ventilation. Such action results from the direct mechanical actions (i.e., intermittent elevation of intrathoracic pressure and the resultant decrease in venous return to the heart), the lessening of the sympathomimetic actions of $Paco_2$, or both.

f. **Carbon dioxide** has three pharmacologic actions important to these considerations: an increased $Paco_2$ directly depresses the heart and smooth muscle of the peripheral blood vessels (i.e., dilation) and indirectly (via sympathetic nervous system) stimulates circulatory function. In sympathetically intact animals, the stimulatory actions of $CO_2$ usually predominate, so increased CO and arterial blood pressure usually accompany an increase in $Paco_2$, becoming lower when $Paco_2$ is normalized.

g.   **Noxious stimulation** during anesthesia modifies the circulatory effect of inhalation anesthetics via stimulation of the sympathetic nervous system. Anesthetic doses that block the response are in the range of 1.5 to 2.0 MAC.

4.   *Renal System*
All inhalation anesthetics reduce **renal blood flow** and **glomerular filtration rate** in a dose-related manner. This action is a common finding regardless of the species studied. During anesthesia, healthy animals produce small volumes of concentrated urine. Accordingly, attendant intravenous fluid therapy and prevention of a marked reduction in renal blood flow will lessen or counteract the tendency for reduced renal function.

a.   **Methoxyflurane** is the most nephrotoxic of the inhalation anesthetics. It causes renal failure that is characterized not by oliguria but by a large urine volume unresponsive to vasopressin. This is caused by the biotransformation of methoxyflurane and the release of free fluoride ion that in turn causes direct damage to the renal tubules.

b.   With the possible exception of **enflurane** and **sevoflurane,** the breakdown of other inhalation anesthetics does not pose a risk of fluoride-induced nephrotoxicity.

c.   **Sevoflurane** is degraded by $CO_2$ absorbents such as soda lime and baralyme. **Olefin,** a nephrotoxic compound, is produced. In humans, a minimum of 2 L oxygen flow is recommended to minimize sevoflurane degradation by absorbent.

5.   *Hepatic System*
Depression of hepatic function and hepatocellular damage may be caused by the action of volatile anesthetics. Effects may be transient or permanent and may be by direct or indirect action. A reduction in intrinsic hepatic

clearance of drugs along with anesthetic-induced alteration of other pharmacokinetically important variables
(e.g., reduced hepatic blood flow) fosters a delayed drug
removal or an increase in plasma drug concentration
during anesthesia.

a.   All of the potent inhalation anesthetics are capable
     of causing **hepatocellular injury** by reducing liver
     blood flow and oxygen delivery. Available data sug-
     gest, however, that of the six contemporary volatile
     anesthetics, isoflurane is least likely to produce liver
     injury, even when administered for prolonged peri-
     ods. The two new agents, sevoflurane and desflurane,
     are nearly similar to isoflurane; whereas halothane
     produces the most striking adverse changes. Local-
     ized hypoxia may damage the hepatocyte directly
     and/or perhaps result in the production of reactive
     intermediary compounds from agent (most notably
     halothane) biotransformation. These compounds
     then act to produce hepatocellular damage via an
     autoimmune-mediated reaction or some other as-
     yet-undescribed process.

6.  *Malignant Hyperthermia*
    **Malignant hyperthermia** (MH) is a potentially life-
    threatening pharmacogenetic myopathy that is most com-
    monly reported in susceptible human patients and swine
    (e.g., Landrace, Pietrain, and Poland China strains); how-
    ever, reports of its occurrence in other species are avail-
    able. Halothane is the most potent triggering agent relative
    to other inhalant anesthetics. The syndrome is character-
    ized by a rapid rise in body temperature that, if not treated
    quickly, causes death. Avoidance of triggering agents and
    prophylactic **dantrolene** given before anesthesia are effec-
    tive in blocking the onset of MH.

## E.   Occupational Exposure: Trace Concentrations of Inhalant Anesthetics

1.  **Operating room personnel** are often exposed to low con-
    centrations of inhalation anesthetics. Contamination of
    ambient air occurs via vaporizer filling, known and un-

known leaks in the patient breathing circuit, and careless spillage of liquid agent. Personnel inhale and retain these agents for some time.

2.  Concern is raised because epidemiologic studies of humans and laboratory studies of animals have suggested that **chronic exposure** to trace levels of anesthetics may constitute a health hazard. Of particular concern are reports that inhaled anesthetics possess mutagenic, carcinogenic, or teratogenic potential. The overwhelming conclusion from both animal and human studies is that there is no carcinogenic risk.

3.  Although the **risk of long-term exposure** to trace concentration of anesthetics for those in operating room conditions appears minimal, current evidence encourages clinicians to reduce exposure to 2.0 parts per million (ppm) for volatile agents and 25 ppm for $N_2O$.

## IV.  MUSCLE RELAXANTS AND NEUROMUSCULAR BLOCK
*L. K. Cullen*

### A.  Physiology of the Neuromuscular Junction

An impulse traveling down the motor nerve causes depolarization of the nerve terminal, triggering the release of acetylcholine, which crosses the junctional cleft to stimulate nicotinic cholinoreceptors on the postsynaptic muscle membrane. If the end plate potential that is established in the muscle is of sufficient magnitude, then muscle fiber contraction ensues. Muscle fiber contraction is part of an all-or-none phenomenon. As the intensity of the stimulus increases, more muscle fibers are depolarized, and the strength of muscle contraction rises until a peak is reached (Fig. 4-13).

1.  *Postsynaptic Cholinoreceptors*
    Acetylcholine released from the nerve terminal crosses the junctional cleft and binds with a receptor before being rapidly hydrolyzed by **acetylcholinesterase.** During normal physiologic function, transmitter destruction is so rapid that acetylcholine does not accumulate from one nerve impulse to another. Although postsynaptic cholinorecep-

tor activity during normal physiologic function is very dynamic, some factors are known to influence it, for example, drugs, temperature, electrolyte balance in surrounding fluids, and changes in fluidity of the surrounding membrane. Acetylcholinesterase is found in high concentrations at the neuromuscular junction, and a single molecule hydrolyzes a few hundred thousand molecules of acetylcholine per minute. The enzyme is synthesized rapidly by nerve and muscle and protects the nerve terminal from persistent depolarization by large concentrations of transmitter.

2.   *Presynaptic Cholinoreceptors*
     When acetylcholine is released from the nerve terminal to trigger postsynaptic receptors, it also activates presynaptic receptors. Evidence indicates that presynaptic receptor stimulation facilitates the mobilization of the reserve store

Anatomy of the Motor End-plate                          Physiology

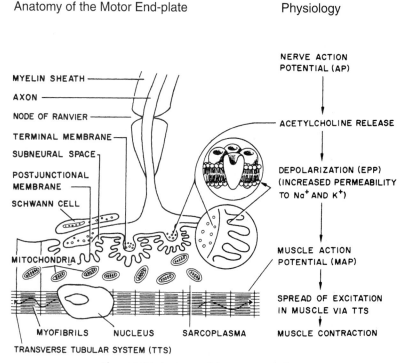

**Figure 4-13.** Anatomy of the motor end plate.

of transmitter in the nerve terminal to the presynaptic membrane, thus keeping it available for demand.

## B. Pharmacologic Actions of Neuromuscular Blocking Drugs

Neuromuscular blocking drugs are classified as **depolarizing** or **nondepolarizing** according to the effects on the acetylcholine receptor.

1. *Depolarizing Blocking Drugs*

   The **succinylcholine** molecule is like two acetylcholine molecules joined back to back. Although acetylcholine is rapidly destroyed in the junctional cleft, succinylcholine molecules remain present for a much longer period and are available to make multiple contacts with receptors. **Depolarization** occurs at the end plate, which then leads to muscle fiber contraction, seen as fasciculations. In addition, succinylcholine depolarizes the motor nerve terminal, producing repetitive discharge of transmitter, which is another cause of muscle fasciculations. Because succinylcholine molecules persist much longer than acetylcholine molecules, end plate depolarization is prolonged, leading to an area of inexcitability on the muscle membrane. The muscle fibers become flaccid, and relaxation ensues.

   a. A single large dose, repeated doses, and a continuous infusion of succinylcholine may result in postjunctional membranes that do not respond normally to acetylcholine, even when postjunctional membranes have become repolarized (desensitization neuromuscular blockade, or phase II blockade). The characteristics of **phase I and phase II blockade** are summarized in Table 4-11.

   b. **Ion channel block** occurs when the receptor ion channels have been opened by an agonist and the neuromuscular blocker, which is a large molecule, physically plugs the channel to stop ion flow. The extent to which this occurs during clinical use of neuromuscular blockers is not clear; however, ion channel block is likely to be of greater significance

---

**Table 4-11. Characteristics of Succinylcholine**

I. Phase I blockade
  A. Decreased single-twitch
  B. Decreased but sustained response to continuous stimulation
  C. Train-of-four ratio > 0.7
  D. Augmentation of neuromuscular blockade by anticholinesterase drugs
II. Phase II blockade (resembles nondepolarizing neuromuscular blockade)
  A. Decreased single-twitch
  B. Fade during continuous stimulation
  C. Train-of-four ratio < 0.7
  D. Antagonism of neuromuscular blockade by anticholinesterase drugs; confirmed with a small dose of edrophonium (0.1–0.2 mg/kg IV)

---

when high doses of relaxants, particularly nondepolarizing blockers, are given.

2. *Nondepolarizing Blocking Drugs*

The nondepolarizing relaxants recognize the acetylcholine receptor, show affinity for it, but do not trigger it. The molecules of the nondepolarizing relaxants are large and prevent acetylcholine from occupying the triggering sites of the receptors. The nondepolarizing neuromuscular blocker molecules react dynamically with receptor recognition sites; they predominantly associate and dissociate with the binding sites, so a characteristic of the block is one of competition. In addition to competing with the transmitter for receptor-triggering sites, nondepolarizing blockers are also likely to cause ion channel block. Blockage of the channel reduces the number of receptors that can be activated.

## C. Monitoring Neuromuscular Function

Neuromuscular function should be monitored with the help of a nerve stimulator whenever possible during the administration of muscle relaxants (Fig. 4-14). Monitoring provides details about the quantity of neuromuscular block required to produce the desired muscle relaxation for surgery and when to administer an antagonist for reversal of the block. The simplest method for assessing neuromuscular function is to electrically stimulate a peripheral nerve and evaluate the evoked muscle contraction. In animals, needle electrodes are positioned so that the active, or negative, electrode is placed over the nerve; the positive electrode is placed proximally. The intensity of the electric stimulus applied during monitoring should be supramaximal to ensure that all muscle fibers are stimulated and there is maximum muscle contraction. The most appropriate time to commence monitoring neuromuscular function is after the animal has been anesthetized and before the relaxant is administered. Prerelaxant evoked muscle responses in the anesthetized animal should be determined and then compared with those obtained after paralysis.

1.  Electric stimulation of the **ulnar, peroneal, tibial,** and **facial nerves** can be evaluated. For a dog, place the animal

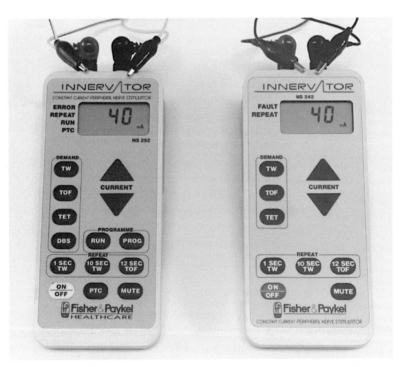

**Figure 4-14.** A small nerve stimulator suitable for monitoring neuromuscular function. These stimulators deliver single-twitch, train-of-four, tetanic, and double-burst stimulation (left stimulator only). The stimulator on the left can be programmed to repeat the stimuli.

# Stimulation Pattern

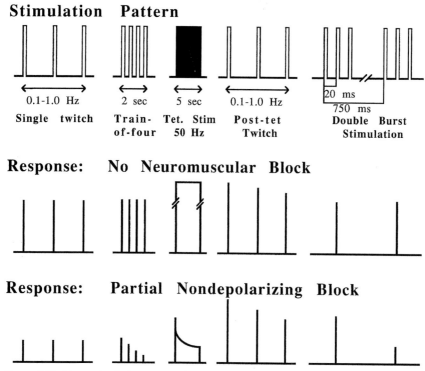

**Figure 4-15.** Nerve stimulation patterns for monitoring neuromuscular activity (*top*). Under each pattern, the characteristics of the evoked muscle responses (measured mechanically) before (*center*) and after (*bottom*) partial neuromuscular block. Train-of-four stimulation is usually repeated in 10-second intervals. See the text for further details.

in lateral recumbency, and stimulate the ulnar nerve on the medial aspect of the elbow, where it lies subcutaneously. Observe the strength of the contraction of the forepaw. For peroneal nerve stimulation, the nerve is stimulated on the lateral aspect of the stifle, and muscle twitch of the hind foot is observed.

2.  Stimulation patterns are **single-twitch, train-of-four, tetanic, post-tetanic single-twitch,** and **double-burst** stimulation. The evoked muscle responses recorded before and after neuromuscular block administration correspond to the patterns of nerve stimulation (Fig. 4-15). Responses can vary according to the onset or recovery from neuromuscular block and the muscle group from which the

evoked responses are recorded. The sensitivity of each stimulatory pattern varies.

a.    **For single-twitch stimulation,** the nerve is stimulated at a frequency of 0.1 to 1 Hz, and the muscle response or twitch is recorded (Fig. 4-15). Onset and recovery from neuromuscular block is evident by decreasing or increasing twitch heights, respectively. Time for return of twitch height (e.g., 25 to 75% of control) gives an indication of the duration of return of neuromuscular function. For recording single-twitch, only 20 to 25% of the functional acetylcholine receptor pool is necessary, or 75 to 80% of receptors require blocking before a single-twitch stimulation shows depression.

b.    **For the train-of-four stimulus,** the nerve is stimulated over 2 s. An interval of 10 s usually occurs between each train, and the pattern is applied either continuously or intermittently. Four muscle responses, or twitches, are measured. In the presence of a partial neuromuscular block with a nondepolarizing relaxant, a progressive decline in the height of the twitches, from one to four, occurs; the fourth is the most depressed (Fig. 4-15). With deepening block, twitches are progressively eliminated; the fourth is eliminated initially. Evaluation of mechanical responses to train-of-four stimulation is a more sensitive assessment of neuromuscular function than that obtained from a single-twitch stimulation. The train-of-four ratio decreases when 70 to 75% of receptors are blocked. Depressed single-twitch heights have shown signs of recovery before there was evidence of a train-of-four ratio increase. Furthermore, different nondepolarizing relaxants have varying ratios at the same stage of block; and fade is usually more pronounced during recovery from neuromuscular block than during onset.

c.    **For tetanic stimulation,** muscle responses to short periods of high-frequency nerve stimulation (up to 200 Hz) are recorded. Nerve stimulation is applied at 50 Hz for 5 s every 5 to 6 min. These rates of stimulation may cause arousal in the lightly anesthetized patient. With a partial nondepolarizing block, reduced tetanic height and tetanic fade occur (Fig. 4-15). Responses to tetanic stimulation provide a more accurate assessment of neuromuscular function than do those from train-of-four stimulation.

d.   The resumption of single-twitch stimulation about 5 s after tetanic stimulation during partial nonde-polarizing block produces twitch heights higher than the pretetanic twitches. This effect, which is called **post-tetanic facilitation,** is transient and is evident when recordings of evoked muscle responses are measured mechanically (tension) or electromyo-graphically. With intense block, post-tetanic facilita-tion may not be evident.

e.   The visual assessment of muscle responses to train-of-four stimulation is inaccurate; therefore, in the absence of recording equipment, **double-burst stim-ulation** is considered to be superior. An initial burst of three impulses to the nerve at a frequency of 50 Hz (one impulse every 20 ms) followed by an inter-val of 750 ms allows visualization or manual detection of small amounts of residual neuromuscular block under clinical conditions (Fig. 4-15). In the absence of muscle relaxation, two short muscle contractions of equal strength are produced. In a partially para-lyzed muscle, the second response is weaker than the first; i.e., the responses fade. Absence of fade in re-sponse to double-burst stimulation means that clini-cally significant residual neuromuscular block does not exist.

## D.   Pharmacology of Neuromuscular Blockers

Neuromuscular blocking agents are **quaternary ammonium compounds.** Relaxants are unlikely to cross lipid membranes such as the blood–brain barrier, placenta, or the renal tubular epithelium to be reabsorbed after being filtered. Muscle relax-ants are unable to penetrate the blood–brain barrier effectively and, therefore, are devoid of sedative, anesthetic, and analgesic properties. Because muscle-relaxant molecules are structurally related to acetylcholine, they are attracted to all cholinergic receptors, those at the neuromuscular junction as well as the

**nicotinic receptors** of the autonomic ganglia and **muscarinic receptors** at postganglionic parasympathetic sites. Their ionization state and hydrophilic nature mean that glomerular filtration is a major route for excretion. Except for pancuronium, vecuronium, pipecuronium, and rocuronium, which have a steroidal chemical structure, neuromuscular blockers rely little on hepatic breakdown.

1. **Succinylcholine** is hydrolyzed by the enzyme **pseudocholinesterase** (plasma cholinesterase) to choline and **succinylmonocholine,** which is further hydrolyzed to succinic acid and choline. Pseudocholinesterase is formed in the liver; and plasma levels of this enzyme are reduced by liver disease, malnutrition, chronic anemia, burns, certain malignancies, cytotoxic drugs, pregnancy, and acetylcholinesterase inhibitors. Some specific drug administrations also inhibit cholinesterase activity; e.g., lithium, echothiophate, metoclopramide, and neostigmine. **Organophosphate insecticides** used as anthelmintics or ectoparasite therapy in animals have a variable effect on succinylcholine activity.

2. **D-Tubocurarine,** or **curare,** is a naturally occurring substance obtained from an Amazonian vine. D-Tubocurarine is a benzylisoquinoline substance, and it is eliminated predominantly in the urine unchanged. A small proportion is excreted in the bile.

3. **Gallamine** is a synthetic trisquaternary compound that relies on renal excretion for elimination.

4. **Pancuronium** is a synthetic steroid molecule that relies on the kidney for elimination of more than half the dose given. Pancuronium neuromuscular block is prolonged in patients with renal failure.

5. **Atracurium** is a synthetic bisquaternary isoquinoline compound that is metabolized by esterases and **Hofmann elimination.** Hofmann elimination spontaneously breaks down atracurium at body pH and temperature to **laudanosine** (tertiary amine) and a monoquaternary acrylate without renal, hepatic, or enzymatic processes. Additional

breakdown is by ester hydrolysis and other metabolic pathways. A decrease in temperature of 5 to 6°C (41 to 44°F) slows the rate of degradation of atracurium to about half that at normal body temperature. Laudanosine at very high concentrations has been shown to cause seizure activity in dogs.

6. **Vecuronium** is the monoquaternary analog of the steroid relaxant pancuronium and was developed to avoid the latter's undesirable actions, namely the ganglion blocking and the indirect sympathomimetic effect. Vecuronium has a potency similar to pancuronium in cats and is less cumulative. Vecuronium is unstable when stored in solution long term and is presented in a lyophilized form that is dissolved in water before clinical use. The solution is stable at room temperature for up to 24 h.

7. **Pipecuronium** is a long-acting bisquaternary steroid neuromuscular blocker. It is an analog of pancuronium and has a higher potency. Renal elimination of the unchanged molecule accounts for about 77% of the injected drug in dogs, and < 5% is excreted in the bile.

8. **Doxacurium,** a benzylisoquinoline compound, is a long-acting nondepolarizing relaxant. It is slightly more potent than pipecuronium and much more potent than pancuronium. This compound is predominantly eliminated unchanged in the urine and bile in cats.

9. **Mivacurium,** a benzylisoquinoline diester compound, is a nondepolarizing relaxant with a potency of one-third to one-half that of atracurium in the monkey. Its short duration of action is caused by rapid hydrolysis by pseudocholinesterase.

10. **Rocuronium** is a derivative of vecuronium but is less potent. It has a rapid onset of action and a duration of effect similar to that for vecuronium in dogs.

**E. Nonneuromuscular Blocking Actions of Relaxants**

Muscle relaxants act predominantly at the **neuromuscular junction,** but because of their structure they recognize cholinoreceptors elsewhere in the body. Undesirable actions of neuromuscular blockers arise from competing with or mimicking acetylcholine at nicotinic autonomic ganglion receptors and muscarinic receptors or by weak actions on sympathetic nerve endings. Most of these actions affect the cardiovascular system. New drugs (e.g., atracurium and vecuronium) have been developed in an attempt to minimize undesirable actions. Additional effects on the cardiovascular system arise through the release of **histamine** by some neuromuscular blockers.

1. *Cardiovascular Effects*

   a. **Vecuronium and atracurium** are nearly free of cardiovascular effects. These are the relaxants of choice if myocardial disease is present, although atracurium has the potential to release histamine.

   b. **Pancuronium** and, to a lesser extent, gallamine weakly stimulate the release of norepinephrine from adrenergic nerve endings in vitro, mechanisms that increase heart rate and blood pressure. Other contributing actions are inhibition of catecholamine reuptake by sympathetic nerve endings. In dogs, pancuronium increases blood pressure, heart rate, and cardiac output.

   c. Because **vecuronium** has no effect on heart rate, arterial pressure, autonomic ganglia, or adrenoceptor or baroreceptor activity in dogs and cats, it has been recommended for patients with myocardial disease.

   d. **Succinylcholine** can stimulate cholinergic receptors to produce either vagal or sympathetic actions. A decrease in heart rate follows direct stimulation of postganglionic cholinergic receptors in the heart or increased vagal tone caused by carotid body sensory receptor stimulation. Sympathetic stimulation increases heart rate and blood pressure. Arterial pressure frequently increases in most animals, though a transient decrease may occur occasionally before the increase. Blood pressure changes that accompany the first dose of succinylcholine usually progressively diminish if successive doses are given. Both bradycardia and tachycardia have been observed.

2. *Histamine Release*
   Histamine release can accompany the administration of some neuromuscular blockers. Of the relaxants that cause histamine release, the higher the dose administered, the greater the potential for release. Anaphylactic or anaphylactoid reactions are rare. Pretreatment with $H_1$- and $H_2$-receptor antagonists are beneficial in avoiding the effects of histamine release. Atracurium releases small quantities of histamine in dogs, but it is of little significance at doses required to cause neuromuscular block.

## F. Nonneuromuscular Blocking Actions of Succinylcholine

Succinylcholine administration is frequently accompanied by **hyperkalemia;** increased intraocular, intragastric, and intracranial pressure; and complications associated with muscle disorders. On occasion, this relaxant is contraindicated because of these actions.

1. In patients with **burns, direct muscle trauma, tetanus, muscle denervation, spinal cord section, brain damage,** and **stroke,** additional acetylcholine receptor sites develop in the extrajunctional area of the muscle fiber, so that the whole muscle fiber membrane becomes sensitive to acetylcholine or succinylcholine. An increased number of ion channels are now available to release potassium during depolarization from succinylcholine, and the increase in serum potassium level is likely to precipitate life-threatening cardiac dysrhythmias. Receptor proliferation along the muscle fiber starts 3 to 15 days after injury and persists for 2 to 3 months after burns or trauma and for 3 to 6 months in patients with tetanus. The dangers of hyperkalemia do not occur in the first 2 days after injury.

2. **Immobilization** of a limb increases the sensitivity of the patient to succinylcholine and raises the potential for complications owing to hyperkalemia. These changes ap-

pear to be the result of the development of perijunctional or extrajunctional receptors. In contrast, muscle immobilization or inactivity increases resistance to the paralyzing effects of nondepolarizing relaxants.

3. **Increased IOP** after succinylcholine administration can cause expulsion of the vitreous humor in patients with penetrating eye injuries. By contrast, nondepolarizing relaxants do not raise IOP.

4. Succinylcholine raises **ICP** in anesthetized cats and dogs. The cause of the change is the accompanying increase in cerebral blood flow after muscle fasciculations. Succinylcholine should not be given to animals with increased ICP.

5. **Muscle fasciculations** are determined by the dose and speed of succinylcholine injection. Fasciculations, which precede relaxation, occur after the initial dose only.

6. **Malignant hyperthermia** is a heritable metabolic disorder of muscles in which there is a defect in the intracellular calcium metabolism. It has been reported in dogs and cats. One of the known triggering drugs of malignant hyperthermia is succinylcholine.

## G.   Use of Muscle Relaxants in Anesthetized Animals

1. **Indications for muscle relaxants** include muscle relaxation without the dangers of deep anesthesia and prolonged recovery. Neuromuscular blockers abolish muscle tone, which improves surgical access. Surgeries for which the most benefit is achieved are laparotomies, fractures, and dislocations. Intraocular and spinal surgery are delicate procedures, and relaxants eliminate the risk of patient movement. Nondepolarizing relaxants maintain the eye in a central position without raising IOP.

2. **The choice of muscle relaxant** depends on the species of animal to be paralyzed, the surgical procedure, the duration of muscle relaxation, and ongoing pathologic processes. Succinylcholine has a variable duration of action in different species. It is contraindicated if hyperkalemia is

present; if intracranial, intraocular, or intragastric pressures are increased; or if the animal is susceptible to certain muscle disorders. Animals in renal failure should not be given gallamine.

a.   **Monitoring of neuromuscular function** during relaxant administration allows the dose to be titrated to effect, thus avoiding overdosing. Small, hand-held nerve stimulators that deliver different stimulation patterns are readily available; and the evoked muscle responses, usually twitches, are easily measured or observed. To avoid relaxant overdose, up to two-thirds or three-quarters of the dose is given initially. The total quantity given is in accordance with the depression of evoked twitches.

b.   **Approximate dose and duration of action** for muscle relaxants given intravenously to dogs and cats are listed in Tables 4-12 and 4-13, respectively. Twitch

**Table 4-12. Use of Intravenous Muscle Relaxants in Canines**

| Drug | Approximate Dose, µg/kg | Approximate Duration, min | Twitch Recovery[a] |
|---|---|---|---|
| Alcuronium | 100 | 70 | 100% |
| Atracurium | 200–400 | 17–28.9 | 50% |
| Doxacurium | 8 | | |
| Gallamine | 400–1000 | 29 | 50% |
| Metocurine | 63 | 109 | 50% |
| Pancuronium | 22–60 | 31–108 | 50–100% |
| Pipecuronium | 3.7–50 | 16–80.7 | 50% |
| Succinylcholine | 300–400 | 22–29 | 10–50% |
| Succinylcholine (Greyhound) | 300 | 38 | 50% |
| ᴅ-Tubocurarine | 130 | 100 | 50% |
| Vecuronium | 14–200 | 15–42 | 50% |

[a]Signifies the end point of duration. Applies to experimental studies that measured evoked muscle contractions after nerve stimulation.

| Table 4-13. Use of Intravenous Muscle Relaxants in Felines | | | |
| --- | --- | --- | --- |
| Drug | Approximate Dose, µg/kg | Approximate Duration, min | Twitch Recovery[a] |
| Alcuronium | 80 | 31 | 100% |
| Atracurium | 250 | 29 | 100% |
| Gallamine | 1200 | 24 | 100% |
| Metocurine | 40 | 42 | 100% |
| Pancuronium | 20–22 | 14–15 | 50–100% |
| Pipecuronium | 2–2.7 | 16.5–24 | 50% |
| Succinylcholine | 3000–5000 (total) | 4–6 | |
| D-Tubocurarine | 200 | 20 | 100% |
| Vecuronium | 24–40 | 5–9 | 75–90% |

[a]Signifies end point of duration. Applies to experimental studies that measured evoked muscle contractions after nerve stimulation.

height, which indicates the end point for recovery, is also listed in the tables. Time for onset of maximum relaxation from a bolus dose of nondepolarizing relaxant that produces 90 to 99% decrease in twitch height takes 5 to 7 min. Faster onset times and a longer period of paralysis are produced by higher doses. The onset time for succinylcholine block is more rapid than that for the nondepolarizing relaxants.

c. **Individual muscles** respond slightly differently to neuromuscular blockers. The diaphragm is usually the last skeletal muscle to be paralyzed, requiring a slightly higher dose of relaxant than that required to paralyze limb muscles. With onset of muscle paralysis, muscle twitches to facial nerve stimulation are initially depressed along with limb muscle twitches.

d. **Multiple doses** or constant infusion of short-acting relaxants have been reported. In dogs, vecuronium at an initial dose of 0.1 mg/kg and incremental doses at 0.04 mg/kg, and atracurium at 0.5 mg/kg and incremental doses of 0.2 mg/kg have been reported.

## H.   Interaction with Other Drugs

1.   **A number of antibiotics** are known to prolong the duration of action of neuromuscular blockers. Antibiotics potentiate nondepolarizing relaxants by different mechanisms of action. Certain antibiotics cause channel block, whereas the **aminoglycosides (streptomycin, neomycin, gentamicin, kanamycin,** and **amikacin**) potentiate relaxants by a postsynaptic action and presynaptically by reducing acetylcholine release. Neostigmine and calcium have been beneficial in reversing block caused by aminoglycosides.

2.   **The polymyxins** have both prejunctional and postjunctional actions, including depression of muscle action potentials. Block is not responsive to calcium or neostigmine. **Tetracycline, lincomycin,** and **clindamycin** (the lincosamides) have a prejunctional action and may directly depress muscle contractility. Calcium and neostigmine may antagonize neuromuscular block enhanced by oxytetracycline and the lincosamides but not tetracycline.

3.   **Local anesthetics, barbiturates, quinidine, procainamide, propranolol, phenytoin,** and **magnesium** compounds also potentiate neuromuscular block. Patients given long-term phenytoin therapy have shown resistance to metocurine, D-tubocurarine, pancuronium, and vecuronium, but not to atracurium.

4.   **Calcium antagonists** used to treat cardiac dysrhythmias prolong nondepolarizing neuromuscular block through a presynaptic action. Dantrolene has a potentiating action of muscle relaxants by blocking muscle excitation–contraction coupling. Diuretics, including furosemide, cause possible presynaptic inhibition of acetylcholine release and hypokalemia. Corticosteroids decrease the potency of nondepolarizing blockers.

5.   Some drugs inhibit cholinesterase enzyme, which prolongs the action of succinylcholine. These compounds include metoclopramide, immunosuppressants (cyclophosphamide, meturedepa, and chlorambucil), ganglion blockers, lithium compounds, and organophosphates.

I.    **Antagonism of Neuromuscular Block**

1.   **Antagonism of a nondepolarizing neuromuscular block** is achieved by increasing the concentration of acetylcholine molecules in the junctional cleft between the nerve terminal and muscle end plate. By giving anticholinesterase drugs, the hydrolysis of acetylcholine is slowed; the number of acetylcholine molecules accumulates to compete for position at the receptor site; and as muscle relaxant molecules are forced away from the neuromuscular junction, normal neuromuscular transmission returns.

2.   Three anticholinesterase compounds, **edrophonium, neostigmine,** and **pyridostigmine,** have been synthesized and are used to inhibit the action of the enzyme. The binding between neostigmine and pyridostigmine and the enzyme is similar to the binding that occurs between acetylcholinesterase and acetylcholine when the substrate is hydrolyzed.

3.   In humans the **onset of action** is 1 to 2 min for edrophonium, 7 to 10 min for neostigmine, and 12 to 16 min for pyridostigmine. The duration of cholinesterase antagonism is similar for neostigmine and edrophonium, whereas for pyridostigmine it is about 40% longer.

4.   **Anticholinesterases** allow the buildup of acetylcholine at nicotinic (neuromuscular junction) and muscarinic cholinoreceptors. Muscarinic receptor stimulation induces bradycardia; increased gastrointestinal motility; increased secretions from salivary glands, the oropharynx, and airways; and bronchiole constriction. Simultaneous administration of an anticholinergic will prevent these adverse effects. Glycopyrrolate has a slower onset of action than atropine; consequently, it should be given about 3 or 4 min before edrophonium. Atropine should be given before edrophonium, whereas it can be given simultaneously with neostigmine and pyridostigmine. Best responses to anticholinesterases are achieved when there is some spontaneous recovery and twitch heights are rising; with the train-of-four stimulation, all four twitches are evident. In monitored patients, at least two twitches of a train-of-four

should be evident before anticholinesterases are administered (Fig. 4-15). When patients are not monitored, obvious diaphragmatic contractions should be present. Anticholinesterase administration is not necessary if all four twitch heights of a train-of-four have returned to prerelaxant heights or there is minimal fade after tetanic stimulation. If anticholinesterase therapy is to be avoided, vecuronium or atracurium are recommended, because spontaneous recovery is fairly rapid.

a.  **In dogs, neostigmine (2.5 mg)** plus atropine can be used to reverse neuromuscular block after atracurium, gallamine, pancuronium, pipecuronium, and vecuronium. **In cats, edrophonium (0.5 mg/kg)** has been used to antagonize vecuronium block. A second dose of anticholinesterase can be given 5 to 7 min after the initial dose if the response is poor. Intravenous calcium can also be tried if response to anticholinesterase injection is poor.

b.  **The patient should be observed closely** after antagonism of neuromuscular block. Short, jerky respirations that suggest the presence of **residual block** or apnea as a result of recurarization may occur. If recovery from muscle relaxation is unduly prolonged, likely causes need to be investigated. These include hypothermia, electrolyte disturbances, excessively deep anesthesia, simultaneous administration of antibiotics, and other compounds known to prolong neuromuscular block.

5.  **Anticholinesterases can prolong the depolarizing block produced by succinylcholine** (Table 4-11). When multiple or high doses of succinylcholine are given or the relaxant has a prolonged action, phase II block develops. Neostigmine reversal of phase II block in dogs should be attempted only when train-of-four twitch heights are measured and the ratio is < 0.4. Without an accurate measurement of the train-of-four ratio, recovery from succinylcholine block should be allowed to occur spontaneously. The patient should be ventilated until it can breathe adequately.

# Chapter 5

---

## Local Anesthetic and Analgesic Techniques

### Introductory Comments

*Local anesthetics make up a group of drugs that reversibly block the propagation of action potentials along nerve axons. They are used to anesthetize a region of the body. These drugs are relatively unique in that they are applied directly at the target site. Absorption into and distribution by the systemic circulation is not necessary to achieve the intended application. Some local anesthetics are employed clinically for purposes other than producing anesthesia (e.g., lidocaine is used to treat cardiac ventricular arrhythmias).*

## Pharmacology of Local Anesthetics
## Local and Regional Anesthetic and Analgesic Techniques

---

## I. PHARMACOLOGY OF LOCAL ANESTHETICS
*James E. Heavner*

### A. Chemistry and Structure–Activity Relationships

Clinically useful local anesthetics have similar physical properties and molecular structures. Most of the drugs are weakly basic tertiary amines. A few, such as hexylcaine and prilocaine, are secondary amines. The basic local anesthetic molecule has three parts: a **hydrophilic end** (imparting water solubility); a **lipophilic end** (imparting lipid solubility); and an **intermediate hydrocarbon chain,** connecting the hydrophilic and lipophilic ends (Fig. 5-1). The aromatic end (lipophilic) is derived from benzoic acid or aniline. The hydrophilic end is less easily characterized, although amino derivatives of ethyl alcohol or acetic acid are

192

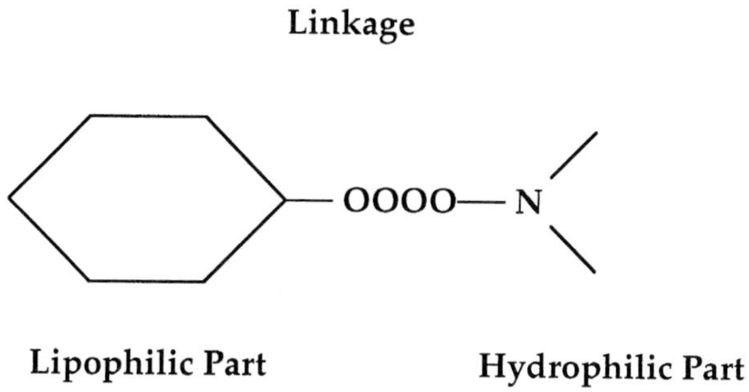

## Linkage

**Lipophilic Part**                    **Hydrophilic Part**

**Figure 5-1.** Basic molecular structure of local anesthetics.

common. Some local anesthetics (e.g., benzocaine) lack the hydrophilic tail and are nearly insoluble in water; thus, they are not suitable for injection but are satisfactory for topical application to mucosal surfaces and open wounds.

The 6- to 9-Å separation of the lipophilic and hydrophilic components by four or five atoms appears to be critical for a molecule to retain local anesthetic activity. Antihistaminics, anticholinergics, and other classes of compounds have a structure similar to that of local anesthetics and often exhibit weak local anesthetic effects.

1.  *Grouping Local Anesthetics*
    Local anesthetics are typically classed as **ester-linked** or **amide-linked**, depending on the structure of the molecule's intermediate chain. Local anesthetics derived from benzoic acid belong to the ester family, and those derived from aniline belong to the aminoacyl or amide family. The nature of the intermediate chain predetermines the course of biotransformation of local anesthetics. Ester-linked local anesthetics, characterized by procaine, are readily hydrolyzed (Fig. 5-2). Amide-linked local anesthetics, characterized by lidocaine, are generally biotransformed by liver microsomal enzymes (Fig. 5-3). Time to onset of effect, potency, and duration of action of local anesthetics basically depend on the physical chemical properties of their molecular structure (Table 5-1). Lipid solubility is a major determinant of intrinsic local anesthetic potency among

drugs. Because axonal membranes are highly lipid in composition, local anesthetics act strongly on these structures.

**Protein binding** is believed to be a primary determinant of local anesthetic duration, presumably because the site of action of local anesthetics involves the protein within the axonal membrane. The greater the binding affinity to axonal protein, the longer anesthetic activity persists.

The **acid dissociation constant (pKa)** is generally thought to determine the speed of action of local anesthetics. Local anesthetic agents exist in solution in both the charged cationic (+) and the uncharged base forms. It is generally thought that the base is primarily responsible for onset of action, because the uncharged form diffuses more readily across the nerve sheath.

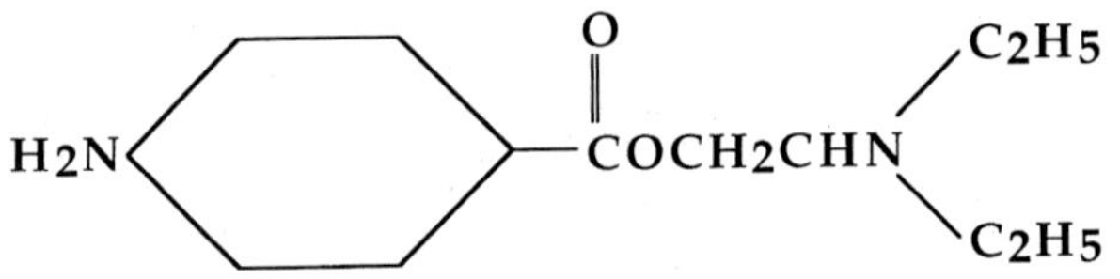

**Procaine**

**Figure 5-2.** Procaine.

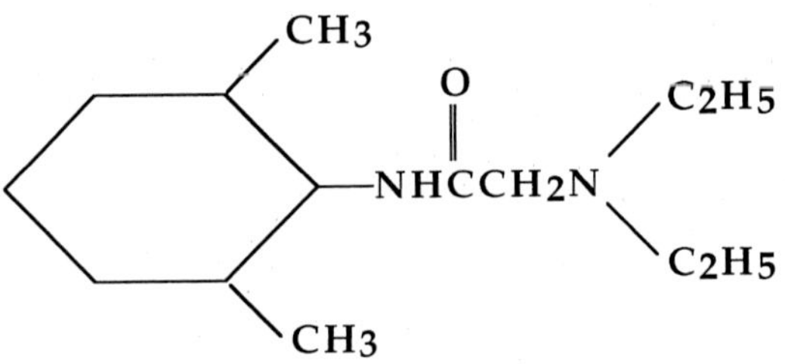

**Lidocaine**

**Figure 5-3.** Lidocaine.

## Table 5-1. Physical, Chemical, and Biologic Properties of Commonly Used Local Anesthetic Agents

| Agent | Lipid Solubility | Relative Potency[a] | pKa | Onset of Action | Plasma Protein Binding, % | Duration, min | Molecular Weight |
|---|---|---|---|---|---|---|---|
| **LOW POTENCY, SHORT DURATION** | | | | | | | |
| Procaine[b] | 1 | 1 | 8.9 | Slow | 6 | 60–90 | 236 |
| Chloroprocaine[b] | 1 | 1 | 9.1 | Fast | 7 | 30–60 | 271 |
| **INTERMEDIATE POTENCY AND DURATION** | | | | | | | |
| Mepivacaine[c] | 2 | 2 | 7.6 | Fast | 75 | 120–240 | 246 |
| Prilocaine[c] | 1 | 2 | 7.7 | Fast | 55 | 120–240 | 220 |
| Lidocaine[c] | 3.6 | 2 | 7.7 | Fast | 65 | 90–200 | 234 |
| **HIGH POTENCY, LONG DURATION** | | | | | | | |
| Tetracaine[b] | 80 | 8 | 8.6 | Slow | 80 | 180–600 | 264 |
| Bupivacaine[c] | 30 | 8 | 8.1 | Intermediate | 95 | 180–600 | 288 |
| Etidocaine[c] | 140 | 6 | 7.7 | Fast | 95 | 180–600 | 276 |

[a]Relative to procaine, the least potent of the local anesthetics in current use.
[b]Ester.
[c]Amide.

## Depolarization

Resting ──►Closed ──►Open ──►Inactivated

## Repolarization

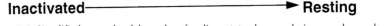

Inactivated ──────────────────► Resting

**Figure 5-4.** Simplified example of the order of sodium state changes during membrane depolarization. Reprinted with permission from Heavner.

2. *Mechanism of Action*

Local anesthetics prevent the rapid influx of sodium into nerve axons, which produces the action potential. Under resting conditions, there is a voltage difference across axonal membranes (the inside is approximately −70 mV relative to the outside). When the membrane receives an adequate stimulus, it depolarizes, producing an action potential that moves in obligatory fashion along the axon (propagated action potential). The influx of sodium ions into the axon is controlled by sodium channels that exist in various states, depending on the transmembrane potential (Fig. 5-4). It is important to note that there are families of channels (i.e., the sodium channels in the heart, brain, and axons are not identical) and that a given tissue may contain a variety of sodium channels. Local anesthetic effects may differ, depending on the kind(s) of sodium channels present in the target tissue; and some local anesthetic effects (e.g., CNS toxicity) may be mediated by actions other than interference with sodium channel function.

3. *Differential Nerve Block*

Analgesia or anesthesia without loss of motor function is frequently desirable and can be achieved with appropriate use of local anesthetics. This suggests that **sensory nerve fibers** might be more readily blocked by local anesthetics than are **large motor fibers.** It is generally agreed that the spread of local anesthetic in a high enough concentration to block three consecutive **nodes of Ranvier** in myelinated axons is the minimum requirement for stopping electric transmission through an axon. Obviously, this does not apply to **unmyelinated C fibers,** which stand apart from **myelinated fibers** with respect to factors that influence local anesthetic block. There is evidence that the frequency with which axons discharge correlates with vulnerability to local anesthetic action. Axons that have a high discharge rate (e.g., C and A-$\delta$ fibers) are more sensitive to local anesthetics than are fibers with lower discharge rates (e.g., A-$\beta$ fibers and frequency-dependent block). Individual variation in response to local anesthetics exists, but the sensation of pain is usually the first sensory modality to disappear, followed by the loss of the sensations of cold, warmth, touch, and deep pressure.

## B.   Pharmacokinetics of Local Anesthetics

1.   *Absorption*
With one exception, local anesthetics are not injected intravascularly to induce anesthesia. The exception is when intravenous regional anesthesia (IVRA) is used to anesthetize an anterior or posterior extremity. Systemic absorption of local anesthetic occurs in the other cases, and the rate of absorption varies directly with the vascularity of the injection site. The faster the absorption rate, the shorter the duration of action of the local anesthetic and the greater the risk of systemic toxicity.

A vasoconstrictor, most commonly **epinephrine,** is added to local anesthetic solutions to reduce local blood flow, thereby prolonging the duration of action and reducing the probability of systemic toxicity. In fact, maximum recommended doses of local anesthetics are increased if a vasoconstrictor is added. The usual concentration of epinephrine is 1:200,000 (5 mg/mL) or 1:400,000 (2.5 mg/mL).

Local anesthetics are generally ineffective when applied to unbroken skin, but they are effective when the skin is broken, when applied to the cornea, or when applied to mucous membranes. A eutectic mixture of local anesthetics (**EMLA cream**) with prilocaine and lidocaine has been marketed that is effective when applied to the skin. The methods of administration of commonly used local anesthetics are summarized in Table 5-2.

2. *Distribution*

    a.   **Distribution of local anesthetic** at the injection site depends on the volume of local anesthetic solution injected and how resistant the tissue is to the spread of the local anesthetic. **Hyaluronidase** is sometimes added to local anesthetic solutions to enhance spread, especially when the local anesthetic is injected into the bony orbit to anesthetize the eye. When a local anesthetic is injected into the subarachnoid space (spinal anesthesia), the specific gravity (baricity) of the solution relative to the specific gravity of cerebrospinal fluid (CSF) influences distribution. **Hyperbaric** solutions prepared by adding glucose (10%) combined with patient positioning are used to direct local anesthetic to specific sites.

    b.   The liver and lungs are major sites for plasma clearance of local anesthetics (**systemic distribution**). The extraction fraction (amount of local anesthetic extracted from the plasma by an organ) is quite high for the liver for most local anesthetics (e.g., 0.75 for lidocaine). A decrease in liver blood flow can, therefore, prolong plasma half-life. Increasing the pH increases the ratio of uncharged to charged molecules in solution. This speeds the onset of block, because the uncharged form readily diffuses to the target site.

3. *Elimination*
Local anesthetics undergo biotransformation and are then excreted from the body via the urine or bile. The liver plays an important role in the metabolism of local anesthetics. It is a source of plasma cholinesterase, which cleaves the ester link, or contains the mixed function oxidases that biotransforms amide-linked local anesthetics.

| Table 5-2. Recommended Methods of Administration of Local Anesthetics | | | | | | |
|---|---|---|---|---|---|---|
| Drug | Topical Anesthesia | Local Infiltration | Peripheral Nerve Block | Intravenous Regional | Epidural Anesthesia | Spinal Anesthesia |
| Procaine | No | Yes | Yes | No | No | Yes |
| Tetracaine | Yes | No | No | No | No | Yes |
| Lidocaine | Yes | Yes | Yes | Yes | Yes | Yes |
| Mepivacaine | No | Yes | Yes | No | Yes | No |
| Bupivacaine | No | Yes | Yes | No | Yes | Yes |
| Etidocaine | No | Yes | Yes | No | Yes | No |
| Prilocaine | No | Yes | Yes | Yes | Yes | No |
| Eutectic mixture | Yes | No | No | No | No | No |

## C.   Local Anesthetic Toxicity

Toxic reactions to local anesthetics are generally not fatal if recognized early and appropriately treated. The most frequent and dramatic reactions observed clinically are acute reactions involving the direct effects of local anesthetics on the cardiovascular system and/or CNS. Bupivacaine affects the heart somewhat differently than do other local anesthetics. The intravenous toxic doses of commonly used local anesthetics are given in Table 5-3, along with the usual doses recommended for peripheral and epidural block procedures.

Acute toxicity is usually associated with accidental intravascular injection of local anesthetics. Numerous strategies exist to avoid intoxication via this mechanism, including incremental dosing, aspiration before injection, and use of test doses or substances. Benzodiazepines apparently have value in aborting seizures, as do ultra-short-acting barbiturates (e.g., thiopental). Evidence from animal studies show that propofol may also be effective in stopping local anesthetic seizures. Cardiac rhythm disturbances and cardiovascular collapse are generally treated symptomatically (e.g., volume expansion, cardiac stimulants, cardioversion, oxygen, sodium bicarbonate).

1.   *CNS Toxicity*

CNS symptoms of local anesthetic toxicity usually occur before cardiovascular changes occur. Data from human and animal studies indicate that local anesthetic-induced seizures originate in the limbic brain. At the neuronal level, local anesthetics appear to produce CNS symptoms via an effect on sodium conductance, possibly via the same mechanism by which they produce conduction block in axons of the peripheral nervous system. Evidence indicates that some of the cardiotoxic effect of local anesthetics, bupivacaine in particular, may actually result from effects of these drugs on the brain.

2.   *Cardiovascular Toxicity*

Local anesthetics can produce profound cardiovascular changes directly by cardiac and peripheral vascular action and indirectly by conduction blockade of autonomic fibers. The primary site of action is the myocar-

**Table 5-3. Commonly Used Local Anesthetic Drugs and Doses for Peripheral and Epidural Block Procedures in Conscious Canines**

| Local Anesthetic | | Concentration, % | Usual Doses, mg/kg | | Toxic Doses, mg/kg IV | | Approximate Onset of Motor and Sensory Block, min | Approximate Duration of Motor and Sensory Block, h | Motor Block |
| --- | --- | --- | --- | --- | --- | --- | --- | --- | --- |
| Generic Name | Trade Name (Manufacturer) | | With Epinephrine | Without Epinephrine | Convulsive | Lethal | | | |
| **ESTER LINKED** | | | | | | | | | |
| Procaine | Novocaine (Withrop) | 1–2 | 8 | 6 | 36 | 100 | 10–15 | 0.5 | ± |
| Chloroprocaine | Nesacaine (Pennwalt) | 1–1.5 | 8 | 6 | | | 7–15 | 0.5–1 | ± |
| **AMIDE LINKED** | | | | | | | | | |
| Lidocaine | Xylocaine (Astra) | 0.5–2 | 7 | 5 | 11–20 | 16–28 | 10–15 | 1–2 | + |
| Mepivacaine | Carbocaine (Breon) | 1–2 | 7 | 5 | 29 | | 5–10 | 2–2.5 | + |
| Bupivacaine | Marcaine (Breon) | 0.25–0.5 | 3 | 2 | 3.5–4.5 | 5–11 | 20–30 | 2.5–6 | ± |
| Ropivacaine | LEA 103 (Breon) | 0.5 | 5 | 3 | 4.9 | | 5–15 | 2.5–4 | + |
| Etidocaine | Duranest (Astra) | 0.5–0.75 | 5 | 3 | 4.5 | 20 | 5–10 | 2–5 | +++ |

±, inconsistent motor nerve block; +, weak motor nerve block; +++, strong motor nerve block.

dium, where decreases in electric excitability, conduction rate, and force of contraction occur. Notable are the cardiac rhythm disturbances associated with local anesthetic cardiotoxicity. High concentrations of local anesthetics dilate blood vessels, but low concentrations may cause vasoconstriction. Inhibition of sodium conductance increase appears to play a major role in the cardiac effects of local anesthetics and probably in the vascular effects as well. There is evidence, however, that potassium channel block may also contribute to the cardiotoxicity of local anesthetics. Recent studies indicate that a host of physiologic changes can affect the cardiotoxicity of local anesthetics, including progesterone (pregnancy), hyponatremia, and diabetes mellitus. Even at the height of CNS symptoms, cardiovascular changes may be minimal, with some increase in pulse rate and a corresponding rise in blood pressure.

3. *Methemoglobinemia*
   Most discussions regarding the propensity for local anesthetics to produce methemoglobinemia focus on prilocaine, the only clinically used local anesthetic that is a secondary amine. Reports, however, implicate prilocaine, benzocaine, lidocaine, and procaine as causative agents. Methemoglobinemia is formed when ferrous iron ($Fe^{2+}$) in hemoglobin is oxidized to the ferric ($Fe^{3+}$) form.

4. *Tissue Toxicity*
   Tissue toxicity includes irritation and lysis of cells. Muscles and nerves are of primary concern, and skeletal muscle appears to be the most sensitive. High concentrations of local anesthetics are clearly cytotoxic.

5. *Allergic Reactions*
   Allergic reactions to local anesthetics may occur; however, the number of documented reactions is small. Reputedly, allergic reactions are more likely to occur with ester-linked local anesthetics than with amide-linked ones. **Methylparaben,** a preservative sometimes added to

local anesthetic solutions, may cause allergic-type reactions.

## II.  LOCAL AND REGIONAL ANESTHETIC AND ANALGESIC TECHNIQUES

*Roman T. Skarda*

### A.   Topical Anesthesia

Many local anesthetics are effective when placed topically on
mucous membranes and may be used in the mouth, tracheo-
bronchial tree, esophagus, and genitourinary tract. Local anesthetics used topically include lidocaine (2 to 5%), proparacaine
(0.5%), tetracaine (0.5 to 2%), butacaine (2%), and cocaine
(4 to 10%). The lowest effective dose of topical anesthetic
should always be used to prevent toxicity from excessive drug
plasma concentrations. Compared to infiltration anesthesia, the
time between application of topical anesthetics and onset of
anesthesia is generally longer and pain relief is less. A 2 to 4%
solution of lidocaine used for topical anesthesia on mucous
membranes produces effects in approximately 5 min and lasts
30 min. Topical anesthesia is safe, is simple to apply, and can be
repeated, although dogs and cats may resent the application of
cold solutions.

Local anesthetic sprays (10% lidocaine, 14 to 20% benzocaine) produce anesthesia of the mucosa up to a depth of 2 mm
within 1 to 2 min after application. Anesthesia lasts 15 to 20 min.
Topical sprays and ointments containing 14 to 20% benzocaine
reproducibly cause dose-dependent methemoglobinemia. Dogs
are usually asymptomatic when concentrations of methemoglo-
bin are < 20%; but they show fatigue, weakness, dyspnea, and
tachycardia at concentrations between 20 and 50%. Laryngeal
sprays containing benzocaine should be used with caution in
cats; and if signs of cyanosis and respiratory distress develop,
methemoglobinemia should be considered.

The cream used most often clinically contains a 5%
eutectic mixture of lidocaine and prilocaine (EMLA), which
overcomes the stratum corneum barrier in humans within 1 h
of topical application without adverse effects. The usefulness of
EMLA cream in dogs, which have a different type of skin than
humans, has not been reported.

## B.    Infiltration Anesthesia

Local infiltration of local anesthetics requires extravascular placement by direct injection, and infiltration may be the most reliable and safest of the local anesthetic techniques. Lidocaine (0.5 to 2.0%) is the local anesthetic most often used for infiltration. Local anesthesia can be produced by multiple intradermal or subcutaneous injections of 0.3 to 0.5 mL local anesthetic solution, using a 2.5-cm, 22- to 25-gauge needle, or by using a longer needle (3.75 to 5 cm) and slowly injecting local anesthetic while advancing the needle along the line of the proposed incision (linear infiltration). Pain is minimal if the needle is advanced slowly into the first desensitized wheal; successive injections are made at the periphery of the advancing wheal.

The amount of local anesthetic used for infiltration anesthesia depends on the size of the area to be anesthetized. From 2 to 5 mg/kg lidocaine or mepivacaine and 4 to 6 mg/kg procaine without epinephrine may be used for infiltration. Alternatively, 5 to 8 mg/kg local anesthetic with epinephrine (1:200,000) may be used for infiltration. The lowest possible concentration of local anesthetic that will produce the desired effect should be administered. For example, an average dog (20 kg) will tolerate approximately 50 mL of 0.5% lidocaine without demonstrating signs of toxicity, whereas only 20 to 30 mL of 1% lidocaine or 10 to 15 mL of 2% lidocaine can be injected. The local anesthetic may be diluted in 0.9% NaCl solution (not with sterile water) to a 0.25% solution, if a large volume of local anesthetic is needed for infiltration of a large operative area. The total dose of drug administered should be reduced by 30 to 40% in older dogs (> 8 years) and sick or cachectic dogs in poor condition. Local anesthetics containing epinephrine should not be injected into tissues supplied by end arteries (e.g., ears, tail) or in thin and dark-skinned dogs (e.g., poodle), because of the risk of severe vasoconstriction, local ischemia, and necrosis.

## C.    Field Block

Field block is a technique for anesthetizing large areas. First, intradermal or subcutaneous linear infiltration is produced around the lesion, as previously described (Fig. 5-5). Local anesthetic is then deposited in the deeper tissues by passing the

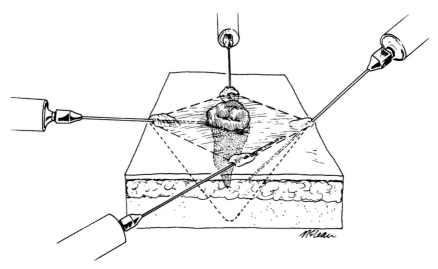

**Figure 5-5.** Field block: the production of walls of anesthesia enclosing the surgical field.

needle through the desensitized skin far enough to infiltrate the deep nerves supplying the area.

### D. Nerve Blocks

Injection of a local anesthetic solution into the connective tissue surrounding a particular nerve produces loss of sensation (sensory nerve block) and/or paralysis (motor nerve block) in the region supplied by the nerves (regional anesthesia). Smaller volumes (1 to 2 mL) of local anesthetic are needed to produce nerve block than are needed to produce field block, thus reducing the danger of toxicity.

### E. Regional Anesthesia of the Head

Administration of local anesthetic drugs around the **infraorbital, maxillary, ophthalmic, mental,** and **alveolar mandibular nerves** can provide extremely valuable and practical advantages over general anesthesia when combined with effective sedation (Fig. 5-6). Each nerve may be desensitized by injecting 1 to 2 mL of a 2% lidocaine hydrochloride solution using a 2.5- to 5-cm, 20- to 25-gauge needle.

The infraorbital nerve is desensitized at its point of emergence from the infraorbital canal. The needle is inserted either intraorally or extraorally, approximately 1 cm cranial to the bony lip of the infraorbital foramen. The needle is advanced to the infraorbital foramen, which can be found between the dorsal border of the zygomatic process and the gum of the upper canine tooth (Fig. 5-6A). Successful injections desensitize the upper lip and nose, the roof of nasal cavity, and the surrounding skin up to the infraorbital foramen.

The maxillary nerve must be desensitized to completely desensitize the maxilla, upper teeth, nose, and upper lip. The needle is placed percutaneously along the ventral border of the zygomatic process, approximately 0.5 cm caudal to the lateral canthus of the eye and is advanced into close proximity of the pterygopalatine fossa (Fig. 5-6B). Local anesthetic is administered at the point at which the maxillary nerve courses perpendicular to the palatine bone, between the maxillary foramen and foramen rotundum.

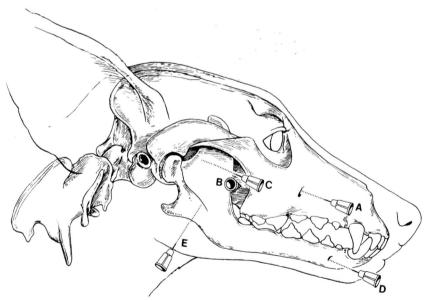

**Figure 5-6.** Needle placement for producing nerve blocks on the head: infraorbital (A); maxillary (B); zygomatic, lacrimal, and ophthalmic (C); alveolar mandibular (D); and mandibular (E) nerves.

1. *Eye and Orbit*

   Anesthesia of the eye and orbit is produced by desensitizing the ophthalmic division of the **trigeminal nerve.** A 2.5-cm, 22-gauge needle is inserted ventral to the zygomatic process at the level of the lateral canthus. The point of the needle should be approximately 0.5 cm cranial to the anterior border of the vertical portion of the ramus of the mandible. The needle is advanced medial to the ramus of the mandible in a mediodorsal and somewhat caudal direction, until it reaches the lacrimal, zygomatic, and ophthalmic nerves at the orbital fissure (Figs. 5-6C and 5-7). Deposition of 2 mL of local anesthetic at this site produces akinesia of the globe, because of the proximity of the abducens, oculomotor, and trochlear nerves to the ophthalmic nerve. Other methods for producing local anesthesia of the eye (retrobulbar anesthesia) run the risk of direct subarachnoid injection, intravascular injection, and systemic absorption.

   The risk of puncturing the globe is minimal if a 7.5-cm, 20-gauge needle is inserted at the lateral canthus through the anesthetized conjunctiva and is advanced past the globe toward the opposite mandibular joint, until the base of the orbit is encountered. The potential for puncturing ciliary and scleral blood vessels is minimal if a 5-cm curved needle (0.5 mm internal diameter), conformed to the roof of the orbit, is inserted through the anesthetized conjunctival sac at the vertical meridian (Fig. 5-8).

   Injection of local anesthetic into the optic sheath can cause respiratory arrest, attributable to the infiltration of local anesthetic into the subarachnoid space of the CNS. The pressure generated by injection into the optic nerve sheath or intrascleral injection is 3 or 4 times that produced by injection into the retrobulbar adipose tissue (135 versus 35 mm Hg). Loss of resistance encountered during retrobulbar block should serve as a warning, mandating redirection of the needle to prevent subarachnoid injection.

2. *Lower Lip*

   The lower lip can be desensitized by percutaneously inserting a 2.5-cm, 22- to 25-gauge needle rostral to the **mental foramen** at the level of the second premolar tooth. Be-

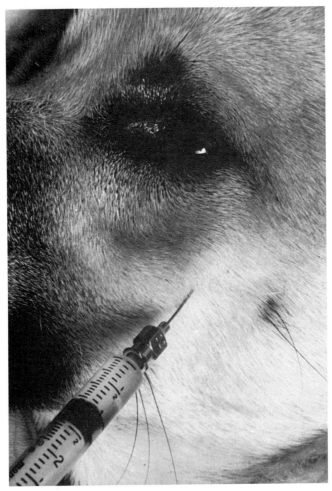

**Figure 5-7.** The site and direction of inserted needle for anesthesia of the ophthalmic nerves.

tween 1 and 2 mL of local anesthetic is deposited in close proximity to the alveolar mandibular nerve (Fig. 5-6D).

3. *Mandible and Lower Teeth*
   The mandible, including cheek, teeth, canine, incisors, skin, and mucosa of the chin and lower lip, can be desensitized by injecting 1 to 2 mL of local anesthetic in close proximity to the inferior alveolar branch of the

mandibular nerve as it enters the mandibular canal at the mandibular foramen (Fig. 5-6*E*). A 2.5-cm, 22-gauge needle is inserted at the lower angle of the jaw approximately 0.5 cm rostral to the angular process and is advanced 1 to 2 cm dorsally along the medial surface of the ramus of the mandible to the palpable lip of the mandibular foramen.

### F.    Anesthesia of the Limb

1.   *Ring Block*
     Local infiltration and field blocks around the distal extremity may be performed with a 2- to 5-cm, 22- to 23-gauge standard needle. Intradermal wheals around a superficial lesion and subcutaneous infiltration around the limb are performed using a short (< 3 cm), fine (23- to 25-gauge) needle.

2.   *Brachial Plexus Block*
     Brachial plexus block is suitable for operations on the front limb within or distal to the elbow. A 7.5-cm, 20- to

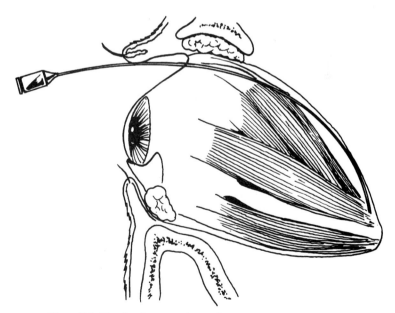

**Figure 5-8.** Needle placement for producing retrobulbar anesthesia.

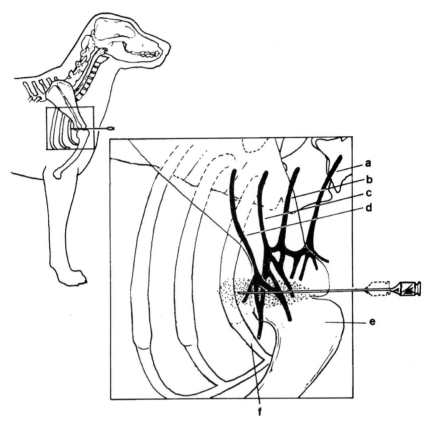

**Figure 5-9.** Needle placement for brachial plexus block of the ventral branches of the (A) sixth, (B) seventh, (C) eighth cervical, and (D) first thoracic spinal nerves; (E) tuberosity of the humerus; and (F) first rib.

22-gauge needle is inserted medial to the shoulder joint and directed parallel to the vertebral column toward the costochondral junction (Fig. 5-9). In larger dogs, 10 to 15 mL of 2% lidocaine HCl solution with 1:200,000 epinephrine is slowly injected as the needle is withdrawn, if no blood is aspirated into the syringe, thereby placing local anesthetic in close proximity to the **radial, median, ulnar, musculocutaneous,** and **axillary nerves.** Gradual loss of sensation and motor function occurs within 10 to 15 min. Anesthesia lasts for approximately 2 h, and total recovery requires about 6 h. Brachial plexus block is relatively simple and safe to perform and produces selective anesthesia and relaxation of the limb distal to the elbow joint (Fig. 5-10). The relatively long waiting period (15 to 30 min) required to attain maximal anesthesia and some occasional failures to obtain complete anesthesia, particularly in fat dogs, are disadvantages of the technique.

3. *Intravenous Regional Anesthesia*

IVRA is a rapid and reliable method for producing short-term (< 2 h) anesthesia of the extremities. The IVRA

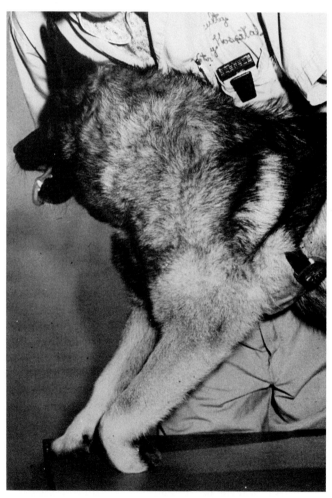

**Figure 5-10.** Anesthesia of the brachial plexus of the left thoracic limb in conscious dogs.

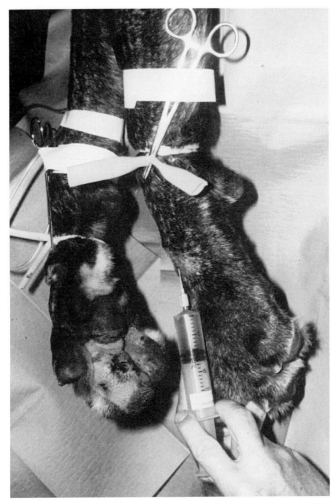

**Figure 5-11.** Injection of 12 mL of 1% lidocaine hydrochloride solution (1.5 mg/kg per leg) into the cephalic veins for regional anesthesia in a sedated, 80-kg bull mastiff in right lateral recumbency for skin biopsies at the palmar paws of both front legs. A rubber tourniquet is placed distal to the carpus (right foot) and proximal to the carpus (left foot). The tourniquets are secured with hemostatic forceps, which are taped to the skin.

technique is also known as **BIER block.** Little information on clinical experiences with IVRA in dogs exists, even though it appears to be a simple, safe, and practical method for providing 60 to 90 min of regional anesthesia in an extremity distal to a tourniquet (Fig. 5-11). The technique is best accomplished in dogs by placing an intravenous catheter in an appropriate and accessible vein (e.g., the cephalic or lateral saphenous vein) distal to the tourniquet. The limb is first desanguinated by wrapping it with an Esmarch bandage. A rubber tourniquet is placed around the limb proximal to the bandage. The tourniquet must be tight enough to overcome arterial blood pressure. Once the tourniquet is secured, the bandage is unwrapped, and 2.5 to 5 mg/kg lidocaine is injected intravenously with light pressure. It takes 5 to 10 min to achieve maximum anesthesia and the surgical procedure can be started. Complications resulting from blood flow deprivation to the limb or the dose of anesthetic used do not occur if the procedure is limited to 90 min.

Once the tourniquet is removed, sensation returns within 5 to 15 min, and residual analgesia remains for up to 30 min. Minimal effects on the heart rate, respiratory rate, and ECG are noted in dogs after removal of the tourniquet. Bupivacaine should not be used for this technique, because of cardiovascular collapse and death associated with its intravenous administration.

## G.   Lumbosacral Epidural Anesthesia

1.   Dogs are generally sedated or tranquilized to reduce fear and apprehension and then are placed either in sternal recumbency (for bilateral anesthesia) or in lateral recumbency (for ipsilateral anesthesia). The hind limbs can be extended cranially to maximally separate the lumbar vertebrae. The anesthetic procedure is not technically difficult when performed by an experienced clinician. Local anesthetic solution is injected through a disposable 2.5- to 7.5-cm, 20- to 22-gauge spinal needle as a single dose or is injected through a catheter that is inserted 1.5 to 2 cm beyond the end of an 18- or 17-gauge Huber-point (Tuohy) or 18-gauge Crawford needle (continuous technique) (Fig. 5-12). A 2.5-cm, 22-gauge spinal needle is used for small dogs; a 3.8-cm, 20-gauge needle for medium dogs; and a 7.5-cm 18-gauge needle for large dogs.

2.   **Important landmarks** for needle placement are easily identified in most dogs. The iliac prominences on either

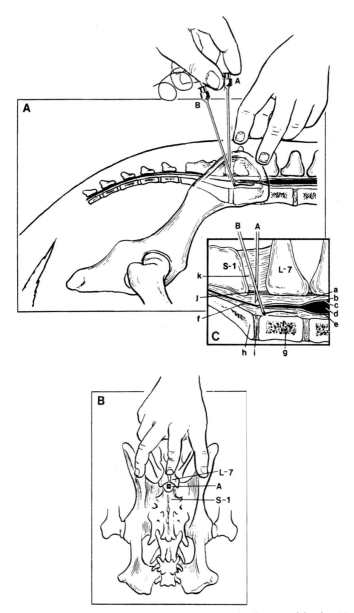

**Figure 5-12. A,** Needle placement into the lumbosacral epidural space of the dog (A) and catheter placement for continuous epidural anesthesia using a local anesthetic and/or analgesia using an opioid (B). **B,** Dorsal view of palpation of the dorsal spinous process of L7 and the dorsoiliac wings. **C,** a, Epidural space with fat and connective tissue; b, dura mater; c, arachnoid membrane; d, spinal cord; e, CSF; f, cauda equina; g, L7; h, S1; i, intervertebral disc; j, interarcuate ligament (ligamentum flavum); k, interspinous ligament.

side of the spine are palpated by using the thumb and middle finger of one hand (Fig. 5-12). The spinous process of the L7 vertebra is located with the index finger. The lumbosacral (L7–S1) interspace should be palpated from both the cranial and the caudal directions by moving the finger on the dorsal spinous processes of L6–7 and S2–1. This helps avoid inadvertent placement of the needle into the L6–7 interspace. The needle must be correctly placed on the midline and caudal to the L7 spinous process and is inserted until a distinct popping sensation is felt as the needle point penetrates the interarcuate ligament. Movement of the tail may indicate that the needle has engaged nerve tissue. The epidural space is best identified by the loss of resistance test, using either an air- or a saline-filled syringe.

3. **The needle or catheter** should be carefully inspected for flow of CSF or blood before the local anesthetic is administered. Presence of CSF indicates inadvertent subarachnoid puncture. Presence of blood indicates penetration of the ventral venous plexus. The possibility of obtaining CSF at the L7–S1 site is minimal, because the subarachnoid space of dogs usually ends cranial to the lumbosacral interspace. A subarachnoid injection may be made if CSF is encountered, with the precaution that only 50% of the intended epidural dose is needed: 1 mL local anesthetic/10 kg body weight injected over a 1-min period. The reduced dose should avoid total spinal anesthesia, with cardiovascular and respiratory depression or collapse. If blood is encountered, the needle is withdrawn and cleansed, and another attempt is made to place it into the epidural space. Intravascular injection of local anesthetic can result in systemic toxicity, which is characterized by convulsions, cardiopulmonary depression, and the absence of regional anesthesia. Inadvertent subarachnoid administration of small amounts (2 mL) of fresh autologous blood aspirated from the venous plexus during attempted lumbar epidural puncture will cause spasm of the pelvic limbs in dogs. The dogs, however, are able to stand unassisted within 20 min after blood injection and demonstrate no signs of meningeal irritation, long-term neurologic sequelae, or neuropathologic changes. It is necessary to administer the

calculated dose of local anesthetic at the body temperature of the dog and slow enough (over 45 to 60 s) to avoid causing pain.

4.  **Local anesthetic dosage** (concentration, volume) depends on the dog's size, the desired extent of anesthesia, and the desired onset and duration of anesthetic effect. A test dose of 0.5 to 1.0 mL of 2% lidocaine hydrochloride solution produces almost immediate dilation of the external anal sphincter, followed by relaxation of the tail and ataxia of pelvic limbs within 3 to 5 min. Approximately 1 mL of 2% lidocaine/4.5 kg body weight will completely anesthetize the pelvic limbs and posterior abdomen caudal to L1 within 10 to 15 min after administration. The flexor pinch reflex of pelvic limbs will be absent in 5 to 10 min after injection. Clinical experience indicates that the disappearance of the toe reflexes is associated with surgical anesthesia from midthorax to coccyx sufficient for abdominal surgery. The latent period is prolonged to 20 to 30 min if 0.75% bupivacaine hydrochloride is administered and is attributable to the drug's low solubility and slow uptake by nervous tissue. Good anesthesia for abdominal and orthopedic surgeries caudal to the diaphragm is generally achieved by administering 1 mL/5 kg (maximum 20 mL) 2% lidocaine or 0.5% bupivacaine, both with freshly added 1:200,000 epinephrine. A reduced volume of 2% lidocaine (1 mL/6 kg) is generally satisfactory for epidural anesthesia in dogs for cesarean section. The reason for the decrease (of approximately 25%) in dose requirement during pregnancy is unclear. It is rarely necessary to inject more than 3 mg/kg lidocaine for epidural anesthesia during cesarean section in dogs.

5.  **Adverse effects** associated with epidural and subarachnoid anesthesia in dogs include hypoventilation secondary to respiratory muscle paralysis, which is attributable to the spread of local anesthetic to the cervical spinal segments; hypotension, Horner's syndrome (Fig. 5-13) and hypoglycemia caused by sympathetic blockade; Shiff–Sherrington-like reflexes; and muscular twitches, coma, convulsion, and circulatory depression owing to

toxic plasma concentrations of local anesthetic. Delay in onset of anesthesia, unilateral hind limb paresis, partial anesthesia of tail or perineal region, and sepsis can result from improper injection technique. Complications can be prevented in most instances by following several basic rules, including careful selection of drugs and dosage,

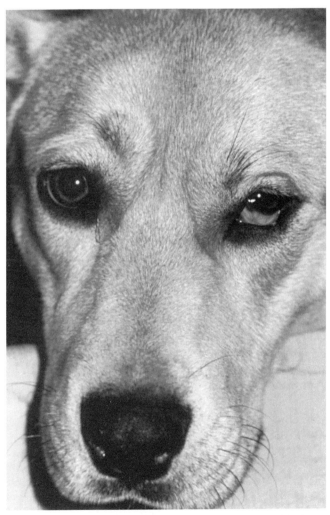

**Figure 5-13.** Unilateral Horner's syndrome (e.g., ptosis, miosis, and enophthalmos) in a 35-kg golden retriever with ipsilateral paresis of the left thoracic limb, after overdosage (12 mL) of the lumbosacral epidural anesthetic.

aspiration before injection (to ensure that the tip of the needle is not in a blood vessel or subarachnoid space), and injection of test doses.

6. **Contraindications** for epidural anesthetic techniques include infection at the lumbosacral puncture site, uncorrected hypovolemia, bleeding disorders, therapeutic or physiologic anticoagulation, degenerative central or peripheral axonal diseases, and anatomic abnormalities that would make epidural anesthesia difficult. Bacteremia, neurologic disorders, and mini-dose heparin therapy are relative contraindications. The benefits of epidural anesthesia often outweigh the risks.

## H.   Continuous Epidural Anesthesia

Despite numerous reports describing continuous epidural anesthesia in dogs, epidural catheters are not used routinely because of technical difficulties; the potential to produce damage of the spinal cord, meninges, and nerves; the risk of infection; and catheter-related problems. Nevertheless, insertion of plastic catheters into the epidural space of dogs is a relatively simple and safe procedure once practiced. **Local anesthetics and/or opioids** may be administered to produce continuous epidural anesthesia by placing a commercially available epidural catheter through an 18- or 17-gauge Huber-point (Tuohy) needle or 18-gauge Crawford needle into the epidural space (Fig. 5-12). Self-prepared sterile 20-gauge catheters (e.g., 160 polyethylene tubing) may also be used. The Tuohy needle is placed into the epidural space between the L7 and S1 intervertebral space, similar to the single-injection epidural block technique. Catheterization is facilitated by first desensitizing the lumbosacral space with a small amount (2 mL) of 2% lidocaine. The Tuohy needle is inserted at a 15°- to 45°-angle from the vertical position with the bevel directed cranially (Fig. 5-12). Catheters with a stylet are preferred. A slight resistance is usually encountered when the catheter passes through the tip of the Tuohy needle. Special markings on the catheter denote the distance the catheter has been advanced. The catheter is advanced at least two to three markings beyond the hub of the needle, which ensures that at least 2 to 3 cm of catheter has entered the epidural space. Flushing the needle with saline, rotating the needle, and advancing the catheter while slowly withdrawing the needle help the catheter thread into the epidural space. If these maneuvers fail, the needle and catheter should be withdrawn together. No attempt should be made to withdraw the catheter back through the needle, because this may sever the catheter. Most authorities believe that no attempt should be made to retrieve severed catheters. Wire-reinforced catheters can be inserted epidurally to the anterior lumbar (L4) or thoracic (T1) vertebrae with minimal resistance and without their coiling, turning on themselves, kinking, or knotting.

## I.    Intercostal Nerve Block

Intercostal nerve blocks may be used for relieving pain during and after thoracotomy, pleural drainage, and rib fractures. They are not recommended for dogs with pulmonary diseases, which impair blood gas exchange, or for dogs that cannot be observed for several hours after injection, because of the chance of clinically delayed pneumothorax. A minimum of two adjacent intercostal spaces both cranial and caudal to the incision or injury site are selectively blocked, because of the overlap of the nerve supply. The site for needle placement is the caudal border of the rib (R3–6) near the intervertebral foramen (Fig. 5-14). Between 0.25 and 1.0 mL of 0.25% or 0.5% bupivacaine hydrochloride/site, with or without epinephrine (1:200,000), is deposited. Small volumes and/or diluted local anesthetic solutions should be used as initial pain therapy so that the total dose does not exceed 3 mg/kg. Small dogs receive 0.25 mL/site; medium dogs 0.5 mL/site; and large dogs 1.0 mL/site. Postthoracotomy pain is generally controlled for 3 to 6 h after a successful block. Prolonged analgesia may be achieved by repeated administrations of local anesthetics, although the patient may not tolerate multiple percutaneous injections.

## J.    Interpleural Regional Analgesia

Pain from lateral and posterior thoracotomies, rib fractures; metastasis to the chest wall, pleura, and mediastinum; mastectomy; chronic pancreatitis; cholecystectomy; renal surgery; abdominal cancer; and posthepatic neuralgesia can be relieved by intermittent or continuous administration of local anesthetic into the pleural space through a catheter, without the systemic

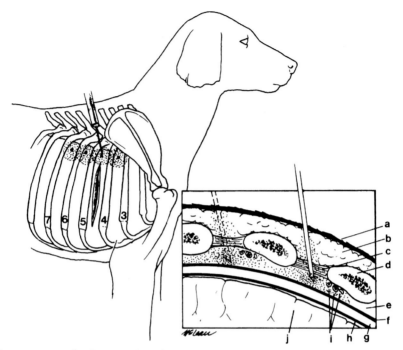

**Figure 5-14.** Needle placement for inducing intercostal nerve block. *a,* Skin; *b,* subcutaneous tissue; *c,* intercostal muscles; *d,* rib; *e,* subcostal space; *f,* pleura costalis and fascia; *g,* interpleural space; *h,* pleura pulmonalis; *i,* intercostal artery, vein, and nerve; *j,* lung.

effects commonly observed after the use of parenterally administered (intramuscularly or intravenously) opioids.

1. The technique requires the insertion of a catheter into the pleural space of a sedated or anesthetized dog. The catheter is placed into the pleural space either percutaneously or before closure of a thoracotomy (Fig. 5-15). The dog should be sedated; and the skin, subcutaneous tissues, periosteum, and parietal pleura over the caudal border of the rib should first be desensitized with 1 to 2 mL of 2% lidocaine solution, using a 2.5- to 5-cm, 20- to 22-gauge needle. A 5 × 1.4-mm (outer diameter), 17-gauge Huber-point (Tuohy) needle is then used for catheter placement. The stylet is removed, and the needle is filled with sterile saline until a meniscus is seen at the needle's hub. The needle is then advanced until a clicking sensation is perceived, as the needle tip perforates the parietal pleura,

or until the meniscus disappears when the needle tip enters the pleural space (hanging-drop technique).

2. Between 1 and 2 mg bupivacaine/kg (0.5%, with or without 5 mg epinephrine/mL) is injected over 1 to 2 min after there has been negative aspiration of air or blood through the catheter. The catheter is then cleared with 2 mL of physiologic saline solution. Bolus interpleural bupivacaine is effective in relieving post-thoracotomy pain for 3 to 12 h. The addition of epinephrine (5 mg/mL) to the local anesthetic solution may or may not increase the duration of analgesia and decrease the plasma concentration of the local anesthetic.

3. **Complications**, such as lung trauma, bleeding, and pneumothorax, are occasionally reported with the blind percutaneous insertion technique in humans. The balloon technique is superior to other methods (e.g., loss-of-

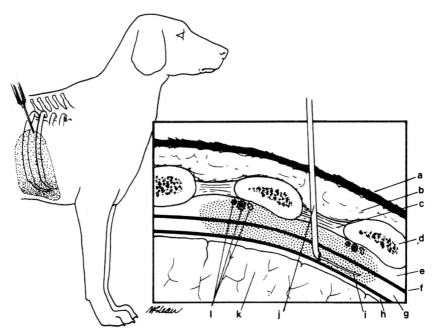

**Figure 5-15.** Interpleural catheter placement. *a*, Skin; *b*, subcutaneous tissue; *c*, intercostal muscles; *d*, rib; *e*, subcostal space; *f*, pleura costalis and fascia; *g*, interpleural space; *h*, pleura pulmonalis; *i*, catheter; *j*, Tuohy needle; *k*, lung; *l*, intercostal artery, vein, and nerve.

resistance technique, low-friction syringe-piston movement, infusion technique).

4. **Catheter placement** in the open chest is accomplished by inserting the Tuohy needle through the skin over the rib at a site that is at least two intercostal spaces caudal to the incision while taking care to retract the lung. The catheter is then passed through the needle and placed 3 to 5 cm subpleurally under direct vision. Local anesthetic is injected in the usual manner. The ventral tip of the catheter is best anchored using one encircling suture of surgical gut (3-0) in the intercostal space at the site of puncture.

5. **Positioning of the catheter** will affect the site of intercostal nerve blockade and is attributable to gravity-induced pooling of the local anesthetic within the interpleural space. Dogs that recover from lateral thoracotomy should be placed with the incision side down. Dogs that have had a sternotomy should be placed in sternal recumbency for approximately 10 min to allow the local anesthetic to pool near the incision and adjacent intercostal nerves. The external portion of the catheter should be anchored with tape, sutured to the skin, and covered with a nonocclusive-type dressing that allows air circulation.

6. The catheter is usually removed 24 h after thoracotomy, when postoperative pain has normally decreased. Long-term use (over several weeks) of an interpleural catheter is possible if the catheter is subcutaneously tunneled.

## K.   Epidural Opioid Analgesia

1. The **major advantages** of selective nociceptive blockade are long-term pain relief without producing muscle paralysis or weakness or significant hemodynamic effects. The physiochemical properties of opioids—particularly their lipid solubility, molecular weight, pKa, and receptor-binding affinity—are important in determining their pharmacokinetic and pharmacodynamic properties and

the onset and duration of analgesia. **Oxymorphone,** for example, is a relatively lipid-soluble opioid that binds relatively rapidly to opiate receptors in the spinal cord and has a small volume of distribution in the CSF (segmental analgesia). In contrast, the relatively hydrophilic **morphine** remains in the CSF for long periods, allowing rostral spread and analgesia distant from the site of injection (nonsegmental distribution of analgesia).

2.  The analgesic efficacy, duration of action, and adverse side effects of epidurally administered morphine are dose related. The most serious adverse effect is respiratory depression, which is biphasic. Respiratory depression is speculated to be caused by absorption of morphine into epidural veins and subsequent circulatory redistribution to the brain (early depression) as well as cephalad movement of morphine in CSF to the brainstem (late respiratory depression).

3.  The administration of $\alpha_2$-**adrenoceptor agonists** (xylazine, medetomidine) alone or in combination with morphine into the epidural space is a relatively new procedure. Morphine (0.11 mg/kg), alone or with medetomidine (5 µg/kg; diluted in sterile 0.9% NaCl solution to make the volume injected 1 mL/4.5 kg) can be epidurally administered at the lumbosacral intervertebral space.

4.  The **therapeutic benefits** achieved after the epidural administration of opioids include profound analgesia, modification of the endocrine-metabolic stress response, improvement in pulmonary function, decreased morbidity, and a comparatively short recovery. Contraindications to epidural opioid analgesia are primarily associated with the technique of epidural catheterization. Side effects are more common when intrathecal injection is performed as opposed to epidural injection, and they can be reversed by a low-dose intravenous infusion of the opioid antagonist naloxone, with minimal effect on the analgesia produced.

**L.   Ganglion Blocks**

Anesthesia of the cervicothoracic ganglion (CTG) and lumbar sympathetic chain in dogs to treat paralysis of the radial, facial, and trigeminal nerves and to treat muscle and joint diseases has been described. Between 5 and 8 mL of procaine HCl solution (0.5%) has been administered in close proximity to the CTG and lumbar sympathetic chain without ill effects.

# Chapter 6

---

## Equipment and Monitoring

---

### Introductory Comments

*An understanding of the anesthetic machine and various inhalation anesthetic delivery systems is essential for their safe use. Determining the proper oxygen flow rates with various delivery systems and appropriately scavenging waste gases are similarly important. Monitoring is an integral part of modern anesthesia. The early detection of anesthetic-induced physiologic derangements increases the safety of anesthesia and enhances the likelihood of an uneventful recovery to consciousness.*

**Equipment**
**Monitoring**

---

## I.   EQUIPMENT
*Sandee M. Hartsfield*

Potent halogenated hydrocarbon anesthetics are vaporized for administration, and should be delivered with accuracy. Nitrous oxide ($N_2O$), a gas, should be administered with adequate oxygen. Generally, machines and breathing systems are required for delivery of inhalant anesthetics. American Society for Testing and Materials (ASTM) standards exist for function and safety of anesthesia machines for human use, but veterinary machines are not required to fully comply.

### A.   Anesthesia Machines

Anesthesia machines are compatible with various breathing systems. They provide a precise, variable gas mixture (oxygen and anesthetic) to a breathing system, which directs those gases

**225**

to the patient, eliminates exhaled carbon dioxide ($CO_2$), and allows controlled ventilation. Sources for oxygen and $N_2O$, a regulator and flowmeter for each gas, and a vaporizer for each anesthetic are basic.

1. **Pressures of gases** vary throughout a machine. The high-pressure area (up to 2200 psi) accepts gases at cylinder pressure and reduces and regulates the pressure (gas cylinders, hanger yokes, yoke blocks, high-pressure hoses, pressure gauges, regulators). The intermediate-pressure area (typically 37 to 50 psi) accepts gases from central pipelines or the machine's regulators and conducts them to the flush valve and flowmeters (pipeline inlets, power outlets for ventilators, conduits from pipeline inlets to flowmeters, conduits from regulators to flowmeters, flow-meter assembly, oxygen flush apparatus). The low-pressure area (variable pressure, ~ 0 to 30 cm $H_2O$) consists of the conduits and components between the flowmeter and the common gas outlet, vaporizer outside the circle system (VOC), piping from the flowmeters to the vaporizer, conduit from the vaporizer to the common gas outlet, conduit from the common gas outlet to the breathing system).

B. **Medical Gases**

Pipeline sources of $N_2O$ and oxygen originate at banks of large (G or H) cylinders; or oxygen may arise from a liquid oxygen source or an oxygen-concentrating system. The latter may not reliably deliver 100% oxygen. Pipeline systems convey gases to station outlets. A noninterchangeable gas-specific connector—threaded diameter index safety system (DISS) or proprietary nonthreaded, noninterchangeable quick connectors—at the station outlet accepts only its corresponding connector, which attaches to the pipeline inlet (a DISS male connector) of the machine through a flexible high-pressure hose.

1. **Gases** move from a cylinder through a brass valve. The valve stem controls flow; a safety relief device (a plug with a low melting point) allows gas to escape to prevent bursting of a cylinder at high temperatures. Threaded outlets of

valve bodies on large cylinders prevent the interchange of oxygen and $N_2O$ at regulators or manifolds. Valve bodies of E cylinders attach directly to hanger yokes (pin index safety system) to prevent interchange of gases. Two pin holes and a port in the valve body correspond to two pins and a nipple on the hanger yoke. Specific spacing of the pins for each gas precludes interchange of gases.

2. The **pin index system** can be defeated. Pins can be removed, broken, bent, or forced into the yoke. The nipple can be stacked with washers, allowing the wrong cylinder to be attached. Yoke blocks coupled to high-pressure hoses will accommodate alternate gas sources. Old yoke blocks may not have pin holes; short blocks can be attached upside down. Older machines should be inspected to ensure the integrity of the pin index system. Small cylinders should be aligned correctly in the hanger yokes to prevent a hazard. Directing the retaining screw into the safety relief device instead of the conical depression may cause rapid cylinder decompression. Each yoke on a machine should be fitted with a cylinder or a yoke plug.

3. An **oxygen cylinder's pressure** is ~ 2200 psi. E cylinders contain about 700 L gaseous oxygen; an H cylinder, about 7000 L. Pressure is proportional to content: An E cylinder at 1100 psi contains ~ 350 L oxygen. Pressure in a full $N_2O$ cylinder is ~ 750 psi at room temperature (liquid and gaseous $N_2O$). Vapor pressure of $N_2O$ varies with temperature and determines the pressure. In a full cylinder, 95% of the volume is liquid; an E cylinder contains ~ 1600 L gaseous $N_2O$; an H cylinder, ~ 16,000 L. As $N_2O$ vaporizes, the cylinder cools, and frosting may occur. The content of a $N_2O$ cylinder is not directly proportional to pressure. As pressure starts to decrease after all the liquid $N_2O$ has vaporized, ~ 25% of the content remains; gas is then depleted based on the rate of flow. A cylinder's true content can be determined by weight. In the United States, the U.S. Department of Transportation (DOT) controls the construction and testing of cylinders. Service pressure (maximum filling pressure at 23°C [70°F]) is typically 1900 to 2200 psi for oxygen. Cylinders are

designated alphabetically (A is smallest); sizes E, G, and H are common.

4.  A **color-coded label** indicates the cylinder's contents (green: oxygen; blue: $N_2O$), warns of hazards (e.g., oxidizing agent), and lists manufacturers or distributors. Signal words are used: **danger,** immediate threat to health or property if gas is released; **warning,** less than immediate threat; and **caution,** immediate hazard to health or property. A diamond-shaped area indicates the hazard class of the gas by words (oxidizer, nonflammable, flammable) and color code (yellow, green, red, respectively). A color-coded tag on the valve body may identify a cylinder's contents. Tags have perforated tabs (full, in use, empty) to track the cylinder's use.

5.  **Cylinders** should not be stored near flammable materials and should be properly secured. It is best to store them in cool, dry, clean, well-ventilated rooms made of fire-resistant materials. Before use, the contents should be identified. Valve ports (pointed away from users) should be opened briefly to clear debris and closed before connecting them to hanger yokes, regulators, or manifolds. Sealing washers should be placed between small cylinder valves and hanger yokes. A valve should be opened slowly to pressurize the regulator and then fully opened. Defective cylinders should not be used.

## C.   Pressure Gauges

Each compressed gas on a machine should have a **pressure gauge** (on regulators for large cylinders and manifolds for banks of cylinders). Gauges indicate the pressure on the cylinder side of the regulator. Usually color-coded, gauges are identified by the gas's chemical symbol or name. The scale indicates units of measure (kilo-Pascals and pounds per square inch); Bourdon tube-type gauges are typical. Early standards required the gauge's full-scale reading to be one-third greater than the maximum pressure and the gauges on one machine to displace a similar arc from lowest to highest readings. Pressure gauges may be used in pipeline systems and on machines to report pipeline pressure.

## D.  Regulators

**Regulators** produce a safe operating pressure, prevent flowmeter fluctuations as cylinders empty, and decrease the sensitivity of the flowmeter's indicator to movements of the control knob. The ASTM standard requires that regulators on machines be set to use pipeline gases preferentially. Regulators may be set at 45 psi (with a power outlet for a ventilator) or at 37 to 42 psi (without a power outlet), because pipeline pressure is usually 50 psi. Older machines may have regulators set at 50 psi; and open E cylinders may flow instead of pipeline gases if no check valve is present, possibly depleting cylinders that should be saved for emergencies. Contemporary machines for humans have additional (second-stage) regulators that deliver gases to the flowmeter at very low pressures (e.g., 12 to 16 psi) to increase the constancy of the flowmeter.

## E.  Flowmeters

Flowmeters are downstream from their regulators. They measure the rate of gas flow and allow precise control of oxygen or $N_2O$ delivery to out-of-system vaporizers and common gas outlets. Gas moves through the flow-control valve to the bottom of a glass tube. Gas flows around a moveable indicator, between it and the tube wall, exiting at the top of the tube. The tube is larger at the top; more gas flows as the indicator rises. The scale shows rate of flow (in milliliters or liters per minute). Some flowmeters have double tapers: a slight taper below for accuracy (in milliliters per minute) and a greater taper above for higher flows. A scale should be on or to the right of the tube (front view), but may be on the left in older machines; operators should know flowmeters' locations.

1.   Flowmeters are **calibrated** at 760 mm Hg and 20°C (68°F); accuracy varies under other conditions. Temperature effects are minimal; a higher flow than indicated may occur at lower barometric pressure (altitude), and a lower flow may occur at a higher pressure (hyperbaric chamber). Because the flowmeter (tube, indicator, scale) is calibrated, parts should not be interchanged. The glass tube, indicator, and scale should be replaced as a unit. The lowest mark on the scale is the first accurate setting; extrapolation is unreliable. The indicator should be read

at the top, except for a ball-type float, which is read at the center. Recent standards require a point of reference on the flowmeter assembly. Flowmeters should be used as originally designed (e.g., vertical).

2.    The **flow-control knob** for oxygen should be as large or larger than the other flow control knobs, have a fluted profile, and project past the controls for other gases so the clinician can feel the gas being set (touch coded). Control knobs are labeled with the gas symbol and are color coded. Good controls have fine threads for accuracy and stops to prevent overtightening and damage to the valves.

3.    The **sizes of indicators** and scales affect accuracy. Floats may be long (> 1 cm); reading the wrong location may affect the flow rate. Incorrect flows to flowmeter-controlled vaporizers can greatly alter the anesthetic concentration. Dirt, static electricity, and damaged floats may cause inaccurate readings. Indicators should move freely; sticking floats should be cleaned or replaced. A sticking float that indicates oxygen flow from an empty cylinder could cause hypoxia.

4.    **Flowmeters should be off** when not in use to prevent sudden pressure on the glass tube and indicator when a cylinder valve is opened. Such pressure may force the indicator upward, damaging it or the stop. Clinicians may not notice that the indicator has jammed at the top. The standard for modern machines requires one flow control for each gas. Two flowmeters for one gas should be in series and controlled with one control knob.

5.    **Flowmeter sequence** is important with multiple gases; oxygen should be downstream. If oxygen enters a manifold upstream, hypoxic mixtures are possible. Canadian and U.S. standards locate the oxygen flowmeter to the right in a cluster. If a flowmeter for a vaporizer is required, it should be to the right of the cluster (10 cm from the oxygen flowmeter). Other arrangements may exist in older machines (oxygen flowmeter located left, right, or center in a cluster); the danger of delivering hypoxic mixtures owing to maladjustment of controls is a consideration

when using both $N_2O$ and oxygen. Flowmeters should be adjusted to meet the patient's oxygen consumption (fraction of inspired oxygen, $FIO_2$, > 0.3) and an adequate concentration of each gas should be provided. Accuracy is especially important when using $N_2O$ and with low-flow systems. Accuracy significantly decreases when flows are < 1 L/min, and it is important to check the $FIO_2$; monitoring oxygen on the inspiratory limb of the breathing system is appropriate. ASTM standards require oxygen analyzers.

## F.  Safety Devices

Machines may be designed to alert the operator to a dangerously low oxygen pressure or flow. When oxygen pressure falls, an alarm may be triggered or the supply of other gases ($N_2O$) may be cut off to prevent hypoxic mixtures. Proportioning devices ensure oxygen flow at a preset minimum portion of the total gas flow. Dupaco machines with oxygen and $N_2O$ had an audible alarm for low oxygen pressure; the Metomatic veterinary machine reduced the flow of other gases if oxygen flow was reduced. Safety mechanisms may malfunction; monitoring the inspired oxygen level is the most reliable safety measure.

## G.  Flush Valves

Oxygen is supplied to the flush valve at ~ 50 psi. It delivers a high flow (35 to 75 L/min) of oxygen to the common gas outlet, or breathing system. Presently, oxygen from the flush valve is not routed through the vaporizer; older machines directed oxygen through the vaporizer with the potential for increased output. At 50 L/min, oxygen can quickly fill a breathing system. Pediatric systems (Bain) should not be filled via the flush valve because of the danger of overpressurization. Current standards require that the valve's actuating device be recessed to prevent inadvertent activation. Problems with flush valves include leaks in the assembly and sticking in the on position.

## H.  Vaporizers

**Concentration-calibrated, variable-bypass vaporizers** (temperature, flow, and back-pressure compensated) are standard in human anesthesia, and recommended for veterinary anesthesia. But a nonprecision, uncompensated vaporizer (Stephens) is marketed as a part of a veterinary machine, and an obsolete vaporizer (Ohio #8 glass bottle without a wick) has been described for delivery of halothane and isoflurane to veterinary patients. Delivery of highly volatile, potent inhalants with nonprecision vaporizers can be risky without instrumental monitoring (e.g., inspired or expired anesthetic concentration).

1. **Carrier gas** (oxygen or oxygen plus $N_2O$) passes through the vaporizer to acquire vapor. Because the saturated vapor pressures of most inhalants are much greater than the partial pressures required for clinical anesthesia—greater than the minimum alveolar concentration (MAC)—the vaporizer should deliver a concentration near that set on the control dial. Otherwise, the concentration of anesthetic should be monitored. Precision vaporizers dilute the high concentration of anesthetic vapor from the vaporization chamber to a clinically usable, relatively safe concentration.

2. The **physics of the vaporizer design** and its structure and function are important. Heat is required for vaporization of liquids; the **latent heat of vaporization** (number of calories required to change 1 g of liquid into vapor) causes the anesthetic to cool during vaporization. The **vapor pressure** is the partial pressure of the anesthetic gas above the liquid at equilibrium; it varies directly with temperature, and cooling limits the vaporizer's output. Substances (e.g., copper) of high **specific heat** (amount of heat required to raise the temperature of 1 g of the substance 1°C) supply heat to the liquid and retard cooling. Materials (e.g., copper) of high **thermal conductivity** (the rate of heat flow through the material) promote the flow of heat inward, from the warmer ambient air, to impede cooling. Certain materials (e.g., **copper, bronze**) have favorable values for specific heat and thermal conductivity. Stainless steel has recently been used. The output of concentration-calibrated vaporizers is expressed as the volume percent of vapor in the gases exiting the vaporizer and is affected by changes in barometric pressure.

3.   Vaporizers have several **compensatory mechanisms** for changes in flow, temperature, and pressure.

a.   Compensatory mechanisms for **temperature variations** in liquid anesthetic include the following. Materials that supply and conduct heat efficiently to the liquid promote a relatively constant temperature; a heat sink promotes thermostability. Automatic changes in flow through the vaporization chamber compensate for temperature variations in Tec (bimetallic strip valves), Ohio calibrated (gas-filled bellows), and Vapor vaporizers (expansion member, silicone cone). Manual adjustments of carrier gas flow are required to compensate for temperature variations in measured-flow vaporizers and older Vapor vaporizers. Some vaporizers are heated (supplied heat; Verni-Trols; Ohio DM 5000). The Tec 6 (desflurane) is electrically heated and thermostatically controlled to 39°C (102°F).

b.   **Differences in carrier gas flow rates** alter the output of uncompensated vaporizers. Modern flow-compensated vaporizers produce relatively accurate anesthetic concentrations over the 250 mL/min to 15 L/min range. The splitting ratio (the ratio of bypass gas flow to the gas passing through the vaporization chamber) sets the output of the vapor, and the resistance to flow through each of the two channels in the vaporizer allows the splitting ratio to be maintained at various rates of flow. At < 250 mL/min and > 15 L/min, output from most vaporizers is variable; performance data outside that range may not exist. Output from older vaporizers (Fluotec 2) may vary significantly from that indicated on the control dial at flows < 4 L/min. Measured-flow vaporizers (Copper Kettle) require adjustments in the flow of oxygen to the vaporization chamber when the total flow of gas is changed.

c.   **Composition of the carrier gas** may alter vaporizer output. Output of anesthetic with oxygen as the carrier may differ from the output with oxygen plus $N_2O$ as the carrier. The magnitude of effect varies, depending on the vaporizer. Newer vaporizers initially deliver inhalant concentrations that are less than that indicated by the control dial setting. With the Tec 3 vaporizer, $N_2O$ has little effect; with the Tec 2 vaporizer, $N_2O$ increases the output of halothane.

d.   **Back-pressure compensation** is needed with use of the flush valve and application of positive pressure ventilation; both may increase the vaporizer output. Newer vaporizers prevent or minimize this pumping effect with small vaporization chambers (Tecs), long spiral tubes at the inlet to the vaporization chamber (Vapor), pressure check valves just downstream from the vaporizer, and/or relief valves at the vaporizer outlet.

4.   **Variations in barometric pressure** ($P_{bar}$)—altitude or hyperbaric chambers—alter vaporizer output (volume percent). A partial pressure of anesthetic (1 MAC) represents the same potency (partial pressure) at any $P_{bar}$. Anesthetic concentration is usually expressed as volume percent, and MAC expressed as volume percent increases as $P_{bar}$ decreases. A change in the $P_{bar}$ alters the viscosity and density of gases flowing through the vaporizers and flowmeters and affects output.

a.   Most **concentration-calibrated vaporizers** (Tec 3) are considered self-compensating and deliver about the same partial pressure, but an increasing volume percent of anesthetic with decreasing $P_{bar}$. So the vaporizer can normally be set in volume percent, despite the inherent inaccuracy of the setting. In theory, a halothane vaporizer at an ambient pressure of 500 mm Hg should deliver twice the concentration on the control dial in volume percent and approximately 1.3 times the dialed concentration in terms of MAC or potency. Because small changes occur in the concentration output owing to variations in the resistance of flow through the vaporizer at differing ambient pressures, the best approach is to measure the partial pressure of anesthetic in inspired or expired gases when working at atypical barometric pressures.

b. For **measured-flow vaporizers,** changes in $P_{bar}$ affect both partial pressure and volume percent of delivered anesthetic. If the $P_{bar}$ is low, output measured in volume percent and as partial pressure increases. When the $P_{bar}$ is high, measured-flow vaporizers deliver a lower anesthetic concentration, expressed as volume percent or partial pressure. Temperature, $P_{bar}$, and vapor pressure affect the final anesthetic concentration; and the greatest effects are on anesthetics with low boiling points and with vapor pressures that are near $P_{bar}$.

c. **Flowmeter function** is affected by $P_{bar}$. Actual flow increases, becoming higher than the flowmeter shows, as $P_{bar}$ decreases. In contrast, the flowmeter will deliver less flow than indicated when the ambient pressure is higher than the calibration $P_{bar}$.

5. There are several **potential problems with vaporizers.** The arrangement of vaporizers on machines and their maintenance affect safety. Filling errors, improper transport, using vaporizers in series, and improperly connecting a vaporizer to a machine may alter output.

a. For **multiple inhalants,** a vaporizer can be filled with the wrong drug, especially with screw-cap filler ports. Keyed filler systems help prevent such accidents, but are inconvenient; screw-cap filler ports with bottle adapters decrease spillage. If an agent-specific vaporizer for a drug with a low vapor pressure (e.g., methoxyflurane) is filled with a potent, highly volatile anesthetic (e.g., halothane), high concentrations may be produced. For Ohio calibrated vaporizers, service is required to replace the paper wicks. For a Tec vaporizer, an option is to drain the vaporizer, flush it with oxygen (5 L/min for 45 min or until no trace of contaminant is present), allow it to stabilize thermally for about 2 h, and refill it with the correct agent. Vaporizers contaminated with a nonvolatile contaminant (e.g., water or thymol) should be drained and serviced.

b. **Filler ports** and sight glasses help limit filling of modern vaporizers, primarily to prevent liquid anesthetic from entering the vaporizer's fresh gas. Recent designs prevent liquid from entering the fresh gas line, even during tipping or inversion. Tipping of certain vaporizers, however, may introduce liquid anesthetic into the bypass channel; a high concentration of anesthetic vapor may be delivered, potentially enough to induce cardiac arrest. Also, moving a vaporizer on a mobile anesthesia machine may alter its output, if the machine is tipped or liquid anesthetic is sloshed. Generally, vaporizers should be emptied before transport.

c.  Single anesthesia machines may be fitted with **multiple vaporizers.** Modern machines for humans are equipped with interlocking mechanisms that prevent two vaporizers being on simultaneously. In-line, non-interlocked vaporizers offer the possibility of operating two vaporizers concurrently, perhaps producing excessive depth of anesthesia. Simultaneous use of multiple vaporizers in series increases the probability of contamination of a vaporizer with an inappropriate agent. The best order for vaporizers in series is methoxyflurane, enflurane, isoflurane, and halothane (upstream to downstream).

d.  **Freestanding vaporizers** are common for pump oxygenators during cardiopulmonary bypass. A freestanding vaporizer is easily tipped. Inadvertently reversing the flow through the vaporizer is possible when connections are changed periodically; forcing oxygen through the vaporizer with the flush valve may occur if it is located downstream from the flush valve. These situations lead to a significant increase in the output concentration.

e.  If concentration-calibrated vaporizers are **connected in reverse,** vaporizer output can potentially be twice that indicated on the control dial.

6.  **Vaporizer classification** is based on six factors (classification systems using only one feature are incomplete, because of the variations among vaporizers).

a.  **Regulation of output** is measured in volume percent. For **variable-bypass** vaporizers, all fresh gas enters the vaporizer; part is directed through and part bypasses the vaporization chamber. The gases rejoin before exiting the vaporizer, to give the concentration set by the control dial. The dial is turned on in a counterclockwise fashion. Concentration-calibrated variable-bypass vaporizers are quite accurate (Tec); uncalibrated variable-bypass units (Ohio #8) are inaccurate. Measured-flow vaporizers are not concentration calibrated; they route oxygen through the vaporizer to be saturated with anesthetic. A second source of oxygen and/or $N_2O$ bypasses the vaporizer, diluting the saturated gas to the desired concentration. Calculations determine the concentration going to the common gas outlet.

b. There are several **methods of vaporization.** A **flow-over** vaporizer directs carrier gas over the surface of the liquid anesthetic; the surface area increases with the use of wicks (which improve efficiency). The **bubble-through** method delivers carrier gas below the surface of the liquid via a diffuser (a sintered bronze disc in a Copper Kettle), which disperses gas bubbles to increase the liquid–gas interface. Efficiency increases when smaller bubbles, deeper dispersion, and slower carrier gas flow are used. **Injection** vaporizers deliver a known amount of liquid anesthetic or vapor into a known volume of gas to produce an accurate concentration.

c. **Vaporizer location** in relation to the breathing system may be outside the circle system (VOC; high resistance) or within the circle system (VIC; low resistance because the patient must inspire through the vaporizer) (Figs. 6-1 and 6-2). Traditionally, highly potent, highly volatile anesthetics have been administered with VOCs, but use of VICs for isoflurane and halothane in veterinary patients has been reported.

d. **Temperature compensation** is important because heat is required to vaporize liquids. To compensate for cooling, which slows vaporization, heat must be supplied or the carrier gas flow must change to account for the changing rate of vaporization. Heat may be supplied from the vaporizer itself (thermostable material; high specific heat and thermal conduc-

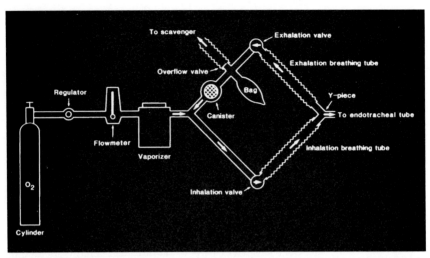

**Figure 6-1.** A VOC system and its relationship to the other basic components of the anesthesia machine and circle system. Reprinted with permission from Hartsfield SM. Machines and breathing systems for administration of inhalation anesthetics. In: Short CE, ed., Principles and practice of veterinary anesthesia. Baltimore: Williams & Wilkins, 1987.

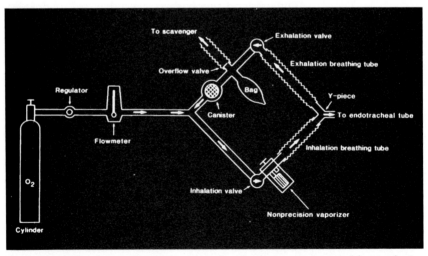

**Figure 6-2.** A VIC system and its relationship to the other basic components of the anesthesia machine and circle system. Reprinted with permission from Hartsfield SM. Machines and breathing systems for administration of inhalation anesthetics. In: Short CE, ed., Principles and practice of veterinary anesthesia. Baltimore: Williams & Wilkins, 1987.

tivity). Heat was supplied by electric heaters and warm-water jackets on older vaporizers; an electric device heats the Tec 6 (desflurane). In other vaporizers, thermostatic mechanisms (e.g., bimetallic strip valve) vary the flow of carrier gas through the vaporization chamber to counterbalance changes in temperature and vaporization. Manual adjustments of flow through the chamber offset variations in temperature for measured-flow vaporizers.

e.   Vaporizers can be **agent specific** (designed for only one inhalant) or multipurpose (designed for any volatile agent). When using a multipurpose vaporizer, label the machine for the agent in use. Be sure to clear the multipurpose vaporizer of the old anesthetic before another is introduced. Draining alone may not eliminate the original anesthetic; servicing may be required. The trend is toward agent-specific, concentration-calibrated vaporizers.

f.   Vaporizers have been classified according to **resistance** to flow. Plenum-type vaporizers are high resistance and designed for a VOC location; high resistance is characteristic of concentration-calibrated, variable bypass vaporizers. Low-resistance vaporizers (Ohio #8; Stephens) are designed for a VIC location.

7.   Ohio #8 glass bottles in the **VIC location** were the basic vaporizers for methoxyflurane on veterinary machines in the 1970s. More recently, the Stephens vaporizer has been advocated for veterinary patients. For safety, VIC machines are best for less-potent (ether, historically) or less-volatile (e.g., methoxyflurane) drugs. For VIC units, inspired anesthetic concentration varies with respiratory minute volume, use of positive pressure ventilation, changes in carrier gas flow rate, and variations in temperature. At a given setting, increased ventilation (spontaneous or positive pressure) and lower fresh gas flows increase the inspired anesthetic concentration. The delivered concentration from an Ohio #8 is unknown and changes unpredictably. Without instrumental monitoring, the anesthetist depends on the patient's responses to determine vaporizer settings, a practice known as qualitative anesthesia in contrast to

quantitative anesthesia (when the concentration of inhalant is known).

a. **The Ohio #8 glass bottle vaporizer** is a variable-bypass, flow-over with a wick, non-temperature-compensated, VIC, low-resistance, and multipurpose vaporizer. The vaporization chamber is glass; a cloth wick increases the surface area. It is not calibrated and is nonprecision; there is no method for temperature control. It is usually on the inspiratory side of the circle. If it is placed on the expiratory limb, the chamber may trap water condensed from the expired gases. Controls adjust from 0 to 10 (0 = no inspiratory flow through the vaporization chamber; 10 = total flow through the chamber). Diversion of gas flow through the chamber makes highly volatile anesthetics dangerous, especially when used with a wick. The delivered concentration is not predictable. In veterinary medicine, the Ohio #8 vaporizer is used for methoxyflurane. It is dangerous to use this machine with a wick for halothane or isoflurane because of the potential for high inspired concentrations. Without a wick, the Ohio #8 vaporizer can be used for isoflurane or halothane only if the clinician is familiar with the guidelines for its use and understands its limitations. The Ohio #8 vaporizer may leak anesthetic into the breathing system when the control is set to off. Eventually, the valves may not seat properly, allowing continuous flow of fresh gases through the vaporization chamber, yielding anesthetic-rich gases.

b. The **Stephens vaporizer** is a variable-bypass, flow-over, non-temperature-compensated, VIC, low-resistance, and multipurpose vaporizer; it is nonprecision. It is usually located on the inspiratory side of a circle system. The vaporization chamber is glass, and a wick is provided for methoxyflurane. The wick should not be used for halothane or isoflurane. It is not calibrated and has no method for controlling the liquid temperature. The control is adjustable from off (no flow though the vaporization chamber) to full-on (complete flow through the chamber) in increments of eighths. The vaporizer is intended for use in a low-flow or closed-circle system.

8. Modern concentration-calibrated vaporizers located outside the circle are precision vaporizers; any volatile anesthetic can be administered safely with a concentration-calibrated, agent-specific **VOC unit.** Older models remain serviceable and may be purchased used. Newer vaporizers are temperature, flow, and back-pressure compensated. The performance of older vaporizers varies with flow, temperature, and back pressure.

   a. **Tec vaporizers** for halothane (Fluotec 3) and isoflurane (Isotec 3) are reliable, and are temperature, flow, and back-pressure compensated under normal conditions. The Tec 3s predecessor, the Fluotec Mark 2, may be available as used equipment; some remain in use. Tec 4, 5, and 6 vaporizers have superseded Tec 3 vaporizers. The **Fluotec Mark 2** vaporizer is a variable bypass, flow-over with wick, VOC, temperature-compensated, high-resistance, and agent-specific machine. Temperature compensation is controlled with a bimetallic strip valve at the outlet from the vaporization chamber. Performance data show that the Mark 2 is imprecise at flow rates < 4 L/min; inaccuracy increases < 2 L/min. **Tec Mark 3** vaporizers (Fluotec Mark 3, Pentec Mark 2, Isotec 3) are variable-bypass, flow-over, temperature-compensated, agent-specific, VOC, and high-resistance machines. Temperature compensation is controlled with a bimetallic, temperature-sensitive element related to the vaporization chamber. Output is almost linear in the range of concentrations and flows typical for veterinary patients (0.25 to 6 L/min). Back-pressure compensation is accomplished in the internal design: a long tube to the vaporization chamber, an expansion area in the tube, and absence of wicks near the inlet of the vaporization chamber.

   **Tec 4 and 5** vaporizers are variable bypass, flow-over with wick, temperature-compensated, agent-specific, VOC, and concentration-calibrated vaporizers. Individual units are made for halothane, enflurane, isoflurane, and sevoflurane. Within limits, they compensate for changes in back pressure, temperature, and carrier gas flow. The Tec 4 can be tipped without changing output; the Tec 5 can be inverted without leakage of liquid into the outlet. Both the Tec 4 and the Tec 5 vaporizers were designed to be used on a manifold with two or more vaporizers in series; an interlocking design prevents the simultaneous use of two or more vaporizers. Typically, Tec 4 or 5 vaporizers on veterinary anesthesia machines are not set up on a manifold with an interlocking system. The Tec 5 offers a larger liquid capacity (300 mL) than the Tec 3 and Tec 4 (125 mL) vaporizers. **Tec 6** vaporizers are injection, temperature-compensated (supplied heat), agent-specific, VOC, concentrated-calibrated vaporizers. The Tec 6 is specifically designed for desflurane and is electrically heated and pressurized. Desflurane has a high vapor pressure (664 mm Hg at 20°C; 68°F); it boils at 23.5°C (74.3°F) near room temperature. The unit has a higher range of control settings to meet the requirements of an agent with a relatively high MAC value (about 7%). Vapor originates in a heated sump (39°C; 102°F) at a pressure of 1500 mm Hg.

b.  **Vapor 19.1 vaporizers** are classified as variable-bypass, flow-over with wick, temperature-compensated, high-resistance, agent-specific, and VOC machines. Specific units are available for isoflurane, halothane, and enflurane. Temperature compensation is automatic, with an expansion member that varies the flow of gas through the vaporization chamber in response to changes in temperature. Pressure compensation is by a long spiral inlet tube to the vaporization chamber. It is accurate at a gas flow of 0.3 to 15 L/min at the lower settings on the control, but complete saturation may not occur at higher settings with higher flows. The vaporizer is designed for operation in the range of 10 to 40°C (40 to 104°F). The **Vapor vaporizer** preceded the Vapor 19 series and has been called semiautomatic, because manual adjustments are required for complete temperature compensation. It is no longer manufactured, but some may be used in veterinary practices. It was made for methoxyflurane and halothane. It is a variable-bypass, flow-over with wick, VOC, high-resistance, agent-specific, temperature-compensated (by manual flow alteration) machine and is considered to be accurate.

c. **Ohio calibrated vaporizers** are variable-bypass, flow-over with wick, automatically temperature-compensated, agent-specific, VOC, and high-resistance vaporizers. The units were made for isoflurane, halothane, and enflurane and were designed for accuracy at variable flows (0.3 to 10 L/min) and temperatures (16° to 32°C; 61° to 90°F). Tilting the machine to 20° while it is in use or up to 45° when it is not in use does not cause problems. Greater tipping may cause high concentrations. The vaporizer has plastic spacers between paper wicks that may react with enflurane or isoflurane (discoloration of liquid), apparently without consequences.

d. **Measured-flow vaporizers** (Verni-Trols; Copper Kettles) are flowmeter-controlled machines. Copper Kettles were the first devices to allow precise vaporization of liquid anesthetics. They are measured-flow, bubble-through, high-resistance, VOC, multipurpose, and temperature-compensated (thermally stable with manual flow adjustments based on temperature of the liquid anesthetic) vaporizers. They have been called saturation vaporizers and are made of copper. Verni-Trols are made of silicon bronze for thermostability, and back-pressure compensation occurs on recent models and can be fitted on older models (check valves). Verni-Trols are available on used machines and can be purchased for veterinary use. Measured-flow vaporizers will accurately vaporize halothane, isoflurane, enflurane, or methoxyflurane. Manual adjustments in flow rates are required to account for variations in total gas flow, day-to-day changes in temperature, and changes in liquid temperature during use, especially with high fresh gas flows. A calculator or slide rule allows the clinician to determine proper flow rates.

Machines with measured-flow vaporizers have oxygen flowmeters for two purposes. One flowmeter routes all of its oxygen through the vaporization chamber, where it is fully saturated with anesthetic; the other supplies oxygen that bypasses the vaporizer and supplies oxygen to meet the patient's requirements. Both sources of gas combine at a mixing valve to achieve the proper anesthetic concentration before the gases enter the breathing system. The output of a measured-flow vaporizer is oxygen that is fully saturated with anesthetic; the concentration of halothane or isoflurane approaches 32%. Dangerously high concentrations of anesthetic can be delivered to the breathing system if flows are set carelessly or if the diluent flow is not on. It is also possible to misread the slide rule and set incorrect flows. Because of potential errors in concentration, continuous monitoring of inspired anesthetic concentration is desirable. The output from measured-flow vaporizers can be calculated or estimated. The vaporization chamber produces an anesthetic concentration equal to the anesthetic's saturated vapor pressure. Thus if halothane's vapor pressure is 243 mm Hg at 20°C (68°F), approximately 32% halothane is delivered to the mixing valve, where it is diluted by bypass gases to an appropriate concentration.

Hazards of measured-flow vaporizers relate to incorrect use (errors in calculations, failure to adjust flowmeters or the vaporizer circuit control valve properly, careless handling during filling and transport). If the machine is tipped, liquid may enter the discharge tube, ultimately delivering very high concentrations of anesthetic to the breathing system. Overfilling is also possible in older models. Older units may not be equipped for back-pressure compensation, and positive pressure ventilation may increase the delivered concentration. Some measured-flow vaporizers, including the Verni-Trol on the Ohio DM 5000 machine and on the Pitman-Moore 980 veterinary anesthesia machine (which was designed for methoxyflurane), are calibrated so the vaporizer flowmeter measures anesthetic vapor instead of oxygen flowing to the vaporizer. If the calculations are used to determine output for Copper Kettle or Verni-Trol machines, the result will be a delivered concentration that is greater than expected. Volatile anesthetics other than methoxyflurane should not be used in the Pitman-Moore 980 vaporizer.

9. **Maintenance** should be performed on a vaporizer if, based on the responses of patients, the dialed anesthetic concentration is suspected to be erroneous or if any parts of the vaporizer function improperly (control dial is difficult to adjust). Servicing, as recommended by the manufacturer, includes an evaluation of operation, cleaning, changing of filters, replacement of worn parts, and recalibration. Halothane and methoxyflurane contain preservatives (thymol and butylated hydroxytoluene, respectively) that do not vaporize and collect in the vaporization chambers and on the wicks, potentially affecting anesthetic output. Vaporizers should be periodically drained to eliminate preservatives. Vaporizers should not be overfilled or tipped when filled. They should be emptied before they are removed from a machine for service. In the past, flushing a vaporizer with ether to dissolve preservatives was recommended. Owing to the flammability and explosiveness of ether, extreme caution should be exercised.

10. **Using an agent-specific vaporizer for an anesthetic for which the vaporizer is not calibrated is problematic,** especially if the introduction of the wrong anesthetic goes unnoticed. A low output of anesthetic is expected if an anesthetic with a low vapor pressure is placed into a vaporizer designed for a drug with a higher vapor pressure. Conversely, a highly volatile anesthetic in a vaporizer designed for a drug with a lower vapor pressure is likely to produce a high, potentially lethal, concentration. The differential potencies of the drugs affect the depth of anesthesia in either situation. When isoflurane was first introduced into veterinary anesthesia, it was commonly administered with agent-specific halothane vaporizers that were not recalibrated for isoflurane. Because the vapor pressures of halothane and isoflurane are similar, the output was not expected to differ greatly from the control

setting. Indeed, halothane vaporizers produce concentrations of isoflurane that are reasonably close to the dial setting for halothane. Nevertheless, current manufacturer recommendations are against the use of isoflurane in halothane-specific vaporizers, and vice versa. Depending on the vaporizer and conditions of operation, isoflurane in a halothane vaporizer may produce 25 to 50% more vapor than expected, and halothane in an isoflurane-specific vaporizer usually yields a delivered concentration that is lower than indicated on the vaporizer dial. If isoflurane is to be used in an agent-specific halothane vaporizer, the vaporizer should be serviced and completely recalibrated. Complete calibration implies testing for accuracy with an anesthetic gas analyzer at various carrier gas flows and temperatures.

I.    **Common Gas Outlet**

The **common gas outlet** is the site from which gases that have passed through the flowmeters and vaporizer (VOC) or flush valve exit the machine on the way to the breathing system. Typically, a 15-mm-internal-diameter (id) opening is fitted to rubber tubing; the other end of which connects to the fresh gas inlet of the breathing circuit. In some simple veterinary machines with VOC units, all gases flow directly from the vaporizer outlet to the fresh gas inlet.

1.   **Disconnections** at the common gas outlet, vaporizer outlet, or fresh gas inlet can impair flow to the breathing system. The ASTM standard requires a retaining device to prevent accidental disconnections at the common gas outlet. Disconnections should be detected during the checkout procedures before each case, but they can occur during use of the machine. A disconnect from the common gas outlet or the outlet of the vaporizer may not be recognized immediately in a spontaneously breathing patient. When using a breathing circle and a VOC, low $F_{IO_2}$, increased respiratory efforts, and light anesthesia are likely. Some circles (Matrx) incorporate an air intake valve (negative pressure relief) to entrain room air if fresh gas flow is inadequate. With a nonrebreathing system and an outlet disconnect, exhaled $CO_2$ will be rebreathed, low $F_{IO_2}$ is

probable, and the patient will appear lightly anesthetized with increased respiratory efforts. An oxygen analyzer for continuous evaluation of inspired gases allows early detection of this problem.

## J.    Breathing Systems

**Breathing systems** deliver anesthetic gases and oxygen, remove $CO_2$ from exhaled gases, and provide a means to support ventilation. Spontaneously breathing patients inhale and exhale through the system, which should supply the patient's peak inspiratory demands. The system adds resistance to gas flow; the diameter of the conduits are a major factor in determining total resistance. Doubling the radius decreases the resistance 16 times. Halving the circuit's length halves the resistance. Changing the direction of flow and restrictive orifices increases turbulent flow and resistance. Breathing systems should be short, with maximum diameters, few bends, and few restrictions to flow. Generally, the endotracheal tube has the smallest diameter of the breathing apparatus; the largest tube that is practical should be selected.

To identify a breathing system, name it, describe its parts, state the fresh gas flow rates, and iterate the patient's body weight and/or oxygen consumption. Circles use chemical absorbents for $CO_2$. They are termed rebreathing systems because part or all of the exhaled gases, after extraction of $CO_2$, return to the patient. In contrast to nonrebreathing systems, rebreathing systems conserve anesthetic, oxygen, heat, and moisture but impart more resistance. Circle systems are relatively costly to buy, but fairly economic to operate.

1.   Pediatric and standard adult (small animal) **circle systems** differ in internal diameter and volume. Arbitrarily in small animal practice, pediatric circles have been used for small veterinary patients (< 6.8 kg; 15 lb) and adult circles for larger patients (6.8 to 135 kg; 300 lb). Choice of circle may be influenced by the species, availability of equipment, type of ventilation, and anesthesiologist's preference. For humans, a pediatric circle usually refers to a standard (adult) absorber assembly, short breathing tubes of small diameter (15 mm id), and a small bag.

a.  All circle systems have the same **basic components,** arranged to move gases in only one direction (Figs. 6-1 and 6-2). Exhaled gases enter the Y piece and flow through the expiratory breathing tube and expiratory one-way valve. Gases may enter the bag before or after going through the absorbent. On inspiration, gases exit the reservoir bag and pass through the inspiratory one-way valve, inspiratory breathing tube, and Y piece.

b.  A circle's **Y piece** is usually constructed of plastic and unites the endotracheal tube connector and breathing tubes. It contributes to mechanical dead space but may incorporate a septum to minimize dead space. The dead space in an adult small animal Y piece may not be much greater than that in a nonrebreathing system. A standard adult Y piece has a 15-mm female port for the endotracheal tube connector, which may accept a mask (22 mm id). The Y piece's 22-mm-outer-diameter (od) male ports connect to the breathing tubes. Disposable systems may have the Y piece and the breathing tubes permanently attached to each other.

c.  **Breathing tubes** are made of rubber or plastic and are flexible, low-resistance conduits between the Y piece and the one-way valves. Corrugations reduce the likelihood of obstructions if the tubes are bent. Breathing tubes add length and volume and increase resistance; they should have an internal diameter larger than the patient's endotracheal tube. Standard adult tubes are 22 mm id and are appropriate for medium-sized small animals (> 7 kg; 15 lb); for smaller patients, 15-mm-id tubes are available. Breathing tubes do not contribute to mechanical dead space if the one-way valves are functional.

d.  **One-way (unidirectional) paired valves** direct gas flow away from the patient on expiration and toward the patient on inspiration, preventing most rebreathing of $CO_2$-rich gases. Gases enter traditional valves from below, raise the disc, and pass under the dome to enter the reservoir bag, absorbent canister, or inspiratory breathing tube, depending on valve location and circle design. One-way valves usually attach to the canister; in older systems, the one-way valves were within the Y piece (and were more likely to become incompetent). Valves add to the resistance of breathing and should be inspected regularly for proper function.

e.  The **fresh gas inlet** is the site at which gases from the common gas outlet or outlet of the vaporizer enter the circle. The inlet is located on the canister near or on the inspiratory one-way valve. Entry of fresh gases into the inspiratory side of the circle minimizes the dilution of fresh gases with exhaled gases when using a VOC, prevents absorbent dust from being forced toward the patient, and reduces loss of fresh gases through the pop-off valve.

f.  The **pop-off valve** (adjustable pressure-limiting, relief, or overflow valve) vents gases to the scavenger system to prevent the buildup of pressure and allows rapid elimination of anesthetics from the circle when 100% oxygen is indicated. The exhaust port (19 or 30 mm od) of the valve diverts gases to the scavenger system. A pop-off valve should vent gases at a pressure of 1 to 2 cm $H_2O$ when fully open. Several types are available; those with a spring-loaded disc are common. The valve is most convenient and relatively conservative of absorbent if it is located between the expiratory one-way valve and the canister. This location limits waste of fresh gases. Pop-off valves are safety features of closed, low-flow, or semiclosed circle systems. They prevent the inadvertent buildup of pressure, and should remain open except during positive pressure ventilation.

g.  The **reservoir bag** is located on the absorber side of the circle, upstream or downstream from the canister, and attaches to the bag port (22 mm od for small animal circles). Gas from the bag supplies peak inspiratory flow and compliance in the system for exhalation. The bag allows controlled ventilation. Bag excursions allow assessment of respiratory rate and tidal volume. If the pop-off valve is closed, the bag provides compliance to slow the buildup of pressure. The ideal minimum bag size is six times the tidal volume; but practically, the volume should exceed the patient's inspiratory capacity; a spontaneous deep breath should not empty the bag. Common bag sizes are 1, 2, 3, and 5 L. An optimal bag allows manual support of ventilation and easy observation of ventilation. A large bag is cumbersome, impairs monitoring, and slows changes in anesthetic concentration when settings on a VOC machine are altered.

h.  **Manometers** are often attached atop the absorber, allowing assessment of inspiratory pressure (in centimeters of water, kilo-Pascals, or millimeters of mercury) during controlled ventilation.

i.  **Air intake (negative-pressure-relief) valves** are located on the domes of inspiratory one-way valves on some machines (Matrx). In emergencies (no fresh gas inflow), they allow room air (21% oxygen) to enter the circle, preventing the patient from inspiring against a negative pressure and becoming hypoxic.

j.  **Vaporizers (Ohio #8; Stephens)** that impart minimal resistance to ventilation can be located in the breathing system.

k.  The **absorber assembly** contains the absorbent for $CO_2$ and is located between the one-way valves, opposite the patient. The canister may be one single or two stacked containers and should allow airspace between the absorbent granules to be equal to or greater than the tidal volume. Intergranular space is about 50% when a canister is filled with absorbent (4 to 8 mesh). Exhaled gases may enter the top or bottom of a canister; baffles or annular rings move gases toward the center to compensate for lower resistance near the canister wall, preventing channeling and inefficient absorption of $CO_2$. Internal tubes for gas return from an absorber may enhance the wall effect and channeling. Some absorbers have a drain for condensate. The absorbent is a source of resistance to ventilation and is changed regularly; failure to create a seal when replacing the canister causes leaks. Normal wear may damage the canister, caustic effects of soda lime may corrode metal, and aging deteriorates gaskets. Soda lime granules on the gaskets can prevent a seal.

2. **Absorption of $CO_2$** is fundamental in a rebreathing system. If fresh gas inflow approximates the patient's oxygen consumption, most exhaled $CO_2$ will be chemically neutralized. $CO_2$ absorption allows lower gas flows, reduces waste, and lowers costs. With higher flows, some $CO_2$ escapes via the pop-off, and dependence on the absorbent decreases.

   a.  **Calcium hydroxide** is the main component of soda lime and barium hydroxide lime, the two common absorbents. Small amounts of sodium hydroxide (NaOH) and potassium hydroxide (KOH) in soda lime activate the reaction; silica and kieselguhr increase granular hardness. Barium hydroxide lime is inherently hard (bound water molecules) and does not require silica. Water (14 to 19%) is required in soda lime for optimal $CO_2$ absorption. Water formed during granular reactions with $CO_2$ can humidify dry gases but does not react in chemical absorption of $CO_2$.

   b.  The overall reaction of $CO_2$ with soda lime includes multiple steps (e.g., $CO_2$ first reacts with water to form carbonic acid) but can be summarized as follows:

$$2NaOH + 2H_2CO_3 + Ca(OH)_2 \rightarrow CaCO_3 + Na_2CO_3 + 4H_2O + Heat$$

   c.  **Granular size** for absorbents is typically 4 to 8 mesh, a compromise between absorptive activity and air flow resistance. Small granules offer more surface area; large granules impose less resistance. Proper packing of a canister prevents gas flow over a single pathway and excessive dead space. Gently shaking the canister avoids loose packing and reduces channeling. Packing too tightly causes dust and more resistance to ventilation.

   d.  **Fresh granules**—$Ca(OH)_2$—are soft and easily crushed; expended granules—$CaCO_3$—are hard. Color indicators of pH are added. Soda lime changes from white to violet with use; the material may revert to white during storage, but the color reappears when the granules are re-exposed to $CO_2$. Absorption of $CO_2$ is exothermic; a heat line should be detectable on the canister if $CO_2$ absorption is effective. In a circle system, inspired $CO_2$ should be near zero. Measuring $CO_2$ in inspired gases (0.1 to 1.0% is acceptable) determines if absorbent is functional. The absorbent should be changed when the color reaction appears in two-thirds of the absorbent.

3. **Fresh gas flow rates** for circle systems are controversial. Semiclosed, low-flow, and closed circles are options, and each has advantages; personal preference usually determines fresh gas flow. The terms *closed, low-flow,* and *semiclosed* refer to the fresh gas inflow compared to the patient's metabolic needs, not to any structural differences or to the pop-off valve.

    a. Closed system anesthesia is a form of low-flow anesthesia in which the fresh gas flow equals uptake of anesthetic gases and oxygen by the patient and system. Thus the flow of oxygen into a **closed circle system** approximates the patient's oxygen consumption, which varies with the patient's metabolic rate.

        i. Metabolic rate and oxygen consumption are affected by body weight, surface area, temperature, state of consciousness, and anesthetic. In anesthetized dogs, oxygen consumption may vary from 3 to 14 mL/kg/min. Suggested gas flows for closed circles in dogs range from 4 to 11 mL/kg/min. In practice, the fullness of the reservoir bag guides the adjustment of fresh gas flow to the patient's uptake of gases.

        ii. Although oxygen consumption guides fresh gas flow for a closed system, the minimum flow for vaporizer accuracy should be considered. Lower flows in a concentration-calibrated vaporizer (VOC) may cause erratic output.

        iii. Generally, $N_2O$ is not used in closed systems; hypoxic gas mixtures may develop. If $N_2O$ is used, monitoring of $FIO_2$ is imperative. Denitrogenation (empty the bag via the pop-off;

refill the system with fresh gas) should be done two to four times during the first 15 min and every 30 min thereafter to prevent exhaled nitrogen from diluting the oxygen. A closed system depends on chemical $CO_2$ absorption; the quality of the absorbent should be ensured. Closed systems are relatively economic, retain heat and humidity, and are relatively safe for the environment.

b. **Low-flow anesthesia** has been defined as an oxygen flow greater than the patient's oxygen consumption (4 to 7 mL/kg/min) but < 22 mL/kg/min (22 mL/kg/min is the traditional flow for a semi-closed circle). Low flow systems are economic, reduce waste gas, and save heat and moisture. A disadvantage of closed and low-flow techniques is inadequate delivery of anesthetic from a concentration-calibrated (VOC) vaporizer during induction or the transition from injectables to inhalants. Higher flows for the first 15 to 30 min followed by a low-flow technique may solve the problem. Changing the depth of anesthesia is slow with low fresh gas flows. To increase the anesthetic concentration in a system set up with a VOC unit, the fresh gas flow should be temporarily increased. To lower the concentration, the vaporizer setting should be decreased and fresh gas inflow should be increased with either a VOC or VIC machine. For small animals, 10 to 15 mL/kg/min is an appropriate flow rate for a low-flow system.

c. **A semiclosed circle system** uses a fresh gas inflow greater than the patient's uptake of oxygen and anesthetic; traditional flows range from 22 to 44 mL/kg/min. Excess gas is eliminated via the pop-off valve. The exact flow rate depends on personal preference; oxygen consumption times three is a common guideline. If a dog's oxygen consumption is 7 mL/kg/min, fresh gas flow is 21 mL/kg/min. The use of $N_2O$ increases the total gas flow requirement. For 50% $N_2O$, both oxygen and $N_2O$ flow would equal 21 mL/kg/min (total fresh gas flow would be 42 mL/kg/min). For a semiclosed circle, nitrogen accumulation is not significant because nitrogen is eliminated via the pop-off valve. $N_2O$ can be safely used, and the inspired anesthetic concentration can be rapidly changed. The dependency on $CO_2$ absorbent is less, because $CO_2$ is partly eliminated through the pop-off valve. A semiclosed circle retains less heat and humidity and is less economical compared to closed and low-flow systems.

4. **Resistance** in a circle is influenced by the pop-off and unidirectional valves and absorbent canister. Resistance varies with gas flow and ventilation. High flows through the pop-off valve increase resistance. The ventilatory pattern affects the flow rate and resistance through the canister and unidirectional valves. Resistance is a reason for not using adult circles for pediatric patients. Circles systems may not be contraindicated for small patients, solely on the basis of resistance; some veterinarians use circles for 2.5- to 3.0-kg patients. Breathing systems that induce the least resistance to gas flow should be chosen for spontaneously breathing patients.

5. **Mapleson systems** use no absorbent for $CO_2$ and depend on high fresh gas flows to flush the exhaled $CO_2$ from the system. They have generally been referred to as nonrebreathing systems, which is technically incorrect because some rebreathing of exhaled gases may occur, especially with lower recommended flow rates. The Mapleson systems are simple and easy to use, are easily cleaned and sterilized, are lightweight and compact, can be positioned conveniently, have few moving parts, are relatively inexpensive, impart little resistance, do not require $CO_2$ absorbents, add minimal dead space, and allow the inspired concentration of anesthetic to be changed rapidly. Their main disadvantage is the requirement for higher flow rates of fresh gas, which decreases economy and promotes hypothermia and drying of the respiratory tract.

   a. **A Magill system** is a Mapleson A system and is characterized by a fresh gas inlet, an overflow valve near the

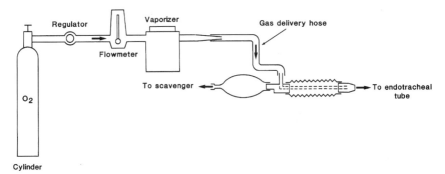

**Figure 6-3.** A Bain coaxial system attached to an anesthesia machine. Fresh gas flows from the outlet of the vaporizer or the common gas outlet of the anesthesia machine to enter the Bain system near the reservoir. Fresh gas move through the Bain's inner tube and is delivered near the patient end of the system. Exhaled gases flow through the corrugated tubing to the reservoir; the overflow is collected by the scavenging system.

patient, and a corrugated tube connecting the patient end of the system to a reservoir bag. Because of the location of the overflow valve, the system is relatively cumbersome during controlled ventilation.

b.  **The Bain coaxial system** is a modified Mapleson D system (Fig. 6-3). It is designed as a tube within a tube. The internal tube (0.7 mm id) supplies fresh gases to the patient end of the system, minimizing dead space. The system accepts an endotracheal connector (15 mm) or a mask (22 mm). The external corrugated tube conducts exhaled gases from the patient to a reservoir. The corrugated tubing may attach directly to the bag, in which case the pop-off valve is built into the bag, or the corrugated tubing may attach to a metal head with drilled channels to accommodate the bag, the overflow valve, and a manometer. Recommendations for total fresh gas flow into a Bain system are variable and are based on minute volume, body weight, and body surface area. During spontaneous ventilation, 200 to 300 mL/kg/min has been recommended for humans, and 100 to 130 or 150 mL/kg/min for veterinary patients. Other authors have suggested 200 mL/kg/min for patients weighing < 7 kg or a range of flow of 220 to 330 mL/kg/min.

The fresh gas flow that will eliminate rebreathing during spontaneous ventilation with a Bain system differs significantly from patient to patient. Most studies recommend fresh gas flows of 1.5 to 3 times the minute volume. Less than 2 to 3 times the minute volume results in some rebreathing of $CO_2$; but end-tidal $CO_2$ concentration may remain normal, even with some rebreathing of $CO_2$. Without regular monitoring of $Paco_2$ or expired $CO_2$ values, flow requirements are difficult to define. Minute volumes for dogs and cats range from 170 to 350 mL/kg/min and 200 to 350 mL/kg/min, respectively. Thus an argument can be made for even higher flows than 660 mL/kg/min. In general, a total fresh gas flow < 500 mL/min or > 3 L/min with a Bain system for animals that weigh < 6.8 kg is not recommended. With controlled ventilation, 100 mL/kg/min is apparently an adequate flow for fresh gases. Higher fresh gas flows are indicated with increased $CO_2$ production, increased dead space, and decreased minute ventilation. Flow rates of 2 to 3 times the minute volume have been recommended for hypoventilating animals in which controlled ventilation was not corrective. During spontaneous ventilation, a Mapleson D system functions identically to a Mapleson F system. The Bain's coaxial design may be effective in reducing loss of heat and humidity, although the overall benefit in small veterinary patients maintained with relatively high fresh gas flow rates is questionable.

c.  **Ayre's T piece and Norman mask elbow systems** equipped with an expiratory limb (corrugated tubing) and reservoir bag are classed as Mapleson F systems. Without a reservoir bag, they are Mapleson E systems.

d.  **Resistance** to ventilation in the Mapleson systems is minimal, which may be an advantage for small patients. Advantages of modern nonrebreathing systems for small patients include decreased resistance to ventilation, better gas exchange, greater control of the depth of anesthesia, and fewer mechanical problems. Hazards of nonrebreathing systems relate primarily to outflow occlusion, development of excessive airway pressure, and barotrauma to the lungs (including pneumothorax).

6. **Systems with nonrebreathing valves** (Stephens-Slater, Fink, Digby-Leigh) were cumbersome and essentially have been replaced by the Mapleson and circle systems. Presently, nonrebreathing valves are used in self-inflating bags for resuscitation or transport of patients requiring manual ventilation. An Ambu bag facilitates resuscitation and transport of apneic or anesthetized patients. Oxygen can be allowed to flow into the reservoir bag to increase $F_{IO_2}$. When the bag is compressed, the pressure closes the exhalation port, and gases enter the patient's respiratory system. When pressure is released, gas flows from the patient through the exhalation port. With spontaneous breathing, the Ambu valve allows the patient to inhale room air only.

7. **Closed containers** are used for oxygenation and inhalant inductions in small patients. Inhalant inductions have decreased in popularity because of difficulty in scavenging waste gases, especially as the patient is removed from the chamber. An effective way to ensure elimination of waste anesthetic gases with this system is use in a fume hood. An advantage of a closed container is reduced physical restraint. Induction is effective for aggressive cats and some laboratory and small wild or exotic species. Most containers for inhalant inductions are made of glass, Plexiglas, or another clear plastic material, allowing observation during induction. Airway obstruction is possible in a closed container, and ventilatory efforts should be monitored. The chamber should be no larger than necessary, but the animal should be able to lie in lateral recumbency without neck flexion. Relatively high flows of fresh gas facilitate inductions in closed containers. The outlet of the chamber should be attached to a scavenger system. Chamber inductions should be done in a well-ventilated area, ideally under a fume hood. Depending on the size of the chamber and patient, total fresh gas flow into the chamber should be 2 to 5 L/min. Low flow rates slow induction and contribute to the development of excitement. Oxygen should be ad-

ministered for about 5 min before the introduction of inhalant anesthetic. Then the concentration of the inhalant
should be increased at 0.5% increments every 10 s until
4 to 4.5% halothane or isoflurane is being administered.
Unless $N_2O$ is contraindicated, it can be used in concentrations of 60 to 70%.

8. **Mask inductions** are facilitated by anesthetic concentrations and fresh gas flows similar to those for closed containers. Masking is smoothest in depressed, sedated, or
tranquilized patients. Masks should fit snugly over the muzzle to minimize dead space, and an appropriately sized
mask should be used. A tight-fitting mask promotes a rapid
induction and minimal loss of waste gases. A clear mask
with a rubber diaphragm allows visualization of the nares
and mouth during induction and creates a good seal
around the muzzle. The mask should be attached to a
breathing system with a reservoir of gases to meet peak
inspiratory flows, which may exceed the inflow of fresh
gases. Most excess gases can be scavenged via the pop-off
valve of the breathing system, but masking should be done
in a well-ventilated area. High fresh gas flows (3 to 5 L/min
for dogs and cats) during masking supply the oxygen demands of the patient, dilute and eliminate exhaled $CO_2$,
and provide anesthetic concentrations for a relatively rapid
induction.

**K.   Scavenging Waste Anesthetic Gases**

Since the 1980s, the exposure of medical and veterinary personnel to waste anesthetic gases has become a significant concern. A
bulletin from the American Veterinary Medical Association's
Liability Insurance Trust indicates that numerous studies in the
United States and abroad have found no conclusive evidence
that waste gases or trace amounts of waste gas cause specific
health problems. There is some evidence, however, to suggest
that removal of gases from veterinary facilities may improve the
occupational health of the veterinary staff.

1. The **Occupational Safety and Health Administration**
(OSHA) has not set limits for exposure to anesthetics, but
OSHA can enforce National Institute for Occupational

Safety and Health (NIOSH) recommendations under the general duty clause: the duty of an employer to provide an environment free from recognized hazards that are likely to cause death or serious physical harm. Recommended exposure limits from NIOSH vary from 2 ppm for halogenated hydrocarbon anesthetics (halothane) to an 8-h time-weighted average exposure to $N_2O$ of 25 ppm. Together, 0.5 ppm for halogenated agents and 25 ppm for $N_2O$ are the limits. The American Conference of Governmental Industrial Hygienists (ACGIH) gives threshold limit values of 50 ppm for halothane and $N_2O$ as 8-h time-weighted averages.

2. **Recommendations for controlling waste gases** have been suggested. Veterinary workers should be aware of risks so that they can minimize exposure to the inhalants. Women in the first trimester of pregnancy, people with hepatic or renal disease, and people with compromised immune systems appear at greatest risk. The following recommendations are important in regard to managing waste anesthetic gases.

   a. All personnel should be educated about potential health hazards of waste gases.
   b. Scavenger systems should be used with all anesthesia machines and breathing systems.
   c. All rooms in which anesthetic gases are used should be well ventilated with an appropriate number of air exchanges (e.g., 15 air changes/h).
   d. Machines and systems should be nearly leak free; leakage tolerances should comply with established criteria (~ 300 mL/min at 30 cm $H_2O$ for circles, pop-off valve closed).
   e. A log documenting the performance and maintenance procedures for anesthesia machines, vaporizers, and breathing systems should be maintained.
   f. Personnel should minimize spillage when filling vaporizers (keyed filling systems).
   g. Periodic monitoring of anesthetic concentrations in induction, operating, and recovery rooms should be done to ensure the efficacy of scavenging.

3. There are several ways to decrease contamination of the occupational environment with anesthetics.

    a. Avoid spills when filling vaporizers.
    b. Start gas flows only after the patient has been intubated.
    c. Use endotracheal tubes with inflated cuffs.
    d. Occlude the Y piece of the circle or the patient end of a Mapleson system if the system is disconnected from the patient.
    e. Use a scavenging pop-off valve.
    f. Discharge all gases through an effective scavenger system.
    g. Flush breathing systems with oxygen before disconnecting the patient.
    h. Use the minimum gas flow that promotes safe anesthesia.
    i. Minimize the use of masks and closed containers. Be sure that masks fit well. Use closed containers only in well-ventilated areas, ideally under a fume hood.
    j. Maintain proper ventilation in work areas and minimize exposure to exhaled gases during the initial phases of the recovery period whenever possible.

4. **Machines and breathing systems** should be properly outfitted and functional to ensure minimal pollution. They should be leak free; each machine–system combination should connect with a functional scavenger system. An efficient scavenging system is the most important factor in reducing trace gases, which can lower ambient concentrations up to 90%.

## L. Scavenging Systems

A scavenging system collects waste gases from the breathing system and eliminates them from the workplace. The scavenging system is composed of a gas-collecting assembly, an interface, and a disposal system; various types of tubing connect these parts.

1. The **gas-collecting assembly** gathers waste gases from the breathing system. At present, the exhaust outlet from the

circle's pop-off valve must be 19 or 30 mm in diameter. Older machines used 22-mm-od connectors, which permitted inadvertent interchange of scavenging hoses and breathing tubes. Depending on the location of the overflow in Mapleson systems, devices connecting to the tail or the side of the reservoir bag serve as the gas-collecting assembly and attach to transfer tubing leading to the interface.

2.  The **interface** is intended to prevent transfer of pressure changes in the scavenging system to the breathing system. The inlet to the interface should be 19 or 30 mm od; the outlet can be of any diameter (not just 15 or 22 mm). An interface should provide positive pressure relief to protect the patient from occlusions of the scavenging system, negative pressure relief to limit the pressure effects of an active disposal system, and a reservoir for excess waste gas for use with active disposal systems. The interfaces may be opened or closed.

3.  **Disposal systems** can be passive or active. Passive systems include nonrecirculating ventilation systems, piping directly to the atmosphere, and absorption devices. Active systems include piped vacuum and active duct systems.

    a.  A **nonrecirculating ventilation system** discharges waste gases through an exhaust vent.

    b.  **Discharging directly to the atmosphere** is suitable for many hospitals, because the distance from the machine to the outside may be short. Such systems should be designed so that water, wind, dust, and insects cannot enter the system.

    c.  **Canisters of activated charcoal** adsorb halogenated hydrocarbon anesthetics with varying efficiency. They are simple and portable. Effectiveness varies with different brands, styles of canister, and rates of flow through the canister. Canisters must be changed regularly, increasing costs; they do not absorb $N_2O$. Other methods are preferable; absorption is reserved for situations in which more reliable methods are not accessible.

d. **Central vacuum systems** are convenient disposal systems for hospitals with such systems in place. The system creates a flow of at least 30 L/min; it functions best when the operator can adjust the flow. A central vacuum for scavenging along with another system for surgical suction is most desirable.

e. An **active duct system** with a high volume of flow and a low negative pressure provides an excellent means of gas disposal. Negative pressure is generated by a fan, pump, or other device in a large duct that is connected to smaller ducts that open at the site of use. These are effective, but regular maintenance is required to ensure that the fan or pump is operational. This system is not affected by wind currents.

## M.  Anesthesia Apparatus: Checkout Recommendations

Evaluation of machines and breathing systems is important for safety of personnel (control of waste gases) and patients (proper oxygen and anesthetic delivery). The FDA published *Anesthesia Apparatus Checkout Recommendations* (1986), which addresses anesthesia gas delivery systems.

1. High-, intermediate-, and low-pressure areas of the apparatus should be evaluated.

    i. **The high-pressure areas** (2200 psi, oxygen; 745 psi, $N_2O$) include gas cylinders, hanger yokes, yoke blocks, hoses, pressure gauges, and regulators. Inspect for loose connections and audible leakage, do pressure checks (loss of pressure with cylinder valves open and flowmeters off), and use soapy water to snoop for leaks (foam or bubbles) at joints.

    ii. **The intermediate pressure areas** (40 to 50 psi) include pipeline inlets, conduits from pipeline inlets to flowmeters, conduits from regulators to flowmeters, flowmeter assembly, and oxygen flush. Tests include visual inspection, listening for leaks, and use of soapy water.

    iii. **The low-pressure areas** (slightly > $P_{bar}$) include vaporizer(s), conduits from flowmeters to the

VOC, conduit from the VOC to common gas outlet, and conduit from common gas outlet to breathing system. Tests include visual inspection and pressure checks with the breathing system. Pressure in the breathing system may affect the low-pressure areas of the machine, but newer machines have check valves near the common gas outlet.

2. **The universal negative-pressure leak test** for the low-pressure areas requires a simple suction bulb (Fig. 6-4). With flowmeters and vaporizers off, the bulb is attached at the common gas outlet and squeezed to create a vacuum. If it reinflates in less than 10 s, a significant leak is present. The test is repeated with the vaporizer on to detect internal vaporizer leaks. This test differentiates between leaks in the low-pressure areas of the machine (vaporizer) and leaks in the breathing system. The test detects leaks as small as 30 mL/min and is considered reliable.

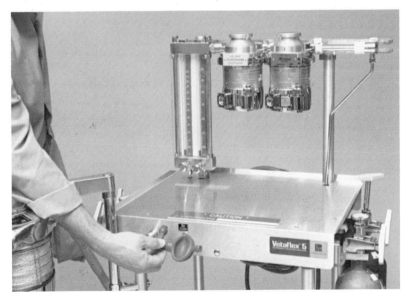

**Figure 6-4.** The universal negative pressure relief test. With all gases off and the vaporizer off, a compressed rubber bulb is attached to the common gas outlet of the anesthesia machine. The bulb should not reinflate in < 10 s. The test should be repeated with the vaporizer control on.

3. **Check machines daily** before the first patient, and recheck the breathing system before each patient. The following FDA recommendations are appropriate for the evaluation of machines and systems before the first case of the day:

a. Check the central oxygen and $N_2O$ supplies for adequacy of gases and pipeline pressures.

b. Inspect flowmeters, vaporizers, gauges, and supply hoses. Ensure correct mounting of cylinders in the hanger yokes; the presence of a wrench for cylinder valves; and a complete, undamaged breathing system with adequate absorbent for $CO_2$.

c. Ensure the connection of the scavenging system to the pop-off valve and its function, using appropriate leak tests. Charcoal canisters, if used, should not be exhausted.

d. Turn off the flow-control valves for the flowmeters.

e. Ensure that the vaporizer is properly filled (filler cap sealed and control dial off).

f. Check the machine's oxygen cylinders. With the pipeline supply disconnected, the oxygen cylinder valve off, and the pressure gauge at zero, slowly open the valve. Pressure (> 500 psi) and the presence of leaks (no drop in pressure) should be evaluated. Check each oxygen cylinder.

g. Check the $N_2O$ supply (if present) as described for the oxygen cylinders. If present, check fail-safe devices to ensure that $N_2O$ cannot be delivered without an adequate amount of oxygen.

h. Test the flowmeters for each gas. When the flow controls are off, the floats should rest at the bottom of the tubes. Over a full range of flow, there should be no sticking or erratic movements.

i. Test the central supplies of oxygen and $N_2O$: small (E) cylinders off, and pipeline inlets connected to the central supply. Adjust the flows to midrange; ensure that supply pressures remain near 50 psi.

j. No anesthetic odor should be present with the oxygen flowmeter on and vaporizer off.

k. Test the circle's unidirectional valves (Figs. 6-5 and 6-6). Wearing a surgical mask, exhale through the exhalation limb to check the exhalation valve; com-

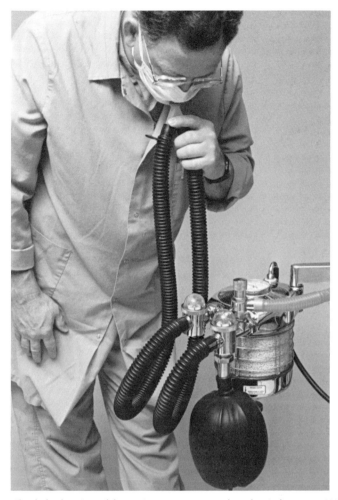

**Figure 6-5.** Check the function of the expiratory one-way valve of a circle system. Wearing a surgical mask, the evaluator exhales through the Y piece and exhales through the expiratory one-way valve to be sure that the valve disc moves appropriately. The reservoir bag should expand as air moves through the valve.

press the reservoir bag (pop-off valve closed; Y piece open) to check the inhalation valve. Valve discs should be present and should rise and fall appropriately.

1. Test for leaks in the circle system and machine (Fig. 6-7). Close the pop-off valve, occlude the Y piece, fill the system with oxygen, and turn the oxygen flow to

5 L/min. As the pressure reaches 20 cm $H_2O$, reduce the flow until the pressure in the system (manometer) no longer rises. The oxygen flow should be negligible; a high leakage rate is unacceptable. Squeeze the reservoir bag to create a relatively high pressure (40 to 50 cm $H_2O$); ensure a tight system.

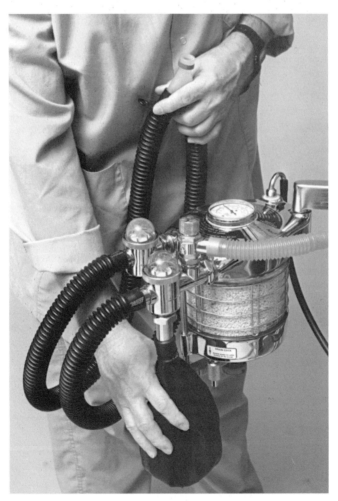

**Figure 6-6.** Check the function of the inspiratory one-way valve of a circle system. With the pop-off valve closed, the reservoir bag is compressed, and the valve disc of the inspiratory one-way valve should move appropriately.

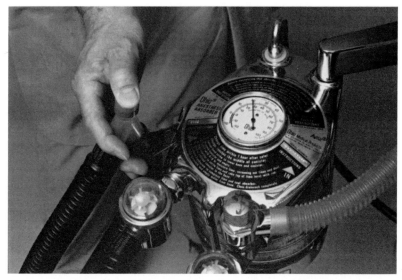

**Figure 6-7.** Evaluate the integrity of a circle breathing system. The pop-off valve is closed, the patient port is occluded, and the system is filled to a pressure of 30 cm $H_2O$ for at least 10 s or the leak as determined by use of the oxygen flowmeter should be < 250 mL/min.

To check the system for leaks, fill the circle (pop-off valve closed; Y piece occluded) to 30 cm $H_2O$; ensure that leakage is < 250 mL/min, that the pressure drop is < 5 cm $H_2O$ in 30 s, or that the pressure remains at 30 cm $H_2O$ for ≥ 10 s. Similar tests may have slightly different values for testing pressures and acceptable leak rates.

m.   Open the pop-off valve slowly; observe the release of pressure. Occlude the Y piece; verify that negligible positive or negative pressure develops at oxygen flows of 0 or 5 L/min.

n.   Ensure that the pop-off valve provides pressure relief when the flush valve is activated.

4.   **Nonrebreathing systems should be tested before use.** For a complete system check of a Bain system (Fig. 6-8), the patient port should be occluded, relief valve closed, and reservoir bag distended. The bag should remain fully distended, and the pressure within the system should not decrease. The complete system check does not ensure a

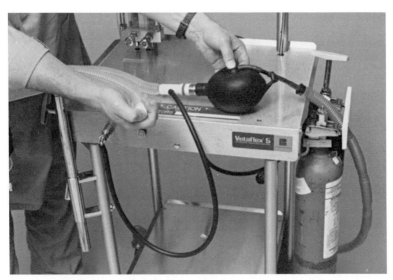

**Figure 6-8.** Evaluate a Bain breathing system and do a complete system check. With all gas flows off, the overflow valve is closed, and the patient port is occluded. The bag is filled with the flush valve to a pressure of 30 cm $H_2O$; a leak-free system should maintain this pressure for at least 10 s. If a leak is present, it can be quantified with the oxygen flowmeter and should not exceed 300 mL/min.

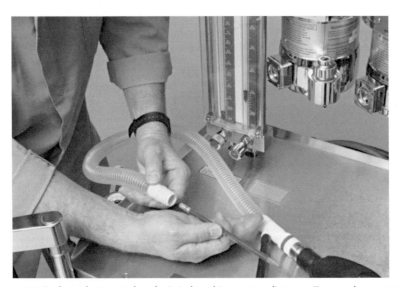

**Figure 6-9.** Evaluate the inner tube of a Bain breathing system: first step. Turn on the oxygen flowmeter. In this example, the flow of oxygen was set at 1 L/min.

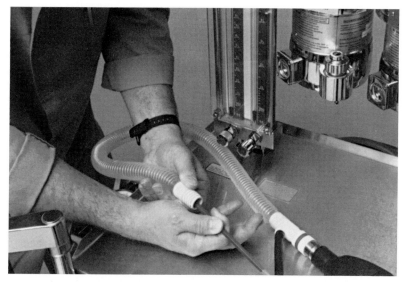

**Figure 6-10.** Evaluate the inner tube of a Bain breathing system: second step. Occlude the patient end of the inner tube. If the inner tube is intact, the oxygen flowmeter's indicator should fall.

leak-free inner tube of the coaxial system. Therefore, the inner tube is evaluated by temporarily occluding the inner tube at the patient end with oxygen flowing at 1 to 2 L/min. Using a plunger of a syringe for occlusion of the inner tube of the system, the float in the oxygen flowmeter should fall (Figs. 6-9 and 6-10). The complete system check will usually suffice for other nonrebreathing systems (e.g., Norman mask elbow; Ayre's T piece).

## II.  MONITORING
*Steve C. Haskins*

The purpose of anesthesia is to provide reversible unconsciousness, amnesia, analgesia, and immobility, with minimal risk to the patient. Anesthetic drugs and adjuvants may, however, compromise patient homeostasis at unpredictable times and in unpredictable ways. Anesthetic crises, unfortunately, tend to be rapid in onset and devastating in nature.

## A. Intraoperative Monitoring

Monitoring helps answer several questions: Is the animal adequately anesthetized or amnesic? Is the animal adequately analgesic and is the autonomic response adequately subdued? Is the animal adequately immobilized? What are the physiologic consequences of the anesthetic state? Are any of the identified intraoperative abnormalities serious enough to warrant treatment?

1.  Anesthesia must provide **unconsciousness** and **amnesia**. With the traditional anesthetics (barbiturates, etomidate, propofol, and the inhalants), unconsciousness is generally achieved at the top of the excitement stage. Because procedures cannot be implemented until spontaneous movement ceases, immobilized patients should be unconscious and amnesic. The signs of anesthetic depth depend, for the most part, on the evaluation of muscular tone and muscular reflexes (see Chapter 1). When the signs of anesthetic depth are unclear and contradictory, the anesthetic depth should be lightened a little until the signs change sufficiently to make it clear that the animal is lightly anesthetized. In normal animals, there is a fairly wide range between cessation of spontaneous movement and serious, drug-induced decompensation, and so some overanesthetization can be done with relative impunity. This range narrows as the patient becomes progressively compromised by disease. It is in these marginal patients that standard anesthetic techniques may cause problems. And it is for this reason that the preanesthetic examination to quantitate the degree of the compromise is so important. Regardless of technique, the problem of awareness or recall during general anesthesia in animals is unresolvable per se and so we are left to extrapolate anesthetic protocols that have been reported to be efficacious in human beings.

2.  If the animal is truly anesthetized (unaware and detached from environmental stimuli), it can be concluded that it is **analgesic** as well (not consciously perceiving pain). If the animal is lightly anesthetized with a traditional anesthetic, reflex or spontaneous movement may occur; however it is extremely unlikely that pain is being consciously per-

ceived. It is a common practice to deepen anesthesia or add an adjuvant drug if there is spontaneous movement, movement in response to surgical stimulation, or a sympathetic response to surgical stimulation. Although probably unnecessary for pain relief, this is an acceptable procedure as long as the patient can tolerate the deeper anesthesia. Opioid-based anesthetic protocols are considered to provide excellent analgesia even though muscular relaxation and CNS depression require reinforcement with adjunctive drugs. Ketamine has been reported to be less efficacious for visceral pain than somatic pain. This does not mean that it is ineffective, only less effective. And it certainly does not mean that it is inappropriate to use ketamine anesthesia for abdominal procedures; only that deeper levels of anesthesia may be required.

3. The required degree of **muscle relaxation** is the amount that is compatible with the completion of the surgical procedure. A little movement, as long as it does not interfere with the surgical procedure, should be acceptable, because it is not generally associated with the conscious perception of pain. Intraocular surgeries clearly constitute an exception to the rule that a little bit of movement is acceptable. In these situations, neuromuscular blocking drugs, rather than very deep anesthesia, should be selected.

4. Animals can experience **adverse physiologic responses** to anesthetic drugs at any anesthetic depth. Although the pharmacodynamic effects of anesthetics vary, the mechanisms by which they cause anesthetic emergencies are usually the same: excessive hypotension, bradycardia, arrhythmias, myocardial depression, vasodilation or vasoconstriction, hypoventilation, hypoxemia, etc. It is the purpose of the monitoring procedures to determine to what extent these problems develop in the perioperative period. It is important to understand the physiologic significance of each monitored parameter so that it is not overinterpreted or underinterpreted. Unless the measurement is extremely low or high, its proper interpretation, clinical importance, and indication of the overall adequacy of the function of the organ system can be assessed

only by correlating its current value with those previously taken (trends) and with other organ system measurements and by considering the patient's recent history.

## B.   Pulmonary Monitoring

The **breathing rate** per se is of limited value without some reference to tidal volume and previous trends, because normal rates can vary so widely. A change in breathing rate is, however, often a sensitive indicator of an underlying physiologic change (Table 6-1). The rhythm, nature, and effort of breathing should be characterized. Arrhythmic breathing patterns indicate a medullary respiratory control problem. Apneustic breathing (inspiratory hold) may be seen in otherwise healthy dogs, cats, and most other species anesthetized with ketamine.

1.   **Ventilation volume** can be estimated by visual observation of the chest or rebreathing bag excursions or measured by ventilometry (Fig. 6-11). Normal tidal volume ranges between 10 and 20 mL/kg. A small tidal volume may be acceptable if the breathing rate is fast enough to accomplish normal alveolar minute ventilation. Normal total minute ventilation ranges between 150 and 250 mL/kg/min. Alveolar minute ventilation is more important than total minute ventilation. Alveolar minute ventilation may be as low as 20% of the total minute ventilation in animals breathing rapidly and shallowly or that have added upper airway dead space, and may be as high as 70% of the total if the animal is breathing slowly and deeply and is endotracheally intubated.

| Table 6-1. Causes of Perioperative Tachypnea | |
| --- | --- |
| Too lightly anesthetized | Atelectasis |
| Too deeply anesthetized | Postoperative recovery phase |
| Hypoxemia | Postoperative pain |
| Hypercapnia | Drug-induced (opioids) |
| Hyperthermia | Individual variation |
| Hypotension | |

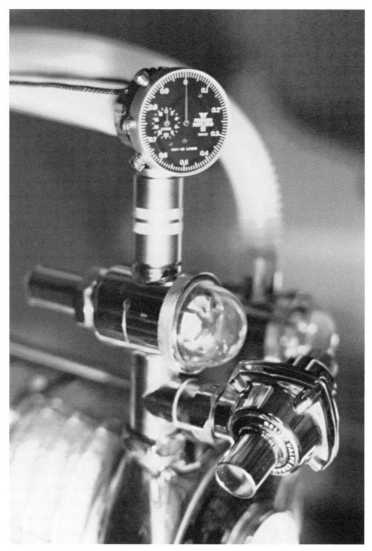

**Figure 6-11.** A ventilometer can be attached to an anesthetic machine to measure expired tidal volume.

2. **Blood gas analysis** of $CO_2$ and oxygen in an arterial blood sample defines pulmonary function. Venous samples interpose a tissue bed between the lungs and the sample site and provide little information about pulmonary function.

a.  **$Paco_2$** is a measure of the ventilatory status of the patient and normally ranges between 35 and 45 mm Hg. A $Paco_2$ < 35 mm Hg indicates hyperventilation; a $Paco_2$ > 45 mm Hg indicates hypoventilation. A $Paco_2$ > 60 mm Hg may be associated with excessive respiratory acidosis and hypoxemia (when breathing room air) and usually represents sufficient enough hypoventilation to warrant mechanical ventilatory support. $Paco_2$ values < 20 mm Hg are associated with severe respiratory alkalosis and a decreased cerebral blood flow, which may impair cerebral oxygenation. Venous $Pco_2$ is usually 3 to 6 mm Hg higher than arterial $Pco_2$ in stable states. It is a reflection of tissue $Pco_2$, which represents some combination of $Paco_2$ and tissue metabolism. $Paco_2$ may also be estimated by measuring the $CO_2$ in a sample of gas taken at the end of an exhalation. The presumption in correlating end-tidal $Pco_2$ with $Paco_2$ is that alveolar and capillary $Pco_2$ are equilibrated. End-tidal $Pco_2$ is usually somewhat lower than $Paco_2$ (1 to 4 mm Hg in humans and dogs). **Capnography** allows the anesthetist to evaluate the adequacy of ventilation, as well as many other problems (Table 6-2). Hypercapnia may be caused by hypoventilation or dead space rebreathing (Table 6-3).

b.  **$Pao_2$** is a measure of the oxygenating efficiency of the lungs. The $Pao_2$ measures the tension of oxygen dissolved in physical solution in the plasma, irrespective of the hemoglobin concentration. Hemoglobin saturation measures the percent saturation of the hemoglobin (Hb) and is related to the $Pao_2$ by a sigmoid curve. The clinical information derived from the measurement of hemoglobin saturation ($Sao_2$) is similar to that obtained from a $Pao_2$ measurement in that they both measure the ability of the lung to deliver oxygen to the bloodstream. The values, however, for identifying hypoxemia differ, as shown in Table 6-4.

c.  **Oxygen content** depends on both hemoglobin concentration and $Po_2$:

$$\text{Oxygen content} = [(\text{Hb} \times 1.34) \times \text{percent saturation}] + (0.003 \times Po_2)$$

| Table 6-2. Potential Causes of Changes in the Capnogram | |
|---|---|
| **End-tidal $CO_2$ Change** | **Potential Causes** |
| Sudden decrease to zero | Airway obstruction; airway disconnect; ventilator failure; capnograph malfunction; obstructed aspirating tube |
| Sudden decrease to low plateau values | Airway leaks |
| Exponential decrease in plateau values | Severe cardiovascular disturbance; inadvertent sudden hyperventilation |
| Slow decrease in plateau values | Hyperventilation; hypothermia; vasoconstriction |
| Low measurement without a good plateau; slow rate of rise | Exhalation not complete before next inhalation (partial obstruction, bronchospasm, rapid breathing rates); low aspirating flow rate; fresh gas contamination |
| Low measurement with a good plateau | Uncalibrated capnograph; large physiologic dead space |
| Increased plateau | Hypoventilation; increased rate of metabolism |
| Increased baseline | Contaminated sample cell |
| Increasing baseline and plateau | Rebreathing |
| Increased $Pa_{CO_2}$–$PA_{CO_2}$ | Dead space ventilation |

Oxygen content is difficult to measure, whereas oxygen saturation and $Po_2$ are easy. Oxygen partial pressure, saturation, and content ($Ca_{O_2}$) are related; but depending on the underlying condition, any one measurement may be misleading (Table 6-5).

3.  A **pulse oximeter** is an ideal perioperative monitor in that it is an automatic, continuous, audible monitor of mechanical cardiopulmonary function. It specifically measures pulse rate and hemoglobin saturation, and requires reasonable pulmonary and cardiovascular function to achieve a measurement. One of the common reasons for poor instrument performance has been peripheral vasocon-

striction; the instrument will not be able to pick up a pulse. Its value as an ongoing monitor in detecting hypoxemia has been established. Accuracy should be verified from time to time with an arterial blood gas measurement. Pulse oximeters attach to a patient externally (tongue, lips, tail, toenail) (Fig. 6-12). For the most part, $Sao_2$ is as informative as $Pao_2$; each is a measure of the ability of the lungs to deliver oxygen to the blood. The two measurements are related via the sigmoid oxygen–hemoglobin saturation curve; if the curve is normal, one can be derived from the other. If the curve is not normal, an extrapolation will be in error to the extent that the curve is shifted to the left or

---

**Table 6-3. Causes of Hypercapnia**

I. Hypoventilation
   A. Neuromuscular disorder
      1. Excessive depths of anesthesia
      2. Intracranial disease
      3. Cervical disease
      4. Neuromuscular junction disorder
   B. Airway obstruction
      1. Big airway
      2. Bronchoconstriction
   C. Thoracic or abdominal restrictive disease

   D. Pleural-space filling disorder
      1. Air
      2. Fluid
   E. Pulmonary parenchymal disease (terminal)
   F. Inappropriate ventilator settings
II. Dead space rebreathing
III. Hyperthermia, increased $CO_2$ production
IV. Recent bicarbonate therapy

---

**Table 6-4. Relationship Between $Pao_2$ and $Sao_2$ with Respect to Hypoxemia**

| $Pao_2$ | $Sao_2$ | Importance |
|---|---|---|
| > 80 | > 95 | Normal |
| < 60 | < 90 | Serious hypoxemia |
| < 40 | < 75 | Very serious hypoxemia |

Table 6-5. Changes Observed in $Pa_{O_2}$, $Sa_{O_2}$, and $Ca_{O_2}$ with Various Diseases and during Anesthesia

| Condition | $Pa_{O_2}$ | $Sa_{O_2}$ | $Ca_{O_2}$ |
|---|---|---|---|
| Anemia | Normal | Normal | Reduced |
| Polycythemia | Normal to reduced | Normal to reduced | Increased |
| Methemoglobinemia | Normal | Reduced | Reduced |
| Severe pulmonary disease | Reduced | Reduced | Reduced |
| Hyperoxemia (anesthesia) | Increased | Normal | Slightly increased |

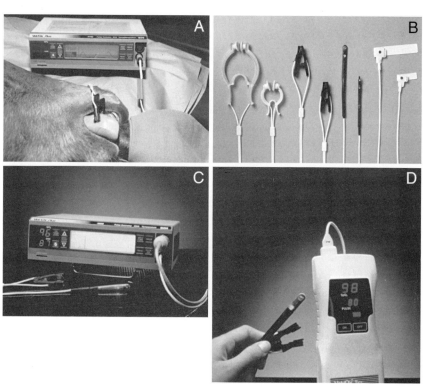

**Figure 6-12.** Pulse oximeters can be attached to the tongue (A), lip, toenail, ear, or tail; any place where the underlying pulse can be detected. Several types of probes (B) and display units (C and D) are available.

right. $Sa_{O_2}$ may not be too discriminating when an animal is breathing an enriched oxygen mixture, because such measurements would most likely be positioned on the upper plateau of the dissociation curve. The difference between a $Pa_{O_2}$ of 500 mm Hg and a $Pa_{O_2}$ of 100 mm Hg in an animal breathing 100% oxygen is very important; the corresponding decrease in $Sa_{O_2}$, from 99 to 98%, would hardly be noticed.

4. **$Pv_{O_2}$** reflects tissue $P_{O_2}$ and bears no correlation to $Pa_{O_2}$. $P\bar{v}_{O_2}$ ranges between 40 and 50 mm Hg. Values < 30 mm Hg may be caused by anything that decreases the delivery of oxygen to the tissues (hypoxemia, low cardiac output, vasoconstriction); values > 60 mm Hg (while breathing room air) suggest reduced tissue uptake of oxygen (shunting, septic shock, metabolic poisons). Venous blood for such evaluations must be from a central vein, such as the jugular, anterior vena cava, or pulmonary artery.

5. **Venous admixture** is the collective term for all of the ways in which blood can pass from the right side to the left side of the circulation without being properly oxygenated (Table 6-6). Venous admixture can be estimated via the alveolar air equation:

$$P_{AO_2} = \text{inspired } P_{O_2} - Pa_{CO_2} \quad (1.1)$$

where

$$\text{Inspired } P_{O_2} = P_{bar} \times 21\%$$

| Table 6-6. Causes of Hypoxemia |
|---|

I. Decreased inspired oxygen concentration
   A. Improper functioning equipment
II. Hypoventilation (while inspiring 21% oxygen)
III. Venous admixture
   A. Low ventilation–perfusion regions (bronchoconstriction)
   B. No ventilation–perfusion regions (atelectasis)
   C. Diffusion impairment (inhalation toxicity)
   D. Anatomical right-to-left shunt

and $1.1 = 1/RQ$, assuming the respiratory quotient (RQ) = 0.9. The difference between the $P_{AO_2}$ and the measured $Pa_{O_2}$ is the $P_{AO_2}$–$Pa_{O_2}$ difference. The normal $P_{AO_2}$–$Pa_{O_2}$ difference is 10 mm Hg when the animal is breathing 21% oxygen and 100 mm Hg when the animal is breathing 100% oxygen. Larger $P_{AO_2}$–$Pa_{O_2}$ differences when breathing room air or 100% oxygen indicate a decreased ability of the lung to oxygenate blood or venous admixture. Patients breathing an enriched oxygen mixture should have an elevated $Pa_{O_2}$. A rough estimate of the expected $Pa_{O_2}$ can be obtained by multiplying the inspired oxygen concentration by 5. A $Pa_{O_2}$ measurement below this value indicates venous admixture. A simplified formula that is relatively independent of inspired oxygen concentration is the a:A ratio ($Pa_{O_2}$:$P_{AO_2}$). An a:A ratio < 0.85 indicates venous admixture.

## C.    Cardiovascular Monitoring

Oxygen delivery to the tissues depends on the coordinated interaction of several physiologic events: The lungs must effectively move oxygen from the environment to the plasma; hemoglobin must be present in adequate amounts; cardiac output must provide sufficient flow of the oxygenated hemoglobin toward the tissues; arterial blood pressure must be adequate to maintain cerebral and coronary perfusion pressure; and vasomotor tone must not be excessive to maintain visceral organ perfusion. This overall perspective of cardiopulmonary function is illustrated in Figure 6-13 and is the focus of cardiopulmonary monitoring and support (Table 6-7). The importance of any one measured parameter to overall function can be determined only by reference to previous measurements of that parameter, to recent therapeutic (or disease-induced) events, and to other measured parameters.

1.  **Abnormal electrical activity** includes bradycardia, tachycardia, and arrhythmias (Tables 6-8 and 6-9). The electrocardiogram does not measure mechanical performance and can appear quite normal in the face of poor myocardial performance and tissue perfusion. The major concern is whether the PQRST wave forms appear to be approximately normal. Ectopic pacemaker activity does

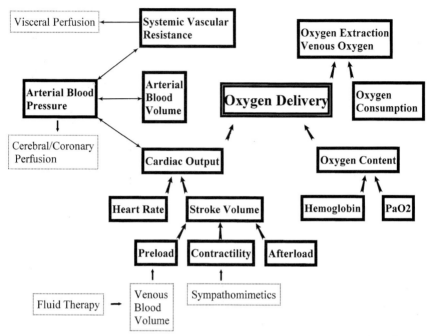

**Figure 6-13.** Proper interpretation of individual cardiopulmonary measurements depends on the integration of the measurement with all other measured parameters. Oxygen delivery is determined by cardiac output (heart rate and stroke volume) and oxygen content (hemoglobin and $Po_2$). Stroke volume is determined by preload, contractility, and afterload. The purpose of preload is to optimize stroke volume, whereas sympathomimetic therapy is used to optimize contractility (and systemic resistance). Arterial blood pressure is determined by arterial blood volume, cardiac output, and peripheral vasomotor tone. Arterial blood pressure is a primary determinant of coronary and cerebral perfusion, and vasomotor tone is a primary determinant of peripheral and visceral perfusion. Venous oxygen is a reflection of the relationship between oxygen delivery and oxygen consumption.

not necessarily require treatment (Fig. 6-14). It indicates the presence of an underlying abnormality that should be identified. Specific treatment is indicated when there is evidence of impaired myocardial performance, cardiac output, or tissue perfusion. Specific treatment is also indicated if there is concern regarding the progression of the arrhythmia to ventricular fibrillation (the rate exceeds the upper limit of normal for the species, when it is multifocal, or when the ectopic beat occurs over the preceding T wave). A simple decrease in the rate or severity of the arrhythmia may be a suitable end point to the titration of the antiarrhythmic drugs.

**Table 6-7. Cardiopulmonary and Oxygenation Parameters in Awake and Anesthetized Canines[a]**

| Parameter | Awake[b] | Ketamine[c] | Oxymorphone[d] | Halothane[e] | Pentobarbital[f] |
|---|---|---|---|---|---|
| Weight, kg | 22 ± 5 | 24 ± 6 | 23 ± 3 | 23 ± 3 | 21 ± 5 |
| Temperature, °C | 38.6 ± 0.5 | 38.9 ± 0.6 | 38.2 ± 0.6 | 38.7 ± 0.1 | 38.5 ± 0.7 |
| Heart rate, bpm | 90 ± 21 | 166 ± 44 | 72 ± 14 | 97 ± 13 | 107 ± 20 |
| Arterial pressure, mm Hg | 104 ± 12 | 139 ± 13 | 112 ± 10 | 64 ± 9 | 118 ± 18 |
| Pulmonary arterial pressure, mm Hg | 15 ± 4 | 17 ± 6 | 21 ± 4 | 10 ± 2 | 17 ± 3 |
| CVP, cm $H_2O$ | 3 ± 4 | 2 ± 4 | 12 ± 4 | 2 ± 1 | NR |
| Wedge pressure, mm Hg | 5 ± 2 | NR | 15 ± 2 | 5 ± 2 | NR |
| Cardiac output | | | | | |
| mL/kg/min | 167 ± 39 | 250 ± 85 | 154 ± 42 | 120 ± 23 | 149 ± 18 |
| L/m²/min | 4.67 ± 1.37 | NR | NR | NR | NR |
| Stroke volume | | | | | |
| mL/beat/kg | 1.86 ± 0.4 | 1.5 ± 0.4 | 2.1 ± 0.3 | (1.2) | (1.4) |
| mL/beat/m² | 52.4 ± 12.1 | NR | NR | NR | NR |
| Systemic resistance | | | | | |
| mm Hg/mL/kg/min | 0.64 ± 0.16 | 0.61 ± 0.21 | 0.65 ± 0.14 | 0.55 ± 0.11 | 0.79 ± 0.13 |
| dyn/s/cm⁵ | 1912 ± 526 | NR | NR | NR | NR |
| Pulmonary resistance | | | | | |
| mm Hg/mL/kg/min | 0.05 ± 0.01 | NR | 0.054 ± 0.031 | NR | NR |
| dyn/s/cm⁵ | 186 ± 69 | NR | NR | NR | NR |

Continued

**Table 6-7. (continued)**

| Parameter | Awake[b] | Ketamine[c] | Oxymorphone[d] | Halothane[e] | Pentobarbital[f] |
|---|---|---|---|---|---|
| $Pao_2$, mm Hg | $100 \pm 6$ | $96 \pm 7$ | $81 \pm 6$ | $540 \pm 46$ | $90 \pm 7$ |
| $Pvo_2$, mm Hg | $50 \pm 5$ | $50 \pm 5$ | NR | $81 \pm 8$ | $51 \pm 3$ |
| $Paco_2$, mm Hg | $40 \pm 3$ | $41 \pm 6$ | $50 \pm 2$ | $45 \pm 8$ | $43 \pm 5$ |
| $P_{AO_2}-Pao_2$, mm Hg | $10 \pm 5$ | $6 \pm 3$ | (14) | NR | $12 \pm 5$ |
| Qs/Qt, % | $4 \pm 3$ | $3 \pm 3$ | $13 \pm 6$ | $6 \pm 1$ | $7 \pm 3$ |
| Hemoglobin, g/dL | $131.1 \pm 1.7$ | $14.9 \pm 1.9$ | $16.3 \pm 1.8$ | $14.0 \pm 2.2$ | $14 \pm 1$ |
| $Do_2$ | | | | | |
|   mL/kg/min | $29 \pm 9$ | $47 \pm 16$ | (30) | $23.7 \pm 5.9$ | (28) |
|   mL/m²/min | $811 \pm 252$ | NR | NR | NR | NR |
| $Vo_2$ | | | | | |
|   mL/kg/min | $8 \pm 2$ | $11.9 \pm 4.6$ | NR | $4.5 \pm 0.7$ | $5.3 \pm 1.5$ |
|   mL/m²/min | $217 \pm 71$ | NR | NR | NR | NR |
| $O_2$ extraction, % | $25 \pm 3$ | (25) | NR | $20 \pm 4$ | (19) |

[a]Data expressed as ±1 standard deviation. Numbers in parentheses were not reported but were calculated from the relevant mean values. NR, not reported.
[b]$n = 60$; unmedicated, untrained, left lateral recumbency, breathing room air.
[c]$n = 18$; 15 min after ketamine, 10 mg/kg IV.
[d]$n = 10$; 75 min after oxymorphone, 0.4 mg/kg IV, followed by 0.2 mg/kg at 20, 40, and 60 min.
[e]$n = 11$; 40 min after first exposure to halothane via mask; approximately 30 min after intubation.
[f]$n = 7$; 40 ± 18 min after pentobarbital induction.

2. **Perfusion** of visceral and other peripheral organs is primarily regulated by vasomotor tone. Vasodilation improves peripheral perfusion but, if excessive, causes hypotension. Vasoconstriction may increase blood pressure but decreases peripheral perfusion. Vasomotor tone is assessed

---

**Table 6-8. Causes of Bradycardia**

Anesthetic drugs: opioids, $\alpha_2$-agonists or excessive doses of any general anesthetic

Excessive vagal tone, which may be caused by pharyngeal, laryngeal, or tracheal stimulation by foreign bodies; by pressure on the eyeball or rectus muscles; by visceral inflammation or distention

Hypoxia, as a terminal event

Exogenous toxemia: digitalis, organophosphates

Endogenous toxemia: hypothermia, hypothyroidism, hyperkalemia, or visceral organ failure

Sick sinus syndrome

---

**Table 6-9. Causes of Paroxysmal, Persistent Atrial, or Ventricular Ectopic Pacemaker Activity**

Endogenous release of catecholamines secondary to any stress, exogenous catecholamine therapy

Hypoxia or hypercapnia

Hypovolemia or hypotension

Digitalis toxicity (potentiated by hypokalemia and hypercalcemia)

Hypokalemia (potentiated by respiratory or metabolic alkalosis, glucose, or insulin therapy)

Hyperkalemia (potentiated by acidosis, hypocalcemia, or succinylcholine or may be iatrogenic)

Some anesthetics lower the threshold to endogenous or exogenous catecholamines (inhalants, xylazine, thiamylal, thiopental)

Myocardial inflammation, disease, or stimulation (intracardiac catheters, pleural tubes)

Thoracic and nonthoracic trauma

Congestive or hypertrophic heart failure

Visceral organ disease (gastric volvulus or torsion)

Intracranial disorders (increased pressure, hypoxia)

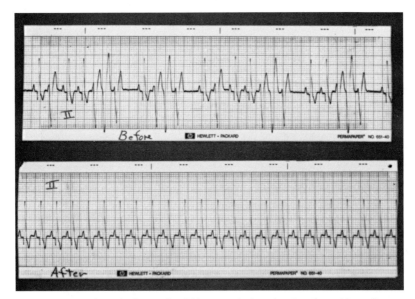

**Figure 6-14.** Ventricular arrhythmias should be treated when they interfere with cardiac output or are sufficiently severe to threaten ventricular fibrillation as seen in upper strip.

by mucous membrane color, capillary refill time, urine output and toe web to core temperature gradient.

3. **Central venous pressure** (CVP) is the luminal pressure of the intrathoracic vena cava (Fig. 6-15). Peripheral venous pressure is variably higher than CVP, is subject to unpredictable extraneous influences, and is not a reliable indicator of CVP. Catheters are usually positioned via the jugular vein into the anterior vena cava. Contact with the endocardium of the right atrium or ventricle should be avoided, because this may stimulate ectopic pacemaker activity. Verification of a well-placed, unobstructed catheter can be ascertained by observing small fluctuations in the fluid meniscus within the manometer that are synchronous with the heart beat and by observing larger excursions that are synchronous with ventilation. A horizontal line drawn between the estimated level of the end of the catheter (the manubrium or thoracic inlet) and the manometer establishes the zero reference level. The vertical difference between the zero level and the meniscus of fluid in the column manometer represents the CVP.

a.     The **normal CVP** in small animals is 0 to 10 cm $H_2O$. Low-range and below-range values indicate relative hypovolemia and suggest that a rapid bolus of fluids might be administered. Above-range values indicate relative hypervolemia and that further fluid therapy should be conservative. CVP is a measure of the relative ability of the heart to pump the venous return; it should be measured when a component of heart failure is suspected.

b.     **Preload** is defined as end-diastolic muscle stretch which, in vivo, is most closely related to end-diastolic volume. CVP is a measure of pressure, not volume, and thus may not truly be representative of preload in diseases associated with reduced ventricular compliance (hypertrophy, tamponade, fibrosis). Diastolic performance (relaxation) is adversely affected by some anesthetics.

c.     CVP measurements are used to determine whether there is room for additional fluid therapy. CVP is an estimate of the relationship between blood volume and blood volume capacity; it should be measured as

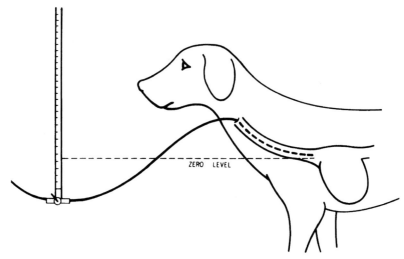

ZERO LEVEL

**Figure 6-15.** The pressure in a central vein depends on venous blood volume, venous vessel tone, and cardiac output. Filling pressure is used as an estimate of preload volume.

an end-point to very large fluid infusions. Subcutaneous edema is not an indication that fluid therapy has been excessive (only that crystalloid therapy has been excessive) and is not an indication of an effective circulating blood volume. Edema may occur in the face of hypovolemia if the patient is hypoproteinemic or if there is increased vascular permeability.

4. **Arterial blood pressure** is the product of cardiac output, vascular capacity and blood volume. Adequate arterial blood pressure establishes a perfusion pressure for the brain and the heart. Because anesthetic drugs and operative procedures can greatly compromise cardiovascular homeostases and because excessive hypotension is not an uncommon cause of perioperative mortality, the measurement and support of arterial blood pressure in patients at risk is extremely important.

   a. **Digital palpation** of the quality of the pulse amplitude in a peripheral artery reflects stroke volume and may bear little correlation to the arterial blood pressure. The weak, thready pulse that occurs with hypovolemia is the result of a small stroke volume; such patients may actually be normotensive, depending on other cardiovascular changes.

   b. **Indirect sphygmomanometry** involves the application of an occlusion cuff over an artery in a cylindrical appendage (Fig. 6-16). The width of the occlusion cuff should be about 40% of the circumference of the leg to which it is applied. The occlusion cuff should be placed snugly around the leg. If it is applied too tightly, the pressure measurements will be erroneously low, because the cuff itself will partially occlude the underlying artery. If the cuff is too loose, the pressure measurements will be erroneously high, because excessive cuff pressure will be required to occlude the underlying artery. Inflation of the cuff applies pressure to the underlying tissues and will totally occlude blood flow when the pressure exceeds the systolic blood pressure. As the cuff

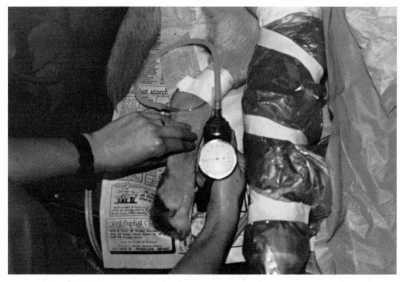

**Figure 6-16.** Systolic arterial blood pressure can be estimated via an occlusion cuff that is placed snugly around a peripheral appendage. The pulse can be detected with a finger, Doppler blood flow detector, or oscillometer.

       pressure is gradually decreased below the luminal systolic pressure, blood will begin to flow intermittently.

c. **Doppler instrumentation** involves the application of a small piezoelectric crystal over an artery. Energy is transmitted into the underlying tissue. The energy frequency reflected from moving tissues is shifted slightly from that which was transmitted, and this frequency difference is converted electronically to an audible signal. Some Doppler instruments measure blood flow and are used for the measurement of systolic blood pressure; other instruments generate signals from the movement of the arterial wall and can be used to measure both systolic and diastolic blood pressures.

d. **Oscillometric technology** simply involves the placement of a cuff around an appendage. The changes in intracuff pressure caused by the changes in appendage size associated with each pulse wave as the cuff is slowly deflated are measured and computed; then systolic, mean, and diastolic blood pressures and the heart rate are digitally displayed. All of these instruments are easily confused by motion artifact. Notwithstanding motion and variation of cuff application, when the instrument can make a measurement, repeat measurements should be within about 20%.

e.  **Direct measurements** of arterial blood pressure are more accurate and continuous compared to indirect methods but require the introduction of a catheter into an artery by percutaneous or cut-down procedure. The dorsal metatarsal artery in dogs and cats is commonly used for percutaneous catheterization. The subcutaneous tissues around these arteries are relatively tight, so that hematoma formation at the time of catheter removal is rarely a problem. The measuring device can be an aneroid manometer (Fig. 6-17). Water or blood must not be allowed to enter the manometer. The manometer can be attached to the catheter by sterile extension tubing. Sterile saline is injected into the tubing toward the manometer via

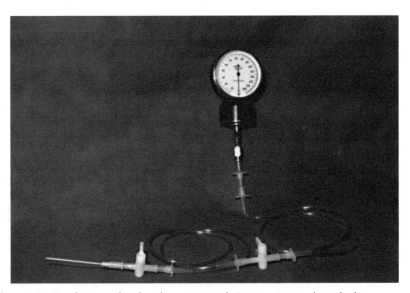

**Figure 6-17.** A catheter can be placed percutaneously into an artery and attached to an aneroid manometer or transducer. Aneroid manometer is shown and provides mean blood pressure data.

a three-way stopcock until the compressed air increases the registered pressure to a level above that of mean blood pressure. The pressurized manometer system is then allowed to equilibrate with the mean blood pressure of the patient. The arterial catheter can also be attached to a commercial transducer and recording system, which is much easier to use for continuous pressure measurement. With modern patient monitors, the transducer can be placed anywhere in reference to the patient, as long as its relative vertical position does not change (in which case the transducer needs to be rezeroed) and the stopcock that is opened to room air is at the level of the heart. The patient monitor will compensate internally with an off-set pressure for any vertical differences between the patient and the transducer and for transducer variances. With older patient monitors without this offset feature, the transducer and the zeroing stopcock should be placed at the level of the heart.

f. **Normal systolic, diastolic, and mean blood pressures** are 100 to 160, 60 to 100, and 80 to 120 mm Hg, respectively. Systolic pressures < 80 and mean pressures < 60 are assumed to result in inadequate cerebral and coronary perfusion and warrant therapy. Hypotension may be caused by hypovolemia, peripheral vasodilation, or reduced myocardial contractility. Hypovolemia (vasodilation causes a relative hypovolemia as well) is the most common cause and should be treated with crystalloids and colloids. The immediate management of heart failure may require sympathomimetic therapy in addition to correction of the underlying systemic disease. A sympathomimetic agent that causes minimal peripheral vasoconstriction should be used for prolonged support (dobutamine or dopamine).

5. **Cardiac output** is a flow parameter and is more relevant to systemic perfusion than is a pressure parameter. Arterial blood pressure may be normal in the face of very low cardiac output and very high peripheral vascular resistance and, therefore, is not the best definition of cardio-

vascular function. Changes in pulse quality (height and width of the pulse pressure wave) provide a rough clinical index to stroke volume. Cardiac output may be reduced by insufficient venous return and end-diastolic ventricular filling volume (hypovolemia, positive pressure ventilation, or disease-induced or surgical inflow occlusion); by ventricular restrictive disease (hypertrophic or restrictive cardiomyopathy, pericardial tamponade, or pericardial fibrosis); by decreased contractility; by excessive bradycardia, tachycardia, or arrhythmias; by regurgitation (retrograde flow) of part of the end-diastolic blood volume owing to insufficient atrioventricular valves; or by outflow tract obstruction (stenosis). Poor cardiac output should be improved before inducing anesthesia by correcting the underlying problem when possible. The dose of anesthetic should be optimized (the least amount that will allow the completion of the surgical procedure). Preload should be optimized. Sympathomimetic therapy is indicated when fluid therapy alone has failed to restore acceptable arterial blood pressure, cardiac output, or tissue perfusion. Adequate blood volume restoration may be functionally defined as a CPV of 5 to 10 cm $H_2O$.

6.  **Oxygen delivery** is the product of cardiac output and blood oxygen content (Fig. 6-13). It is the bottom line of cardiopulmonary function. Disease becomes life-threatening when, despite compensatory mechanisms, oxygen delivery is reduced below the critical level for the patient. Therapeutic intervention is adequate when oxygen delivery is adequate to meet the oxygen consumption needs of the patient. Oxygen consumption is generally reduced during general anesthesia in association with muscular inactivity and hypothermia. A low $Pvo_2$ or a high oxygen extraction calculation suggests either that oxygen delivery is impaired or that oxygen consumption exceeds the amount delivered. When cardiac output is not measured, the adequacy of oxygen delivery must be extrapolated from measured parameters, such as pulse quality, capillary refill time, urine output, toe-web to core temperature gradient, base deficit, $Pvo_2$, and blood lactate concentration.

### D.  Renal Function

The presence of **urine output** is used as an indirect measure of renal blood flow; which in turn can be used as an indirect measure of visceral blood flow. Urine output can be assessed by serial palpation of the urinary bladder or by actual measurement after the aseptic placement of a urinary catheter. Normal urine output should be 1 to 2 mL/kg/h.

### E.  Overall Evaluations and Treatment

Certain parameters, including packed cell volume or hemoglobin; total protein, albumin, and colloid oncotic pressure; platelets and coagulation parameters; and core temperature may be altered during and immediately after the operative period and should be monitored at regular intervals in patients at risk. Most parameters do not merit specific treatment when they are only slightly abnormal. All such abnormalities, when carried to an extreme, however, may harm the patient and thus warrant specific therapy. There is much patient-to-patient variation and a generic definition of a critical point is probably not possible. A heart rate of 60 bpm, for instance, is a commonly recommended critical point; however the actual heart rate at which oxygen delivery becomes insufficient depends on the interplay of all of the other determinants of oxygen delivery. Heart rates of about 50 bpm are not necessarily associated with unacceptable cardiovascular function. For most parameters, there is no critical point but rather a critical range. Specific therapy is warranted if the abnormal value indicates negative overall performance of the organ system or if the performance of the organ system could be improved by specific therapy. If the potential for improving overall organ system performance outweighs the risks and disadvantages of the therapy, it should be given strong consideration.

# Chapter 7

## Airway Management and Ventilation

### Introductory Comments

*Safe anesthesia includes establishing a patent airway, adequate ventilation, and oxygenation. If spontaneous ventilation is insufficient, assisted or controlled ventilation is indicated. If hypoxemia develops, supplemental oxygen is needed.*

**Endotracheal Intubation**
**Techniques for Administration of Oxygen**
**Mechanical Ventilation**
**Guidelines for Mechanical Ventilation**
**Anesthesia Ventilators**
**Guidelines for Use of Anesthesia Ventilators**
**Anesthesia Ventilators for Small Animals**
**Respiratory Assist Devices and Manual Resuscitators**

*Sandee M. Hartsfield*

## I.   ENDOTRACHEAL INTUBATION

Indications for endotracheal intubation include maintenance of a patent airway, protection of the airway from foreign material, application of positive pressure ventilation, application of tracheal or bronchial suction, administration of oxygen, and delivery of inhalant anesthetics. Correct endotracheal intubation reduces anatomic dead space. For inhalant anesthesia, the tube should create a seal with the trachea to prevent leakage of the anesthetic gases. An endotracheal tube is basic, but ancillary equipment may be required. Intubation can be through the oral cavity, nasal passages, an external pharyngotomy, or a tracheostomy.

## A.    Endotracheal Tubes

1.    **A Murphy tube** has an opening, a Murphy eye (side hole), in the wall opposite the bevel; it allows gas flow, if the end hole is occluded. A cuffed Murphy tube is shown in Figure 7-1.

2.    **Cole tubes** are uncuffed and characterized by a shoulder near the distal end (Fig. 7-2). The diameter of the distal end is smaller than the rest of the tube. Only the smaller

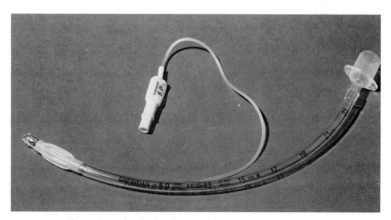

**Figure 7-1.** A Murphy endotracheal tube designed for humans, but commonly used for small animals. Numbers and markings indicate the internal and external diameters (5.0 and 8.0 mm, respectively), the length of the tube from the patient end (13, 15, 17, 19, 21, and 23 cm), the manufacturer (Sheridan), and an indication of tissue toxicity testing (Z79). The internal diameter (5.0 mm) and manufacturer are also shown on the pilot balloon.

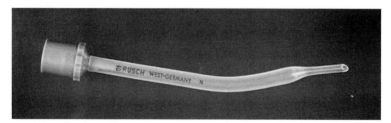

**Figure 7-2.** French–Cole endotracheal tube, appropriate for small veterinary patients. Note the smaller diameter of the laryngotracheal portion of the tube (distal end of the tube, to the *right*).

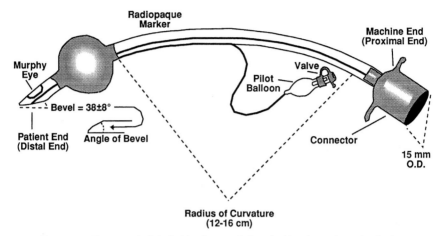

**Figure 7-3.** The parts and desirable characteristics of a Murphy endotracheal tube.

portion fits into the larynx and trachea. Fitting the shoulder against the arytenoid cartilages creates a seal, but excess pressure against the laryngeal cartilages and within the lumen may be deleterious.

3. Endotracheal tubes are made from **polyvinyl chloride,** rubber, silicone, and other plastic or rubberized materials. Endotracheal tubes should be clear to allow inspection for cleanliness and obstructions. Red rubber tubes are opaque, prone to cracking, and difficult to clean and disinfect; they are not recommended.

4. **The components** of a cuffed endotracheal tube include a connector to the breathing system (15 mm outside diameter; od), the tube itself, and a cuff system (inflating valve, inflating tube, pilot balloon) (Fig. 7-3). Some tubes include the size (od) in French units (French size is equal to the od in millimeters times $\pi$). Radiopaque markers are present in some tubes.

5. **Inflating the cuff** applies pressure to the tracheal mucosa (perfusion pressure ranges from 25 to 35 mm Hg). A cuff

pressure of 20 to 25 mm Hg usually does not interfere with mucosal blood flow; but higher pressures may cause ischemic injury, perhaps leading to tracheal strictures in serious cases. The cuff should be inflated with the smallest amount of air that will be effective.

6. **Armored or reinforced endotracheal tubes** are designed with helical wire or plastic implanted within the walls to prevent kinking of the tube and obstruction of the airway when the patient's head and neck are flexed (Fig. 7-4). Such tubes are useful for ophthalmic surgery, cervical spinal taps, myelograms, oral surgery, and head and neck surgery.

7. Providing an airway through a **tracheostomy or an external pharyngotomy** may be necessary for obtaining a patent airway. Cuffed tracheostomy tubes with 15-mm-od connectors are available (Fig. 7-5).

8. Direct application of a **local anesthetic** (e.g., lidocaine) to the larynx may prevent laryngeal spasms in susceptible animals, e.g., cats (Fig. 7-6). The local anesthetic can be sprayed into the larynx, applied with a cotton swab, or squirted from a syringe and hypodermic needle. When spraying local anesthetic onto the larynx, the clinician can easily exceed the toxic dose for small patients.

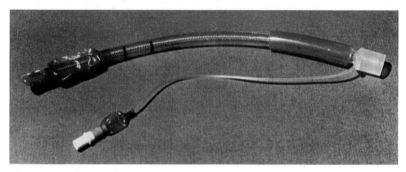

**Figure 7-4.** An armored endotracheal tube with a spiral wire embedded in the wall. The endotracheal tube connector, bite guard near the proximal end of the tube, inflatable cuff, pilot balloon, inflation line, and self-sealing inflation valve are present.

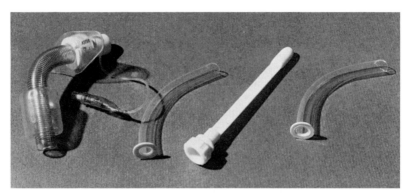

**Figure 7-5.** A cuffed tracheostomy tube (*far left*) designed for humans but applicable to veterinary patients. *Left to right:* cuffed tracheostomy tube with inflation line and pilot balloon, removable lumen for the tube, obturator to facilitate insertion, and another removable lumen.

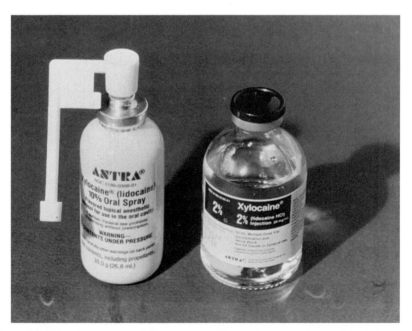

**Figure 7-6.** Lidocaine as a spray (*left*) or as a liquid (applied with a cotton swab or delivered by squirting it with a syringe and needle) can be applied topically to the larynx to facilitate endotracheal intubation in some species. With either method of delivery, the anesthetist should make sure the total dose of lidocaine remains below the toxic dose for the patient and species involved.

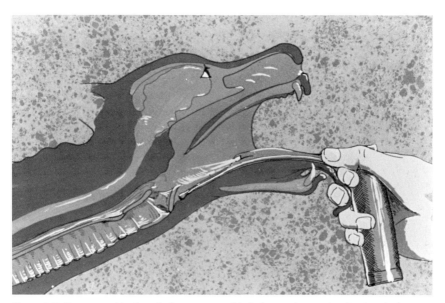

**Figure 7-7.** Correct positioning of a laryngoscope blade for maximum visualization the larynx. Note that the dog's mouth is opened widely, the tongue is extended from the mouth maximally, and the tip of the laryngoscope blade is positioned at the base of the epiglottis.

9. After use, endotracheal and tracheostomy tubes should be scrubbed with a soft brush, rinsed, dried, and **sterilized or disinfected.** If ethylene oxide– or hydrogen peroxide–based sterilization is not available, chemical disinfectants (e.g., glutaraldehyde) can be used. After disinfection, tubes should be rinsed thoroughly and dried.

10. **Laryngoscopy** is required for endotracheal intubation of some species. The laryngoscope's light source may be the main benefit, but the blade can be used to manipulate the tongue, soft palate, and epiglottis to view the glottis (Fig. 7-7). Useful blades include the Miller, McIntosh, and Bizarri-Guiffrida (Fig. 7-8).

## B. Techniques of Endotracheal Intubation

1. *Dogs*
   Dogs are positioned in **sternal recumbency** for intubation. An assistant holds the head with one hand, placing a finger and thumb beside the maxillary canine teeth and

pulling the lips upward to create the best field of view. With the other hand, the assistant opens the dog's mouth widely and extends its tongue. In small patients, dogs with oral or pharyngeal lesions, and brachycephalic dogs, a laryngoscope facilitates intubation and should be available if difficulty should arise.

a.   **Sizes of endotracheal tubes** for dogs range from 1.5 to 15 mm internal diameter (id). Breed differences preclude generalizations about the choice of tube diameter based on body weight. For example, a 25-kg (55 lb) English bulldog usually accepts only about a 7.5-mm-id tube, but a 25-kg (55 lb) mixed breed dog may easily accept a 10-mm-id tube. Most tubes designed for humans are too long for dogs and should be cut proximally to fit (Fig. 7-9).

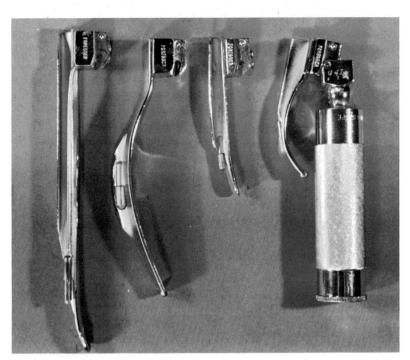

**Figure 7-8. Left to right:** adult Miller laryngoscope blade, adult Bizarri-Guiffrida blade, pediatric Miller blade, and pediatric Bizarri-Guiffrida blade on a laryngoscope handle. The Bizarri-Guiffrida blades allow the maximum field of view without the interference of a flange.

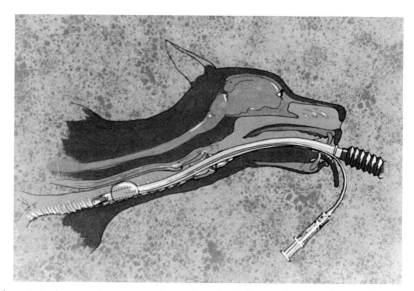

**Figure 7-9.** The correct placement of an endotracheal tube in a dog. Note that the connector is located near the incisors to minimize mechanical dead space and that the cuffed end of the tube is in the cervical trachea near the thoracic inlet.

b. **Extubation** should be done when oral and pharyngeal reflexes have returned. The tube should be pulled directly between the upper and lower incisors.

2. *Cats*

Intubation in most cats requires an endotracheal tube and light source; however, a laryngoscope, stylet to stiffen the tube, guide tube (canine polyethylene urinary catheter), sterile water-soluble lubricant, mouth speculum, and local anesthetic may be useful. Inadequate depth of anesthesia is probably the most common reason for difficult intubation.

a. **Sizes of tubes** for domestic cats range from 1.5 to ~ 5.5 mm id; most adult cats readily accept 4.0- to 4.5-mm-id tubes, allowing optimal internal diameter with minimal difficulty in intubation. An option is to use a Cole tube.

b. The cat should be positioned in **sternal recumbency.** Local anesthetic (0.5% lidocaine) applied to the larynx may desensitize the arytenoid cartilages and epiglottis, facilitating intubation and preventing laryngospasm. An assistant holds the head with one hand, placing a finger and thumb beside the cat's maxillary canine teeth and pulling the lips upward to create the best field of view (Figs. 7-10 and 7-11). With the other hand, the assistant extends the tongue. With a good light source, most cats can be intubated without a laryngoscope, but a laryngoscope is helpful. The blade should not touch the arytenoid cartilages or the epiglottis, because that may cause active closure of the glottis. A laryngoscope should always be available for a difficult intubation (e.g., oral or pharyngeal lesions). The routine use of a guide tube (5- to 8-Fr canine urinary catheter) that extends past the cuffed end of the endotracheal tube for a distance of 2 or 3 cm makes feline intubation very easy. As the endotracheal tube is advanced toward the glottis, rotating it from 0° to 90° or more will facilitate its passage.

c.  **Extubation** should be done when oral and pharyngeal reflexes have returned. The tube should be pulled directly between the upper and lower incisors.

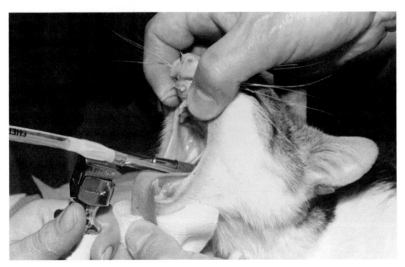

**Figure 7-10.** An excellent method of positioning a cat for endotracheal intubation. Note the secure grip on the maxilla with the index finger and thumb caudal to the canine teeth. The tongue is extended, maximizing the field view.

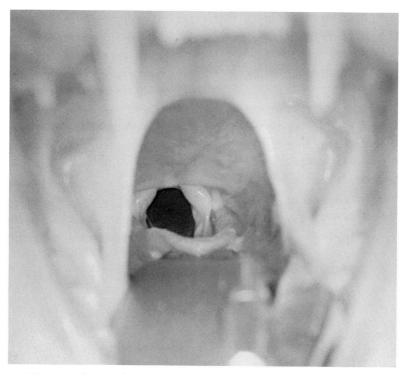

**Figure 7-11.** View of a cat's glottis using the restraint and positioning shown in Figure 7-10. The laryngoscope blade is placed on the tongue, with the tip just ventral to the epiglottis.

3.  *Rabbits and Small Laboratory Animals*

    Most techniques for intubation of rabbits and small labora-
    tory animals include the use of a laryngoscope or a modi-
    fied otoscope to expose the glottis, a catheter or stylet for a
    guide tube, small-diameter lubricated endotracheal tube,
    and lidocaine to desensitize the larynx. Laboratory rabbits
    weighing about 3.0 kg (6.6 lb) usually require 3.5-mm-id,
    14-cm-long tubes.

    a.  Rabbits should be intubated in **sternal recumbency,**
        with the head and neck extended and the fleshy
        tongue gently withdrawn from the mouth (Fig. 7-12).
        The head can be held with a piece of rolled gauze
        placed caudal to the maxillary incisors. A size-0
        Miller laryngoscope blade (75 mm long) is used to
        expose the glottis; the blade is carefully manipulated

lateral to the maxillary incisors; into the mouth; and over the base of the tongue to expose the soft palate, epiglottis, and glottis. Then a guide tube (5-Fr canine urinary catheter) can be passed through the larynx and into the trachea, about 2 cm past the glottis. The guide tube should not be forced; the trachea is easily torn, leading to subcutaneous emphysema, pneumothorax, pneumomediastinum, pneumoabdomen, and death. The endotracheal tube is passed over the guide tube, through the larynx, and into the trachea (Fig. 7-12). The cuff should be inflated minimally, the pilot balloon should remain soft, and a leak around the cuff should occur at an inspiratory pressure of ~ 15 cm $H_2O$. Alternatively, in large rabbits, a blind approach to intubation is often successful when the head and neck are maximally extended and the endotracheal tube is advanced into the remiglottis. Intubation of the trachea is expedited by listening for air movement through the tube while gently advancing it into the trachea.

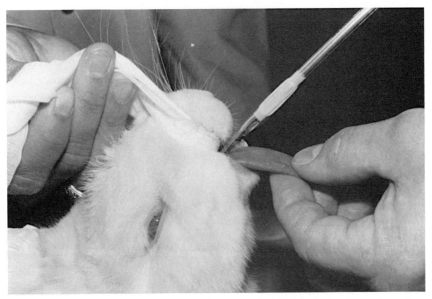

**Figure 7-12.** Endotracheal intubation in a rabbit. The endotracheal tube is advanced over the guide tube and into the mouth. The distal end of the guide tube is located 2 cm caudal to the cricoid cartilage.

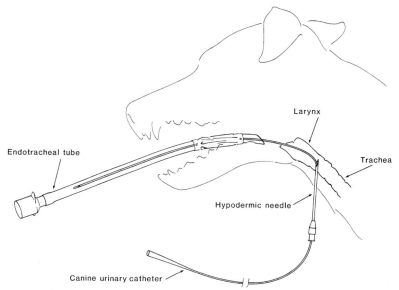

**Figure 7-13.** The placement and use of a retrograde guide tube for passage of an endotracheal tube. This technique is reserved for patients that cannot be intubated by other methods. Reprinted with permission from Hartsfield SM. Alternate methods of endotracheal intubation in small animals: emphasis on patients with oropharyngeal pathology. Tex Vet Med J 1985;47:25.

4.  *Birds and Reptiles*
    Intubation of birds and reptiles that commonly undergo anesthesia is relatively easy. The glottis is usually located on the midline at the base of the tongue and is readily apparent when the mouth is opened. Appropriately sized tubes should be selected. In small birds and reptiles, mucus may collect in the distal end of the tube.

## C.  Special Techniques for Endotracheal Intubation

1.  Use of a **retrograde guide tube** or wire involves passing a hypodermic needle through the skin of the neck and into the trachea at the junction of the second and third tracheal rings. A guide wire is then maneuvered through the needle cranially into the larynx, pharynx, and oral cavity until it can be used as a guide for passage of an endotracheal tube (Fig. 7-13). The cuff should be located

caudal to the puncture site of the hypodermic needle to avoid forcing gases subcutaneously or into the mediastinum during positive pressure ventilation.

2. Intubation by **external pharyngotomy** may be appropriate for selected patients that require oropharyngeal surgery or orthopedic procedures of the mandible or maxilla. Major advantages are improved visualization within the operative field during oropharyngeal surgery and normal dental occlusion to aid in the proper reduction of mandibular or maxillary fractures. Hemostats are bluntly passed through the skin incision into the caudal part of the pharynx. After removing the adapter, the clinician grasps the adapter end of the tube and pulls it from the pharynx, through the subcutaneous tissue and skin incision. The adapter is replaced, and the tube is reconnected to the breathing system. The tube should be secured to the skin with tape and several sutures.

3. Laryngoscopy with a flexible **fiber-optic endoscope** can be useful for intubation in patients with abnormal anatomy or disease processes involving the larynx, pharynx, or head and neck. Depending on the species and the specific conditions, the endoscope can be placed inside the endotracheal tube to directly guide intubation or passed orally beside the endotracheal tube.

4. A temporary **tracheostomy** may be the only reasonable option for intubation in certain cases, and some patients arrive in the induction room with a tracheostomy tube in place. A tracheostomy tube with a replaceable lumen should be used if available, but standard endotracheal tubes are satisfactory.

## D. Extubation of the Trachea

1. Extubation is performed after patients regain the ability to swallow and protect their airways. When the cuff is deflated, the endotracheal tube is removed slowly and deliberately; take care to avoid damaging tissues with the endotracheal tube and damaging the cuff as the tube passes the teeth. The pharynx should be inspected visually, and any

debris should be removed after extubation. Animals anesthetized for gastrointestinal surgery are prone to passive movement of fluid into the pharynx (e.g., gastric dilation and volvulus in a dog). The patient's head should be positioned to allow drainage of fluid from the pharynx and mouth before the cuff of the endotracheal tube is deflated. It may be prudent to remove the endotracheal tube with the cuff inflated for patients that have had fluid in the pharynx during surgery. The anesthetist should be prepared to manage the airway at the time of extubation, knowing that complications can impair ventilation and oxygenation. In some cases of postextubation airway obstruction, reanesthetizing the patient and reintubation may be the only feasible option.

## II.  TECHNIQUES FOR ADMINISTRATION OF OXYGEN

**Supplemental oxygen** in anesthetized and critical patients increases the partial pressure of oxygen in arterial blood ($Pa_{O_2}$) and promotes delivery of oxygen to the tissues. When a patient breathes room air, values for $Pa_{O_2}$ < 80 mm Hg indicate the potential for hypoxemia. If the $Pa_{O_2}$ decreases < 60 mm Hg, supplemental oxygen is indicated. Several **techniques** can be used to administer oxygen to anesthetized and critically ill patients.

### A.  Masks for Delivery of Oxygen

Masks require constant attention, and some patients will not accept a mask unless sedated. Both factors limit the effectiveness of masks in awake patients. Indeed, some patients object to a mask vigorously, increase their oxygen consumption, and nullify the benefits of a greater $F_{I_{O_2}}$.

1.  **Flow rates** for increasing $F_{I_{O_2}}$ when using masks are variable, usually ranging from 3 to 5 L/min in dogs and cats.

2.  A mask should be used with a **breathing system with a reservoir** that is capable of supplying tidal volume demands or with a valved system that allows room air to be entrained. For example, a dog with a tidal volume of 300 mL and an inspiratory time of 1 s has a peak inspiratory gas flow of approximately 18 L, which exceeds the practical flow rate for oxygen during masking. High inspiratory

flow rates can be provided if the mask is attached to a circle breathing system with a reservoir bag. In addition, a breathing system has an overflow valve to prevent the buildup of excessive pressure with a tight-fitting mask.

### B.    Nasal Insufflation of Oxygen

1.    **Insufflation** involves delivery of oxygen into the patient's airway at relatively high flow rates (Fig. 7-14). The patient inspires both oxygen and room air; their relative proportions of the gases are determined primarily by the oxygen flow rate and the rate of gas flow during inspiration.

2.    Insufflation can be accomplished by a variety of methods. For most awake veterinary patients, oxygen is insufflated through a **nasal catheter,** the tip of which is positioned in the nasopharynx. The catheter is usually made of soft rubber, and the tube should have several fenestrations to prevent jetting lesions from developing in the nasopharyngeal mucosa. For awake small animals, instilling 2% lidocaine into the nasal passage with the patient's head and neck extended and held upward may facilitate passage of

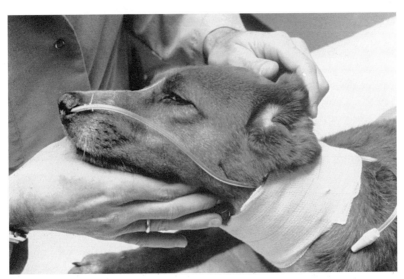

**Figure 7-14.** A nasal catheter for administration of oxygen in dogs. The tube is secured to the muzzle with suture.

the tube. The external portion of the catheter is secured to the patient's head with tissue adhesive, tape, and/or sutures.

3. The **flow rate requirements** for oxygen during insufflation are quite variable; the patient's ventilation and the desired $F_{IO_2}$ are two important factors. In small animals, flow rates of 1 to 7 L/min are typical. To prevent mucosal drying, oxygen should be flowed through a bubble-type humidifier.

## C. Tracheal Insufflation of Oxygen

1. An **intratracheal catheter** placed percutaneously through the cricothyroid membrane or between tracheal rings near the larynx can be used to insufflate oxygen to a compromised patient.

2. An intratracheal catheter should be placed aseptically, should be of the over-the-needle type with a relatively large bore, should have several smooth fenestrations to prevent jet lesions, and should be positioned with the tip near the bronchial bifurcation. **Oxygen should be humidified,** and flow rates should approximate those for nasal insufflation.

## D. Oxygen Cages

1. Oxygen cages regulate oxygen flow, control humidity and temperature, and eliminate carbon dioxide. Typically, the flow rates of oxygen are <10 L/min, cage temperature is 22°C (72°F), and cage humidity is 40 to 50%. With such flows, most cages produce an oxygen concentration of 40 to 50%. The effectiveness of an oxygen cage diminishes as body size increases. Thus nasal insufflation of oxygen has supplanted oxygen cages in many instances.

2. **Smaller patients** can be managed relatively easily in oxygen cages, but temperature and humidity are more difficult to control with larger dogs. A major disadvantage of an oxygen cage is that the animal must be removed from the cage for examination and treatment.

### E.   Oxygen Toxicity

Oxygen toxicity develops with prolonged exposure to high oxygen concentrations. It leads to the deterioration of pulmonary function, pulmonary edema, and death. Significant species and individual variability exists in the development of oxygen toxicity. In dogs, microscopic and early pulmonary effects of oxygen toxicity develop within 24 h of exposure to 100% oxygen. As a guideline, **40 to 50% oxygen is generally safe.**

## III.   MECHANICAL VENTILATION

### A.   Hypoventilation

Essentially all anesthetized patients hypoventilate; they may not maintain $Paco_2$ values near 40 mm Hg. Although controlled ventilation is not always necessary, various circumstances may compel the anesthetist to employ **intermittent positive pressure ventilation** (IPPV). The absolute indication for IPPV is apnea; but IPPV should be instituted if hypoventilation becomes significant, if neuromuscular-blocking drugs are employed, or if intrathoracic surgery is performed.

### B.   Carbon Dioxide

Normalizing **arterial carbon dioxide tensions (35 to 45 mm Hg)** is a goal of mechanical ventilation in anesthetized patients. Controversy exists about routine use of IPPV in anesthetized patients, simply to keep the $Paco_2$ near 40 mm Hg. Because IPPV may reduce cardiovascular function and moderate increases in $Paco_2$ are associated with improvement in some cardiovascular variables, IPPV for every anesthetized patient is not universally accepted or practiced. Inotropic drugs may be necessary to improve cardiovascular function during surgical anesthesia in mechanically ventilated animals.

### C.   Hypercapnia

**Inhalant anesthetics** and epidural or spinal anesthesia reduce the circulatory responses to $CO_2$. Hypercapnia has been related to enhanced vagal responsiveness, bradycardia, and even cardiac arrest. Hypercapnia may not stimulate vagal activity directly, but may predispose the patient to cardiac arrest with vagal stimulation. Carbon dioxide produces narcosis in dogs. Hypercapnia and the associated increases in circulating catecholamines have been linked to the development of cardiac arrhythmias, especially when the heart has been sensitized by halogenated inhalant anesthetics.

### D. Mechanical Ventilation

**Mechanical ventilation** may impede venous return to the right heart, leading to decreases in stroke volume, cardiac output, and arterial blood pressure. In the anesthetized, mechanically ventilated patient, a reduction in blood pressure and damping of the pressure waveform is not uncommon, especially in a critically ill patient with a marginal blood volume. The negative effects of mechanical ventilation on cardiovascular function can be exacerbated by prolonging inspiratory time, holding positive pressure in the lungs at the end of inspiration, retarding exhalation, applying positive pressure during the expiratory phase, and employing an excessively rapid respiratory rate. Fortunately, these negative effects can often be overcome by the appropriate expansion of extracellular fluid volume and administration of inotropic drugs.

## IV. GUIDELINES FOR MECHANICAL VENTILATION

Guidelines for mechanical ventilation include values for inspiratory time, respiratory rate, inspiratory to expiratory time ratio, and tidal volume. Variations exist owing to differences in body size, species, condition of the lungs and thorax, and existing disease processes.

### A. Tidal Volume

For IPPV, the **tidal volume** set on the ventilator is usually greater than the spontaneous tidal volume to compensate for pressure-mediated increases in the volume of the breathing system and airways. The recommended setting for tidal volume in small animals is 20 mL/kg.

### B. Inspiratory Time

**Inspiratory time** compared to the time of the entire expiratory phase is the **I:E ratio**. That ratio should be 1:2 (I:E) or less for mechanical ventilation. Ratios approaching 1:1 result in a long duration of positive intrathoracic pressure, interfering with cardiovascular function. If respiratory rate is 10 breaths/min and the inspiratory time is 1.5 s, the I:E ratio equals 1:3.

### C.     Peak Inspiratory Pressure

Tidal volume and inspiratory time affect the development of **peak inspiratory pressure.** In general, 15 to 30 cm $H_2O$ will expand the lung; 15 to 20 cm $H_2O$ is the common range for peak inspiratory pressure for small animals with normal lungs. Excessive or sustained pressure during IPPV can cause disruption of the alveolar membrane. Peak inspiratory pressure should not exceed 30 cm $H_2O$.

### D.     Respiratory Rate

The appropriate **respiratory rate for IPPV** varies with the species and the tidal volume selected. Commonly, dogs are ventilated at 8 to 14 breaths/min, and cats at 10 to 14 breaths/min. In patients requiring smaller tidal volumes to avoid excessive inspiratory pressures (e.g., diaphragmatic hernia, gastrointestinal distension), respiratory rates should be increased to maintain minute ventilation.

### E.     Discontinuing Mechanical Ventilation

When **controlled ventilation is discontinued,** the return of spontaneous ventilation may be impaired. If $Paco_2$ is low, spontaneous ventilation may not resume. During controlled ventilation, the $Paco_2$ should remain relatively normal, avoiding hypocarbia in most cases. In general, the $Paco_2$ must increase to stimulate spontaneous ventilation, or the patient must regain a level of consciousness that promotes spontaneous ventilation. Reducing the rate of controlled ventilation usually increases the $Paco_2$ enough to stimulate spontaneous breathing as the animal regains consciousness. Generally, the patient is mechanically or manually ventilated at a rate of 1 to 4 breaths/min until spontaneous ventilation resumes. After spontaneous breathing begins, assisted ventilation and oxygen should be provided until the respiratory rate and tidal volume normalize.

## V.     ANESTHESIA VENTILATORS

Anesthesia ventilators provide mechanical ventilation for patients being maintained with inhalant anesthetics. An **anesthesia ventilator** is a reservoir bag (a bellows) in a closed container (housing) that can substitute for the reservoir bag of a breathing system. Within limits, the ventilator drives its bellows to produce a specific tidal volume or a specific inspiratory pressure at a preselected rate. It performs the job of the anesthetist who squeezes the breathing system's reservoir bag to ventilate the patient. Anesthesia ventilators are usually double-circuit units with two gas sources: the driving gas circuit (outside the bellows), which compresses the bellows, and the patient gas circuit (inside the bellows), which originates at the anesthesia machine and provides oxygen and anesthetic to the breathing system (Fig. 7-15). The classification and characteristics of some small animal ventilators are given in Table 7-1.

## A.  Terminology

1.  *IPPV*

    With **IPPV,** airway pressure is maintained above ambient pressure during inspiration, and falls to ambient pressure to allow passive expiration. Assist-control mode ventilation (**AMV**) provides a preset tidal volume from the ventilator in response to patient-initiated attempts to inspire; the ventilator delivers a preset frequency if the patient fails to initiate breathing. The term *intermittent positive pressure breathing* (IPPB) is synonymous with IPPV.

2.  *Positive End-Expiratory Pressure*

    With positive end-expiratory pressure (**PEEP**), airway pressure at end expiration is maintained above the ambient pressure. The term PEEP is applied when positive pressure is maintained between the inspirations delivered by a ventilator.

3.  *Continuous Positive Airway Pressure*

    The term *continuous positive airway pressure* (**CPAP**) (instead of PEEP) is used if airway pressure remains above the ambient pressure during spontaneous breathing.

4.  *Intermittent Mandatory Ventilation*

    Intermittent mandatory ventilation (**IMV**) is the periodic sigh that the anesthetist provides manually during spontaneous ventilation to expand the lungs and decrease collapsed alveoli in anesthetized animals. It is used for

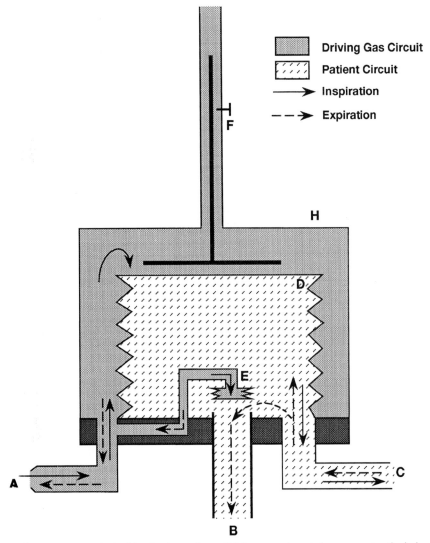

**Figure 7-15.** A generic double-circuit ventilator. Driving gas enters at *A*, compressing the bellows and forcing the gas in the patient circuit toward the breathing system and the patient's respiratory system (*C*). Overflow gas from the patient circuit exits through the pop-off valve (*E*) and flows into the scavenger system (*B*). Also shown are the tidal volume adjustment (*F*), the bellows (*D*), and the bellows housing (*H*).

**Table 7-1. Classification and Characteristics of Anesthesia Ventilators**

| Ventilator | Power Source | Drive Mechanism | Cycling Mechanism | Bellows | Type of Ventilation |
|---|---|---|---|---|---|
| Drager SAV | Pneumatic | Pneumatic | Time fluidic | Ascending | Controlled |
| Hallowell EMC 2000 | Pneumatic and electronic | Pneumatic | Time electronic | Ascending | Controlled |
| Mallard 2400 | Pneumatic and electronic | Pneumatic | Time electronic | Ascending | Controlled |
| Ohio Metomatic | Pneumatic | Pneumatic | Time fluidic | Descending | Assisted and controlled |
| Ohmeda 7000 | Pneumatic and electronic | Pneumatic | Time electronic | Ascending | Controlled |
| Anesco SAV 2500 | Pneumatic and electronic | Pneumatic | Time electronic | Ascending | Controlled |
| ADS 1000 | Pneumatic and electronic | Pneumatic | Time electronic | None | Controlled |

ventilatory support and for weaning patients from ventilators. The patient breathes spontaneously, but mechanical breaths are inserted at a preset volume and frequency.

5.  *Assisted Ventilation*

    **Assisted ventilation** can be performed manually by the anesthetist, who synchronizes compression of the breathing bag with the patient's spontaneous breath to augment the tidal volume. When a ventilator is used, assisted ventilation is patient initiated (negative pressure on inspiration), and the ventilator delivers a preselected tidal volume.

6.  *Controlled Ventilation*

    During **controlled ventilation** (defined for CMV), inspiration is initiated by the ventilator, and a preset respiratory rate is maintained. The ventilator controls frequency, tidal volume, and minute volume. Controlled ventilation is necessary if the patient is unable to initiate an adequate number of breaths. Controlled ventilation can be provided manually by the anesthetist, who uses the reservoir bag of the breathing system to establish rate, tidal volume, and minute volume.

7.  *Assisted-Controlled Ventilation*

    **Assisted-controlled ventilation** has been defined as assisted ventilation (patient-controlled rate with ventilator-controlled tidal volume) with a preset minimum acceptable respiratory rate. If the patient-initiated rate falls below the preset rate, the ventilator cycles at the minimum preset rate. Assisted-controlled ventilation has been suggested for the transition period between controlled and spontaneous ventilation.

## VI.  GUIDELINES FOR USE OF ANESTHESIA VENTILATORS

The controls on most anesthesia ventilators include settings for tidal volume, inspiratory time, inspiratory pressure, respiratory rate, and I:E ratio (either adjustable or preset). Other controls may be present. The setting for tidal volume is usually between 10 and 20 mL/kg, and the inspiratory pressure is normally between 12 and 30 cm $H_2O$. The respiratory rate should be set between 8 and 14 breaths/min. Inspiratory time should be short compared to expiratory time, so that positive interpleural pressure will minimally interfere with venous return and cardiac output. Inspiratory time should be 1 to 1.5 s. Therefore, the I:E ratio should be 1:2 or less (e.g., 1:3 or 1:4), depending on the respiratory rate.

## VII. ANESTHESIA VENTILATORS FOR SMALL ANIMALS

The following ventilators are appropriate for small animals. Some were designed specifically to support anesthetized veterinary patients; others were designed for human use but are applicable to veterinary patients. Before use, the proper connections to the gas supply and scavenger system should be made, and the appropriate pre-use checkout should be done.

### A. Drager SAV

The **Drager SAV small animal ventilator** was marketed as an optional component for the Drager Narkovet 2 anesthesia machine and was available on a mobile stand (Fig 7-16). It is not being manufactured but remains in use for veterinary anesthesia.

### B. Hallowell EMC Model 2000

The **Hallowell EMC Model 2000 small animal veterinary anesthesia ventilator** is designed for use with standard small animal anesthesia machines and breathing systems (Fig. 7-17); the connections to the breathing system, scavenger, and driving gas are shown in Figure 7-18. Three sizes of interchangeable bellows and housings are available (Fig. 7-19). Tidal volume can be set from 20 mL to 3 L; spontaneous ventilation from the bellows is allowed when the ventilator is not in operation.

### C. Mallard Medical Model 2400V

The **Mallard Medical Model 2400V anesthesia ventilator** was originally designed for anesthetized pediatric and adult human patients (Fig. 7-20). For veterinary use, it is a stand-alone unit for use with a breathing system and anesthesia machine. Two sizes of bellows are available. The adult bellows provides tidal volumes ranging from 200 to 2200 mL; the pediatric bellows produces volumes ranging from 50 to 300 mL.

*Text continued on p. 320.*

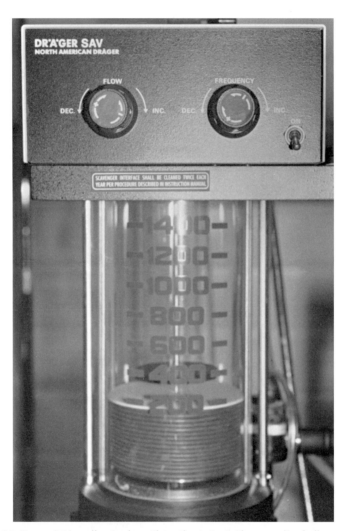

**Figure 7-16.** Drager SAV small animal ventilator (front view). The ascending bellows and the bellows housing with the tidal volume marked in milliliters are shown at the *bottom;* and the inspiratory flow control knob (*left*), frequency control knob (*center right*), and power switch (*far right*) are shown at the *top.*

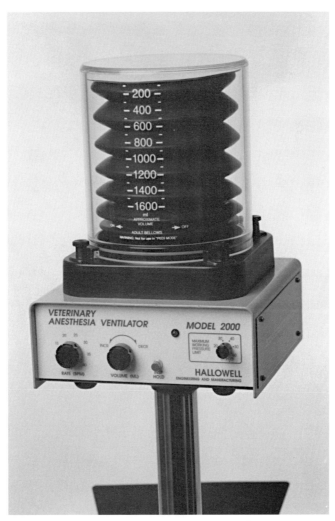

**Figure 7-17.** Hallowell EMC Model 2000 small animal veterinary anesthesia ventilator (front view). The bellows shown is the medium-sized bellows for tidal volumes between 300 and 1600 mL, and the basic control knobs and alarm indicator light are on the front panel. Courtesy of W. Stetson Hallowell.

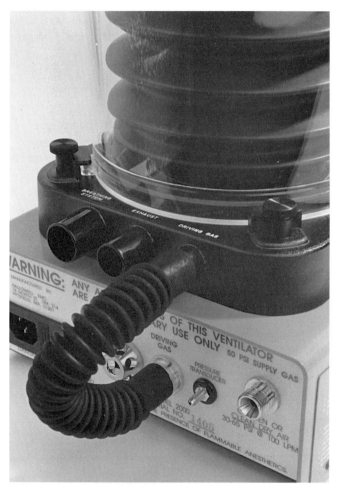

**Figure 7-18.** Hallowell EMC Model 2000 Small animal veterinary anesthesia ventilator (rear view). Note the connectors on the bellows housing for the breathing system, scavenger system (exhaust), and driving gas. The port for connecting the pressure transducer to the breathing system, the diameter index safety system connector for the driving gas supply, and the electric connector (*left*) are shown. Courtesy of W. Stetson Hallowell.

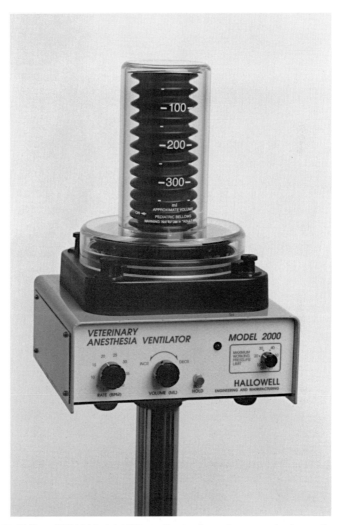

**Figure 7-19.** Hallowell EMC Model 2000 small animal veterinary anesthesia ventilator (front view). The smallest bellows, for tidal volumes between 0 and 300 mL, is shown. The basic control knobs and alarm indicator light are on the front panel. Courtesy of W. Stetson Hallowell.

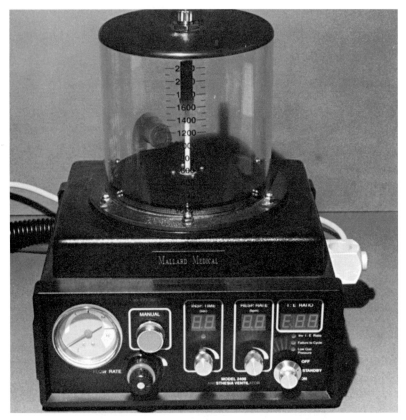

**Figure 7-20.** Mallard 2400V small animal anesthesia ventilator. The bellows is collapsed on the floor of the bellows housing. The tidal volume control is set at ~ 1600 mL. See the text for details.

### D.   Metomatic

The **Metomatic veterinary ventilator** was designed to ventilate anesthetized small animals being maintained with circle systems (Fig. 7-21). It is no longer being manufactured, but many units are still in operation in veterinary hospitals.

### E.   Ohmeda 7000

The **Ohmeda 7000** is a double-circuit ventilator with an ascending bellows that is pneumatically driven and electronically controlled with a preset minute volume (Fig. 7-22). It is specifically designed as an anesthesia ventilator and can be fitted with either an adult or a pediatric bellows. The 7000 and upgraded models are readily applicable to small animal anesthesia. The Ohmeda 7800 series of ventilators is an advanced group of machines. The 7800 is available as a stand-alone unit and potentially could be applied to small animal patients. A major difference between the 7000 and the 7800 units is that tidal volume, rather than minute ventilation, is selected, which appears to be a significant advantage.

**F.    Anesco SAV 2500**

The **Anesco SAV 2500 small animal anesthesia ventilator** was designed, according to the manufacturer, to be easy to use and particularly effective in the area of anesthesia ventilation. The ventilator can be mounted on an anesthesia machine, or it can be prepared as a portable ventilator for use with multiple anesthesia machines. It is intended to provide controlled ventilation and has an ascending bellows.

**G.    Vet-Tec SAV-75**

The **Vet-Tec SAV-75 anesthesia ventilator** is designed for small animal anesthesia. The bellows ascends on expiration and is

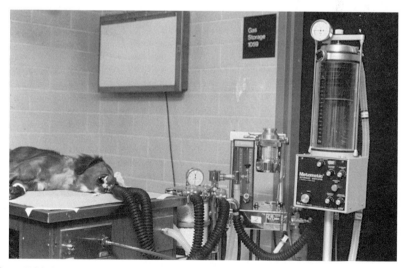

**Figure 7-21.** Metomatic veterinary ventilator. The ventilator's bellows is connected by a corrugated breathing tube to the reservoir bag port of the circle breathing system, allowing controlled ventilation.

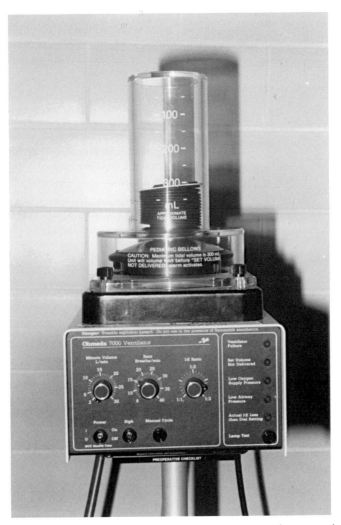

**Figure 7-22.** Ohmeda 7000 ventilator. The control module is shown with six controls on the left two-thirds of the panel and six warning indicators on the right two-thirds of the panel. This ventilator is equipped with a pediatric bellows assembly for a tidal volume of 0 to 300 mL.

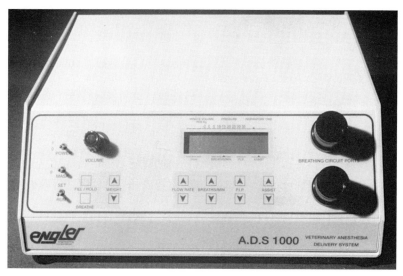

**Figure 7-23.** ADS 1000 veterinary anesthesia delivery system and critical care ventilator. The ports for the breathing hoses are located on the right side of the ventilator, and the controls for the ventilator are located on the front panel of the console.

pneumatically driven by a Bird ventilator. Used without a bellows, Bird ventilators are classed as single-circuit ventilators, but the SAV-75 performs as a double-circuit unit. This ventilator can be used in assist, control, or assist-control modes. The Bird ventilator supplies gas to pressurize the space between the bellows and the bellows housing (canister) to force the bellows downward, which delivers gases from the bellows through the interface hose (corrugated breathing tube) to the breathing system.

## H.   ADS 1000

The **ADS 1000 veterinary anesthesia delivery system and critical care ventilator** is a microprocessor-controlled ventilator that is marketed either for use with a vaporizer or for patients not requiring an anesthetic (e.g., critical care patients). The ventilator–anesthesia system functions as a nonrebreathing circuit, does not incorporate a bellows assembly, and does not include a canister for chemical absorbent for carbon dioxide (Fig. 7-23). It is not intended for use with another breathing system. The microprocessor determines values (based on body weight) for the ventilatory parameters provided by the ventilator.

### I.   Hazards Associated with the Use of Ventilators

With ventilators, some contact is lost between the anesthetist and the patient. Without a hand on the reservoir bag, the anesthetist may miss disconnections in the patient circuit, variations in respiratory resistance and compliance, and changes in the rate of spontaneous ventilation. Ventilators are mechanical and may malfunction, and many veterinary ventilators are not equipped with alarm systems.

The hazards of mechanical ventilation are associated with malfunctions of equipment and inappropriate or inadvertently altered control settings. The operator should select a ventilator capable of meeting the patient's respiratory requirements. Hazards include hypoventilation, hyperventilation, excessive airway pressure, negative pressure during expiration, and failure of alarms.

## VIII. RESPIRATORY ASSIST DEVICES AND MANUAL RESUSCITATORS

Several types and brands of respiratory assist devices are available. Some are manual in operation (resuscitation bags with one-way valves); some use compressed gas (oxygen) to assist ventilation (demand valves). A manual resuscitator is appropriate for IPPV in small animals. The basic components of a resuscitator are a compressible self-re-expanding bag, a bag refill valve, and a nonrebreathing valve (Figs. 7-24 and 7-25). Some resuscitators can be attached to a source of oxygen to enrich the inspired gases. Manual resuscitators can be fitted with a reservoir to serve as a source of oxygen when the flow does not meet the filling demands of the resuscitator. A reservoir, however, makes the resuscitator more cumbersome.

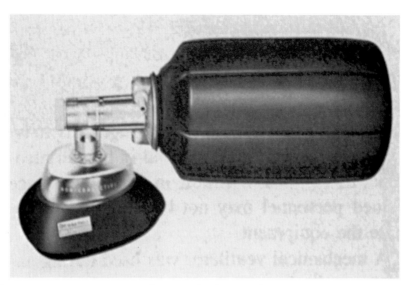

**Figure 7-24.** A Hope resuscitator. This unit is fitted to a mask, but can be attached to an endo-tracheal tube to support ventilation. Reprinted with permission from Lumb WV, Jones EW. Oxygen administration and artificial respiration. In: Lumb WV, Jones EW, eds. Veterinary anesthesia. 2nd ed. Philadelphia: Lea & Febiger, 1984.

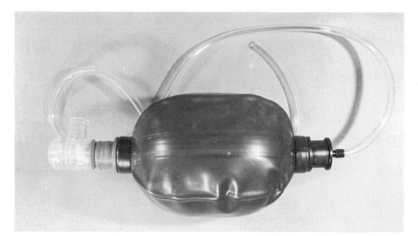

**Figure 7-25.** A manual resuscitation bag. Plastic tubing, which may be connected to an oxy-gen flowmeter, is attached to the bag refill valve to facilitate the addition of oxygen to inspired gases. The components of the resuscitation bag include the clear elbow (*left*), which is a nonrebreathing valve, the black self-inflating bag, and a refill valve (black apparatus on the right end of the bag). The nonrebreathing valve may be connected to a mask or to an endotra-cheal tube.

# Chapter 8

Acid–Base Balance and Fluid Therapy

## Introductory Comments

*Central to the concept of good medical care is the maintenance of normal acid–base physiology and body fluid balance in both healthy and diseased patients. Stress associated with disease and hospital care can alter normal fluid intake and homeostatic mechanisms, whereas anesthetic drugs and surgical manipulations may further impair compensatory physiologic processes responsible for maintaining acid–base and fluid balances. This chapter provides a brief, up-to-date review of commonly encountered acid–base, fluid, and electrolyte disturbances and their treatment.*

## Acid–Base Balance
## Fluid and Electrolyte Therapy

---

## I. ACID–BASE BALANCE

W. W. Muir and H. S. A. de Morais

All schemes of acid–base balance are based upon the understanding that normal oxygen-dependent metabolism of food (carbohydrates, lipids, and proteins) results in the predictable production of work, heat, and waste. Indeed, normal metabolic processes are responsible for the production of thousands of millimoles of carbon dioxide ($CO_2$; volatile acid) and potentially hundreds of milliequivalents of nonvolatile hydrogen ions (fixed acid) daily. The $CO_2$ that is produced is combined with water and is catalyzed by carbonic anhydrase (CA) to form carbonic acid ($H_2CO_3$). The formation of carbonic acid from $CO_2$ and $H_2O$ and the subsequent generation of $H^+$ and $HCO_3^-$ serves as the focal point for almost all discussions of acid–base balance:

$$CO_2 + H_2O \xleftrightarrow{\text{ca}} H_2CO_3 \leftrightarrow H^+ + HCO_3^-$$

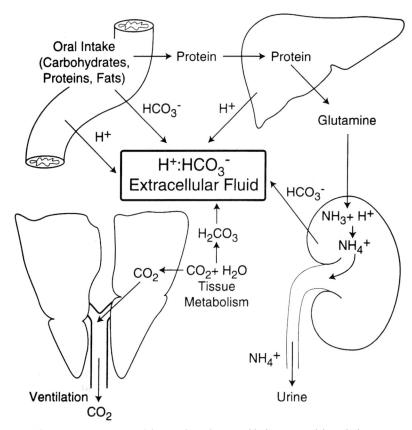

**Figure 8-1.** Integration of the gut, liver, lung, and kidney in acid–base balance.

Acid–base homeostasis ($H^+$ regulation) involves the integrated normal activity of the lungs, kidney, and liver. The lung removes $CO_2$, the kidneys remove $H^+$ as fixed acid, and the liver metabolizes protein, generating 1 mmol $H^+$/kg body weight daily (Fig. 8-1).

## A.    The Henderson–Hasselbalch Equation

The work by Sorensen on the pH concept combined with the theory of acid–base balance proposed by Henderson and the methods of measuring pH in blood introduced by Hasselbalch led to the development of the Henderson–Hasselbalch equation and the characterization of **acid–base disturbances** as being either **respiratory** or nonrespiratory (**metabolic**) in origin. Henderson used the concentration of dissolved molecular $CO_2$ instead of $H_2CO_3$, because carbonic acid could not be measured. Hasselbalch then introduced $P_{CO_2}$ into Henderson's equation and put the equation into logarithmic form, producing the now universally applied **Henderson–Hasselbalch equation:**

$$pH = pK_a + \log_{10} \left( \frac{[HCO_3^-]}{[S \times P_{CO_2}]} \right)$$

Where pH is $-\log_{10} [H^+]$, $pK_a$ is $\log_{10} K_a$, and $S$ is the solubility of $CO_2$. This equation is frequently rewritten for explanatory purposes as:

$$pH = pK_a + \log \left( \frac{base}{acid} \right) = \left( \frac{kidney\ function}{lung\ function} \right)$$

### B.    Mechanisms for Buffering Changes in $H^+$

The body uses **three principal mechanisms** to minimize or **buffer** changes in $[H^+]$. **Chemical buffers** act within seconds to resist or reduce changes in $[H^+]$ and are the first line of defense against changes in pH. The **respiratory system** responds within minutes to resist changes in $[H^+]$ by regulating $P_{CO_2}$ (physiologic buffering) and eliminating excess $CO_2$ molecules caused by an increase in $H^+$ production (chemical buffering) (Fig. 8-2).

$$\uparrow H^+ + HCO_3^- \rightarrow H_2CO_3 \rightarrow H_2O + CO_2$$

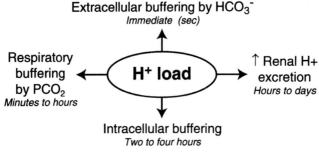

**Figure 8-2.** Rate of response of the body's buffering mechanisms.

Finally, $H^+$ that is produced by nonrespiratory mechanisms (metabolic or nonrespiratory acidosis) are excreted by the **kidney** in the urine over a period of hours or days.

1. **Chemical buffers** are compounds that minimize changes in the $[H^+]$ or the pH of a solution when an acid or base is added. A **buffer** solution consists of a weak acid and its conjugate base and is most effective when the pH is within 1.0 pH unit of its $pK_a$. Alterations in blood, interstitial, and intracellular $[H^+]$ are immediately modified by chemical buffer systems. Approximately 60% of the body's chemical buffering capacity is accomplished by **intracellular phosphates and proteins. Proteins** are by far the most important intracellular buffers.

   a. **Hemoglobin** contributes ~ 80% of the nonbicarbonate buffering capacity of whole blood and, with other intracellular proteins, is responsible for three-quarters of the chemical buffering power of the body.

   b. **Plasma proteins,** particularly albumin, also contain histidine and α-amino groups. They are collectively responsible for 20% of the nonbicarbonate buffering capacity of whole blood.

2. The **respiratory system** offers an alternative route by which $[H^+]$ can be regulated by varying the $Pco_2$.

   a. Changes in blood $CO_2$ also have important consequences for **hemoglobin affinity** for **oxygen** and its buffering capacity.

      i. Increases in $Pco_2$ increase blood $[H^+]$ and decrease hemoglobin affinity for oxygen (**Bohr effect**). This change in oxygen affinity is advantageous in tissues, allowing hemoglobin to release more oxygen for metabolism.
      ii. **Unoxygenated hemoglobin** in turn can transport more carbon dioxide in the form of hemoglobin-contained carbamino compounds ($H^+$ Prot) to the lungs (**Haldane effect**).

3. The synthesis of new $HCO_3^-$ and the excretion of excess $H^+$ emphasize the **role of the kidneys** as both **a chemical and a physiologic buffer system** (Fig. 8-3).

    a. Although relatively slow (hours, days), compared to the lungs (minutes) and chemical buffering (seconds), the kidney serves as the principal means by which acids produced by metabolic processes (not owing to $CO_2$ production but rather fixed acids) are ultimately eliminated.

    b. All $H^+$ produced by metabolic processes are excreted in the urine in combination with weak anions, primarily phosphate and ammonium salts.

    c. It is important to note that **potassium loss** from cells can lead to **intracellular $H^+$ or $Na^+$ accumulation** to maintain electric neutrality.

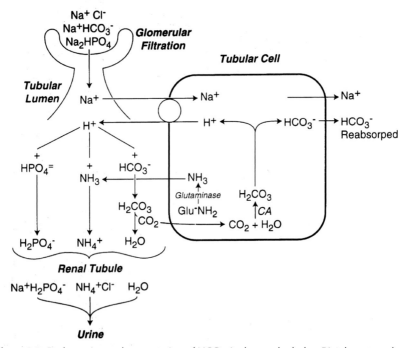

**Figure 8-3.** Reabsorption and regeneration of $HCO_3^-$ in the renal tubules. Bicarbonate reabsorption in the proximal tubule coincides with $H^+$ secretion. Bicarbonate regeneration in the renal tubules coincides with titration of phosphate by $H^+$ and ammonium formation.

| Table 8-1. Effect of Temperature on $P_{O_2}$, $P_{CO_2}$, and pH | | | |
| --- | --- | --- | --- |
| Temperature, °C | $P_{O_2}$ | $P_{CO_2}$ | pH |
| 39 | 90 | 44 | 7.37 |
| 37 | 80 | 40 | 7.40 |
| 30 | 54 | 30 | 7.50 |

    i.    This effect in renal tubular cells can lead to increased $H^+$ excretion (aciduria) and $HCO_3^-$ reabsorption (alkalemia and paradoxical aciduria). Alkalemia and paradoxical aciduria are known to occur in ruminants, but their importance in dogs and cats is questionable.

    ii.    Hyperkalemia has the opposite effect on acid–base balance.

  4.  Increases and, more routinely, decreases in **body temperature** are frequently encountered in patients subjected to anesthesia and surgery.

    a.    Changes in body temperature affect the $[H^+]$ of all body fluids. Increases in body temperature decrease pH and vice versa; blood pH changes by 0.015 to 0.02 units/1°C.

        As body temperature decreases, the $pK_a$ and blood solubility of $CO_2$ increase, producing an increase in pH and decrease in $P_{CO_2}$ (Table 8-1).

    b.    From a practical standpoint, however, pH and $P_{CO_2}$ do not need to be corrected for temperature. Measurements of a blood sample taken from a hypothermic (37° or 38°C) patient permit the clinician to make appropriate therapeutic decisions.

## C.   Acid–Base Disturbances

The **Henderson–Hasselbalch equation** characterizes all acid–base disturbances as being either respiratory or metabolic because of the body's production and elimination of volatile (dissolved $CO_2$; $H_2CO_3$) and nonvolatile or fixed (lactic and phosphoric) acids, respectively.

1. Therefore, only **four primary acid–base abnormalities** are possible: respiratory acidosis, metabolic acidosis, respiratory alkalosis, and metabolic alkalosis (Table 8-2).

2. Clinically, the terms *respiratory* and *metabolic* have been used to imply the involvement of the lung and kidney in acid–base regulation:

$$pH = \frac{HCO_3^-}{Pa_{CO_2}} = \frac{\text{kidney function (fixed acids)}}{\text{lung function (volatile acids)}}$$

3. The term **nonrespiratory** frequently replaces the term **metabolic** in many discussions of acid–base imbalance, because the word *metabolic* is not totally descriptive and is somewhat misleading, implying that all fixed acids are produced by cellular metabolism. The term *nonrespiratory* incorporates all mechanisms responsible for acid–base imbalance other than the production of carbon dioxide and carbonic acid. These mechanisms include alterations in the $P_{CO_2}$, concentrations of strong (fully dissociated) ions and strong ion difference (SID), nonvolatile plasma buffers ($A_{tot}$; primarily serum proteins), and the ionic strength ($pK_a$) of the solution. These four factors used to describe these changes in $[H^+]$ are collectively referred to as **independent variables,** because each of them is regulated or changed independently of the others. It should be

| Table 8-2. Characteristics of Primary Acid–Base Disturbances | | | | |
|---|---|---|---|---|
| **Disorder** | **pH** | **[H⁺]** | **Primary Disturbance** | **Compensatory Response** |
| Nonrespiratory acidosis | ↓ | ↑ | ↓ $[HCO_3^-]$ | ↓ $P_{CO_2}$ |
| Nonrespiratory alkalosis | ↑ | ↓ | ↑ $[HCO_3^-]$ | ↑ $P_{CO_2}$ |
| Respiratory acidosis | ↓ | ↑ | ↑ $P_{CO_2}$ | ↑ $[HCO_3^-]$ |
| Respiratory alkalosis | ↑ | ↓ | ↓ $P_{CO_2}$ | ↓ $[HCO_3^-]$ |

noted, however, that changes in temperature can affect all the independent variables, a consideration that has special importance during surgery and anesthesia.

### D. Primary Abnormalities

**Primary abnormalities** in acid–base balance can arise from disturbances in any one or several of the independent variables.

1. **Simple acid–base abnormalities** are said to occur only when one independent variable is responsible for the disturbance.

2. **Mixed acid–base abnormalities** are caused by disturbances in two or more of the independent variables. Mixed acid–base abnormalities may be additive (respiratory and nonrespiratory acidosis) or **offsetting** (respiratory alkalosis and metabolic acidosis) in regard to their ability to influence $[H^+]$ measured as pH. The following observations suggest a mixed acid–base disturbance:

   The presence of a normal pH with abnormal $P_{CO_2}$ and/or $[HCO_3^-]$.
   A pH change in the opposite direction from that predicted by the known primary disorder.
   $P_{CO_2}$ and $[HCO_3^-]$ changing in opposite directions.

   Mixed acid–base disorders can be classified based on their effect on the patient's pH in additive combinations, offsetting combinations, and triple disorders (Table 8-3). The final pH reflects the dominant of the two offsetting disorders in offsetting combinations.

### E. Secondary Abnormalities

**Secondary** or **compensatory** (adaptive) acid–base changes frequently occur in response to most primary acid–base abnormalities and help buffer or minimize changes in plasma $[H^+]$. **Respiratory acid–base abnormalities,** for example, are generally **compensated** for by controlled, oppositely directed changes in nonrespiratory function. In simple acid–base abnormalities, such as primary respiratory acidosis caused by hypoventilation, the kidney compensates by producing nonrespiratory alkalosis.

| Table 8-3. Classification of Mixed Acid–Base Disorders | |
|---|---|
| **Classification** | **Effect on pH** |
| **MIXED RESPIRATORY** | |
| Acute and chronic respiratory acidosis | Additive |
| Acute and chronic respiratory alkalosis | Additive |
| **MIXED RESPIRATORY AND NONRESPIRATORY** | |
| Respiratory and nonrespiratory acidosis | Additive |
| Respiratory acidosis and nonrespiratory alkalosis | Offsetting |
| Respiratory alkalosis and nonrespiratory acidosis | Offsetting |
| Respiratory and nonrespiratory alkalosis | Additive |
| **MIXED NONRESPIRATORY** | |
| Nonrespiratory acidosis and alkalosis | Offsetting |
| Normal plus high anion gap nonrespiratory acidosis | Additive |
| Mixed high anion gap nonrespiratory acidosis | Additive |
| Mixed normal anion gap nonrespiratory acidosis | Additive |
| **TRIPLE DISORDERS** | |
| Nonrespiratory and respiratory acidosis plus nonrespiratory alkalosis | Function of relative dominance of acidifying and alkalinizing processes |
| Nonrespiratory and respiratory alkalosis plus nonrespiratory alkalosis | Function of relative dominance of acidifying and alkalinizing processes |

1. When analyzing secondary changes in a given acid–base disorder, it is important to remember that, with the exception of chronic respiratory alkalosis, compensation does not return the pH to normal. Overcompensation does not occur; and sufficient time must elapse for compensation to reach a steady state, when the expected compensation can be estimated using the formulas given in Table 8-4.

2. **Respiratory compensation** in metabolic acid–base disorders is obtained by changing alveolar ventilation and, therefore, changing $CO_2$ excretion by the lungs.

a. **Nonrespiratory acidosis** is characterized by an increase in $[H^+]$, a decrease in blood $[HCO_3^-]$ and pH, and a decrease in $P_{CO_2}$ caused by secondary hyperventilation.

b. **Nonrespiratory alkalosis** is characterized by a decrease in $[H^+]$, an increase in blood $[HCO_3^-]$ and pH, and an increase in $P_{CO_2}$ owing to compensatory hypoventilation.

**Table 8-4. Expected Compensatory Responses in Primary Acid–Base Disorders**

| Disorder | Primary Change | Expected Range of Compensation |
|---|---|---|
| Nonrespiratory acidosis | $\downarrow [HCO_3^-]$ | $P_{CO_2}$ = last 2 digits of pH × 100 |
| | | $\Delta P_{CO_2} = 1 - 1.13\ (\Delta[HCO_3^-])$ |
| | | $P_{CO_2} = [HCO_3^-] + 15$ |
| | | $P_{CO_2} = 0.7\ [HCO_3^-] \pm 3$ (canines) |
| Nonrespiratory alkalosis | $\uparrow [HCO_3^-]$ | $P_{CO_2}$ = variable increase |
| | | $P_{CO_2}$ = increases of 0.6 mm Hg for each 1 mEq/L increase in $[HCO_3^-]$ |
| | | $P_{CO_2} = [HCO_3^-] \pm 3$ (canines) |
| Respiratory acidosis | | |
| Acute | $\uparrow P_{CO_2}$ | $[HCO_3^-]$ = increase 1 mEq/L and pH decreases 0.05 unit for each 10 mm Hg increase in $P_{CO_2}$ |
| | | $[HCO_3^-] = 0.15\ P_{CO_2} \pm 2$ (canines) |
| Chronic | $\uparrow P_{CO_2}$ | $[HCO_3^-]$ = increases 3.5 mEq/L and pH decreases 0.07 unit for each 10 mm Hg increase in $P_{CO_2}$ |
| | | $[HCO_3^-] = 0.35\ P_{CO_2} \pm 2$ (canines) |
| Respiratory alkalosis | | |
| Acute | $\downarrow P_{CO_2}$ | $[HCO_3^-]$ = decreases 2 mEq/L and pH increases 0.1 unit for each 10 mm Hg decrease in $P_{CO_2}$ |
| | | $[HCO_3^-] = 0.25\ P_{CO_2} \pm 2$ (canines) |
| Chronic | $\downarrow P_{CO_2}$ | $[HCO_3^-]$ = decreases 5 mEq/L and pH increases 0.15 unit for each 10 mm Hg decrease in $P_{CO_2}$ |
| | | $[HCO_3^-] = 0.55\ P_{CO_2} \pm 2$ (canines) |

**F.**    **Analyzing Abnormalities**

A common question when **analyzing** simple **acid–base abnormalities** that demonstrate both respiratory acidosis and nonrespiratory alkalosis is, Which is primary and which is secondary or compensatory? The answer is not always obvious, although simple primary acid–base abnormalities change pH in the direction of the primary disorder.

**G.**    **Nonrespiratory Acidosis**

Because **nonrespiratory acidosis** is so frequently associated with disease processes in animals, indices of acid–base balance have evolved that permit the quantitative evaluation of the nonrespiratory component of acid–base abnormalities.

    1.   The **standard bicarbonate** is the concentration of bicarbonate in plasma after the whole blood sample has been equilibrated to a $P_{CO_2}$ of 40 mm Hg at 38°C.

    2.   Similarly, the **base excess** (BE) quantitates the number of milliequivalents per liter of acid or base required to titrate 1 L blood to pH 7.40, while the $P_{CO_2}$ is held constant at 40 mm Hg at 38°C. The base excess has a normal value of $0 \pm 3$ and is changed only by nonvolatile acids, thereby indicating nonrespiratory acidosis. The numerical magnitude of the base excess is a guide to therapy:

$$\text{Base } (Na^+HCO_3^-) \text{ needed} = 0.3 \cdot BW_{kg} \cdot \text{base excess}$$

where 0.3 is the percent body weight (BW) that is extracellular water (adult animal).

**H.**    **Anion Gap**

The **anion gap** (AG) is a useful tool to assess mixed acid–base disorders. Chemically, there is no anion gap because electroneutrality must be maintained and the anion gap actually is the difference between the unmeasured anions ($UA^-$) and unmeasured cations ($UC^+$). When applied in the clinical setting:

$$AG = ([Na^+] + [K^+]) - ([Cl^-] + [HCO_3^-]) = [UA^-] - [UC^-]$$

    1.   Every time there is a decrease in $[HCO_3^-]$, either $[Cl^-]$ or $[UA^-]$ must increase to maintain electroneutrality.

2. When titrated $HCO_3^-$ is replaced by $Cl^-$ in nonrespiratory acidosis, the difference $([UA^-] - [UC^+])$—and consequently the AG—will remain the same (**hyperchloremic or normal AG acidosis**).

3. When titrated $HCO_3^-$ is replaced by $UA^-$, the difference $([UA^-] - [UC^+])$—and consequently the AG—will increase while $[Cl^-]$ remains the same (**normochloremic or high AG acidosis**).

4. Usually an **increase in the AG** implies an accumulation of organic acids in the body.

5. An increase in AG also occurs in **alkalemia** caused by an increase in the net negative charge on serum proteins or in situations when concomitant nonrespiratory alkalosis or respiratory alkalosis overrides a high AG nonrespiratory acidosis.

6. **Hypoalbuminemia** is probably the only important cause of a **decrease in the AG,** and each decrease in albumin concentration by 1 g/dL has been associated with a decrease of 3 mEq/L in the AG.

## I.   Strong Ion Difference

A new theory of acid–base regulation (SID) has been proposed. According to this theory $[HCO_3^-]$ and pH $([H^+])$ depend on $P_{CO_2}$, the total concentration of plasma weak nonvolatile acids $([A_{tot}]$, composed mostly of albumin and inorganic phosphates), and the difference between the strong cations and strong anions (Fig. 8-4).

1. As noted, strong ions are substances that are completely dissociated in plasma at body pH. The **most important strong ions** in plasma are $Na^+$, $K^+$, $Ca_2^+$, $Mg_2^+$, $Cl^-$, lactate, $\beta$-hydroxybutyrate, acetoacetate, and $SO_4^{2-}$.

2. **Changes in SID are recognized by changes in $[HCO_3^-]$ or BE.** A decrease in SID is associated with nonrespiratory acidosis, whereas an increase in SID is associated with nonrespiratory alkalosis. There are three general mecha-

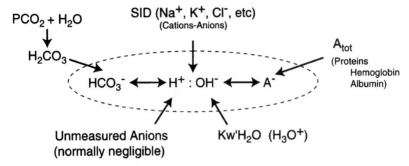

**Figure 8-4.** The influence of independent variables on the acid–base balance. *Dashed line,* encloses the dependent variables ($H^+$ and $OH^-$).

---

| Table 8-5. Disorders of SID |
| --- |

I. Free water abnormalities
  A. Increase in $[Na^+] \rightarrow$ concentration alkalosis
  B. Decrease in $[Na^+] \rightarrow$ dilution acidosis
II. Chloride abnormalities
  A. Decrease in $[Cl^-]$ corrected $\rightarrow$ hypochloremic alkalosis
  B. Increase in $[Cl^-]$ corrected $\rightarrow$ hyperchloremic acidosis
III. Unmeasured strong anions abnormalities
  A. Increase in $[XA^-] \rightarrow$ organic acidosis

$[XA^-]$, unidentified strong anion.

---

nisms by which SID can change: free water abnormalities, chloride abnormalities, and unmeasured strong ion abnormalities (Table 8-5). Changing the **water content** of the various body fluid compartments will dilute or concentrate both strong anions and strong cations. Consequently, SID will change by the same proportion.

3. Accumulation of **metabolically produced organic anions** (e.g., lactate, acetoacetate, citrate, β-hydroxybutyrate) or addition of exogenous organic anions (e.g., salicylate, glycolate from ethylene glycol poisoning, and formate from methanol poisoning) will cause nonrespiratory acidosis, because these strong anions decrease SID.

**Treatment of organic acidosis** should be directed toward the primary disorder and stabilization of the patient. Sodium bicarbonate should be used cautiously, because metabolism of accumulated organic anions will normalize SID and increase $[HCO_3^-]$. The initial goal for patients with severe organic acidosis is to raise the systemic pH to 7.2.

**J.    Evaluations of Acid–Base Balance**

1.   A stepwise approach should be followed in all animals with suspected acid–base disorders.

    a.    After obtaining the samples, the first step is to determine the pH and the nature of the primary disorder from the blood gas.

    b.    The possibility of a mixed respiratory and nonrespiratory acid–base disorder should be assessed by calculating the expected compensation (Table 8-4).

2.   **Two quantitative clinical approaches** for assessment of nonrespiratory acid–base disturbances have been proposed, one based on the use of BE and the other based on a mathematical relationship to estimate SID.

    a.    Base excess has been used to assess changes in the nonrespiratory component, because SID is synonymous with buffer base.

    b.    Base excess is a measurement of the deviation of buffer base (and therefore SID) from normal values.

    c.    Formulas to estimate changes in base excess owing to changes in SID and $[A_{tot}]$ are listed in Table 8-6. These formulas help the clinician understand complex acid–base disorders in domestic animals.

## II.   FLUID AND ELECTROLYTE THERAPY
*David C. Seeler*

At birth, **total body water** is in excess of 75% of body weight. Maturational changes result in reductions of total body water content to 60 to 66% of the adult's body weight. Lower water content can be anticipated to exist in the obese patient. Total body water is made up of intracellular and extracellular compartments. The **intracellular fluid volume** increases slightly with age, and in the mature animal it is equivalent to approximately 40% of body weight. The volume of the **extracellular fluid compartment** decreases with maturation and accounts for 20% of the weight of the adult animal. The extracellular fluid compartment is further divided into the interstitial, plasma or intravascular, and transcellular fluid compartments. The volume of water in the **interstitial compartment** accounts for 15% of the mature animal's weight. **Plasma water volume** constitutes 5% of the body weight and approximately 50% of the total blood volume (Table 8-7). The **transcellular fluid compartment** consists of joint and cerebrospinal fluid (CSF) in addition to water located within the eye and pleural, peritoneal, and pericardial spaces, and approximates 1.0 to 3.0% of body weight.

## A.  Electrolyte Solutions

The term **crystalloid solution** refers to any solution of crystalline solids that are dissolved in water, such as sodium-based

---

**Table 8-6. Estimating Changes in BE Caused by Changes in SID and [$A_{tot}$]**

I. Changes in [$A_{tot}$]
   A. Changes in albumin (Alb) concentration or total protein (TP)
      a. $\Delta Alb$ (mEq/L) = 3.7 × ([Alb] normal − [Alb] patient[a])
      b. $\Delta TP$ (mEq/L) = 3.0 × ([TP] normal − [TP] patient[a])
   B. Changes in inorganic phosphate ($P_i$) concentration
      a. $P_i$ (mmol/L) = P (mg/dL) × (10 ÷ 30.97)
      b. $\Delta P$ (mEq/L) = (1.6 × [$P_i$] patient[b]) + (0.2 × [$P_i$] patient)
II. Changes in SID
   A. Changes in free water
      a. $\Delta$Free water (mEq/L) = $Z^c$([$Na^+$] patient[d] − [$Na^+$] normal)
   B. Changes in chloride ($Cl^-$) concentration
      a. $\Delta Cl^-$ (mEq/L) = [$Cl^-$] normal − [$Cl^-$] corrected[e]
   C. Changes in unidentified anions ($XA^-$)
      a. $\Delta XA^-$ = BE − ($\Delta$free water + $\Delta Cl^-$ + $\Delta Alb$ + $\Delta Pi$)

Modified from de Morais HAS, Muir WW. Strong ions and acid-base disorders. In: Bonagura JD, Kirk RW, eds., Kirk's current veterinary therapy XII. 12th ed. Philadelphia: Saunders, 1995:121–127.
[a]Measured in g/dL.
[b]Measured in mmol/L.
[c]Equals 0.25 for canines and felines.
[d]Measured in mEq/L.
[e]Equals patient [$Cl^-$] in mEq/L after correct for changes in free water.

Table 8-7. Approximate Vascular Fluid Volumes (mL/kg) in Mature Animals

| Species | Plasma Volume | Total Blood Volume |
|---|---|---|
| Bovine | 38 | 57–60 |
| Canine | 50 | 88 |
| Caprine | 53 | 70 |
| Equine | | |
| Thoroughbred | 61 | 100 |
| Other | | 72 |
| Feline | 47 | 68 |
| Ovine | 50 | 60 |
| Porcine | 47 | 50 |

Table 8-8. Electrolyte Distribution across Fluid Compartments (mEq/L)

| Ion | Plasma | Interstitial | Intracellular |
|---|---|---|---|
| $Na^+$ | 142 | 145 | 13 |
| $K^+$ | 5 | 4 | 155 |
| $Ca^{2+}$ | 5 | 3 | 2 |
| $Mg^{2+}$ | 2 | 2 | 35 |
| $Cl^-$ | 106 | 115 | 2 |
| $HCO_3^-$ | 24 | 30 | 10 |
| Phosphates | 2 | 2 | 113 |
| Sulfates | 1 | 1 | 20 |
| Organic acids | 5 | 5 | 0 |
| Protein | 16 | 1 | 60 |

electrolyte solutions and solutions of dextrose in water. If the electrolyte composition of the prepared solution approximates that of extracellular fluid (Table 8-8), then the parenteral fluid is referred to as a **balanced electrolyte solution.**

1. Multiple or balanced electrolyte solutions are formulated based on the concept that the amount of water and

electrolytes that a patient retains depends on intact regulatory mechanisms in the body, not on the amount of water
and electrolytes received. Solutions that are polyelectro-
lytic have value in maintaining or replenishing electrolytes.

2.  Preparations that contain lactate, acetate, or gluconate
    produce an **alkalinizing effect** when the anion is metabo-
    lized to carbon dioxide and water.

3.  Fluids are defined as isotonic, hypotonic, or hypertonic,
    based on their effect on erythrocyte size or volume.

    a.  Administration of **isotonic solutions** to the intravas-
        cular space does not alter the osmolality of the
        extracellular fluid. As a result, there is no net osmotic
        effect, and only the volume of the extracellular fluid
        compartment is expanded.
    b.  Parenteral administration of **hypotonic solutions** re-
        duces extracellular fluid osmolality and results in the
        osmotic movement of water into the intracellular
        compartment.
    c.  **Hypertonic solutions** increase the osmolality of ex-
        tracellular fluids, which results in a fluid shift out of
        the intracellular compartment.

**B.  Maintenance Solutions**

**Maintenance solutions** are designed to meet the water and
electrolyte requirements of patients that are not taking in
amounts sufficient to meet their daily losses.

1.  Daily water loss includes the **insensible loss** of water
    through evaporation from the respiratory system and skin
    as well as **sensible losses** in which there is an associated
    obligatory loss of electrolytes.

    a.  For many domestic species and birds, the **daily
        maintenance** water requirement ranges from 40 to
        60 mL/kg/day.
    b.  The net daily loss of sodium in small animals ranges
        from 35 to 50 mmol/L (35 to 50 mEq/L), and the

daily potassium losses are 20 to 30 mmol/L (20 to 30 mEq/L).

2. To meet these specific daily requirements, **maintenance solutions** have lower sodium and chloride concentrations and a higher potassium concentration than does extracellular fluid.

   a. If the concentration of **potassium** in the parenteral solution is < 20 mmol/L (20 mEq/L), then the maintenance fluid may be supplemented with additional potassium chloride to that level. Infusion rates up to 15 mL/kg/h are safe, as long as the potassium concentration in the parenteral solution is < 30 mmol/L (30 mEq/L).

   b. **Hypotonic** preparations or solutions that contain dextrose provide **free water.** Isotonic salt solutions provide osmolar water, not free water. For solutions containing dextrose, free water is not available until the dextrose has been metabolized.

   c. Maintenance fluids are generally **administered** over a 24-h period. These solutions should not be used in situations in which large volumes might be rapidly infused, because this could result in significant extracellular fluid electrolyte abnormalities.

## C. Replacement Solutions

**Replacement solutions** are isotonic, balanced electrolyte solutions such as lactated Ringer's USP that closely approximate the electrolyte composition of extracellular fluid. These solutions may be administered rapidly, in large volumes, to re-expand the extracellular fluid volume without inducing changes in its electrolytic composition. Because they are isotonic, their use does not induce fluid shifts between the intracellular and extracellular compartments.

1. Balanced electrolyte solutions will rapidly equilibrate across the intravascular and interstitial fluid compartments. As a result, only 20 to 25% of the administered volume remains within the intravascular space after 1 h.

2. When replacement fluids are used to replenish **intravascular losses,** it is necessary to administer a volume equivalent to at least three times the volume of blood lost to replace the vascular deficit.

3. Replacement solutions are often used as maintenance fluids. In this situation, normal renal function should be present to ensure that electrolytes in excess of daily requirements are eliminated.

   a. Long-term management of a patient's maintenance requirements with a replacement solution may result in **hypokalemia.** In this instance, replacement solutions should be supplemented with potassium chloride to provide a final potassium concentration of 20 mmol/L (20 mEq/L).
   b. Replacement fluids that have been supplemented with potassium chloride should not be used in clinical situations in which large volumes may be rapidly infused.

## D.  Other Parenteral Solutions

1. **Isotonic saline** is prepared as a 0.9% solution that contains 154 mmol/L (154 mEq/L) each of sodium and chloride ions and has an osmolarity of 308 mOsm/L.

   a. The use of 0.9% sodium chloride solutions has been advocated for maintenance and replacement purposes.
   b. Isotonic saline is used for rapid expansion of the extracellular fluid volume.
   c. Isotonic saline does not meet the patient's free water and electrolyte needs for maintenance purposes.
   d. Isotonic saline may be used for the correction of hyponatremia and nonrespiratory alkalemia.

2. **Hypotonic saline** solutions are available in several strengths. Commercial preparations of 0.45% saline are hypotonic (osmolarity of 154 mOsm/L) and may be used as a hydrating solution.

a. Hypotonic saline preparations may be used for **maintenance** purposes, particularly when they are supplemented with dextrose and potassium chloride.

b. When 2.5% dextrose is added to 0.45% saline, the resultant solution is isotonic. Upon metabolism of the dextrose, free water is made available for distribution across all fluid compartments.

3. **Hypertonic saline** solutions of 3 and 5% saline have been used in the treatment of patients with severe hyponatremia for which rapid sodium replacement is considered necessary.

a. Recently, hypertonic saline solutions have been used with success in the management of **severe shock,** particularly hemorrhagic shock.

b. Hypertonic saline solutions of 7.5%, although not commercially available, are commonly used for this purpose. The osmolarity of 7.5% saline is 2400 mOsm/L. To **prepare 7.5% saline**, it is necessary to purchase 5% saline in 500-mL bags and 23.4% saline in 30-mL bottles (American Reagent, Shirley, NY; Lyphomed Canada, Markham, ON). Remove 120 mL of 5% saline from the 500-mL bag and inject 60 mL of 23.4% saline solution into the bag to make a 7.5% solution.

c. **Physiologic effects** include improved cardiac output and aortic blood pressure, reduced peripheral vascular resistance, increased plasma volume with hemodilution, and increased interstitial fluid volume.

i. Upon administration, hypertonic saline equilibrates rapidly throughout the extracellular fluid space. Because of the increase in extracellular fluid osmolality caused by the hypertonic solution, water moves out of the intracellular fluid compartment. As a result, the extracellular fluid compartment volume is expanded.

ii. Solutions of 7.5% saline, when infused intravenously into dogs, increase plasma volume 2 to 4 mL for each 1 mL administered.

      iii.    Maximum vascular volume expansion occurs within 30 min of the administration of the hypertonic saline solution. These fluid shifts result in an intracellular water debt and an eventual decrease in total body water because of obligatory water loss associated with natriuresis.

    d.    The **intravenous administration** of 4 to 6 mL/kg of 7.5% saline over 3 to 5 min results in the rapid restoration of hemodynamic parameters with subsequent improvements in tissue perfusion. Concern has been expressed that the hemodynamic effects of 7.5% hypertonic saline are not sustained.

4.   **Dextrose solutions** are commercially available in variety of concentrations, ranging from 2.5 to 50% dextrose in water. $D_5W$ contains 50 g dextrose monohydrate per liter water and exerts an osmolarity of 252 mOsm/L.

    a.    Dextrose solutions provide a source of **free water** for total body distribution once the carbohydrate is metabolized. An additional 0.6 mL water is made available for each gram of dextrose that is metabolized.

    b.    Dextrose solutions are not effective for use as plasma volume expanders.

    c.    $D_5W$ solutions contain 171 Cal/L, which is not capable of meeting the energy requirements of domestic animal species.

        i.    **Hypertonic dextrose** solutions are generally used for the purpose of caloric supplementation of parenteral maintenance fluids.

        ii.    Long-term infusions of $D_5W$ or the infusion of hypertonic dextrose solutions may result in the development of **thrombophlebitis.** Care should be taken to ensure that hypertonic preparations in particular are infused via the caudal or cranial vena cava.

        iii.    The **administration rate** of dextrose solutions should be carefully regulated. Glucose solutions should not be administered at a rate > 0.5 g/kg/h so as to not induce a glucosuria.

5. **Sodium bicarbonate** solution is a preparation of sodium bicarbonate ($NaHCO_3^-$) in sterile water for injection. Sodium bicarbonate solution is administered intravenously, either in another parenteral solution or undiluted in emergencies. An isotonic solution can be obtained by adding a 50-mL vial of 7.5% sodium bicarbonate to 200 mL of water for injection.

   a. Sodium bicarbonate is indicated in the treatment of **metabolic acidosis.**

   b. **Overcorrection** of the bicarbonate deficit produces metabolic alkalosis with a rise in blood pH. Administration of sodium bicarbonate is generally contraindicated for patients losing chloride through vomiting and for those with hypokalemia.

   c. Intravenous sodium bicarbonate administration leads to increased $CO_2$ levels in blood and CSF. Because plasma $HCO_3^-$ enters the CSF slowly, a **paradoxical acidosis** in the brain may result. Adequate ventilation of the patient is thus mandatory to prevent these adverse side effects.

   d. Sodium bicarbonate produces sodium retention and should be used with caution in patients with congestive heart failure or other conditions causing edema.

   e. Dosages up to 2 mEq/kg in cats induce minimal changes in the electrolyte status of the animal. Doses in excess of 4 mEq/kg can induce hyperosmolality, hypernatremia, and hyperkalemia.

6. Tromethamine (THAM) is a slightly hypertonic (380 mOsm/L) organic amine buffer used for correction of severe systemic acidosis, such as that which occurs during shock, cardiac arrest, and massive transfusions of acid-citrate-dextrose (ACD) preserved blood. THAM distributes across all body fluid compartments and is an effective **intracellular buffer.** Tromethamine is supplied in 500-mL bottles containing 18 g (150 mEq) of tromethamine and ~ 3 g (50 mEq) of acetic acid. The pH of the formulation is ~ 8.6.

   a. Given intravenously, it acts as an amine **proton acceptor,** attracting hydrogen ions to form salts that are then excreted by the kidneys. THAM's buffering capacity is equivalent to that of sodium bicarbonate, without causing hypernatremia or hypercarbia.

b.    Tromethamine also acts as an osmotic diuretic, increasing urine flow, urine pH, excretion of electrolytes, fixed acids, and carbon dioxide.

c.    Tromethamine is **contraindicated** in anuria and uremia. Large doses may depress respiration owing to pH change and $CO_2$ reduction, with a subsequent increase in blood lactate.

d.    The approximate **intravenous dose** may be estimated from the buffer base deficit:

$$0.3 \text{ M tromethamine (mL) required} = BW_{kg} \times \text{base deficit (mEq/L)} \times 1.1$$

e.    In treatment of **cardiac arrest,** tromethamine solution should be given at the same time as other standard resuscitative measures, including cardiac massage, are being applied. Doses ranging from 3.5 to 6.0 mL/kg have been administered intravenously.

**E.**    **Colloids**

**Colloids** are in effect a suspension of large molecular weight particles. If the average molecular weight of the particles in solution exceeds 50,000, they will tend to remain within the vascular compartment. This results in an increase in intravascular colloid osmotic pressure. Owing to these properties, colloid preparations are effective when used for **vascular volume expansion.** Colloids are also used in acute **hypoproteinemic** states in which plasma albumin levels are < 15 g/L (1.5 g/dL)—or total serum protein levels are < 35 g/L (3.5 g/dL)—to ensure that an effective vascular volume is maintained. **Natural colloids** include plasma, albumin preparations, and whole blood. **Artificial colloids** include dextran, gelatin, and hydroxyethyl starch preparations. Artificial colloids exert a vascular effect similar to that of plasma. Table 8-9 lists types of natural and synthetic colloid solutions and the indications for their most effective use.

1.    **Plasma proteins** play a predominant role in establishing plasma oncotic pressure, which is ultimately responsible for maintaining vascular volume at the level of the capil-

lary beds. Each gram of albumin will retain 17 to 18 mL water within the vascular space.

a.  Plasma must be gradually warmed to 37°C before being administered. Plasma should not be thawed at temperatures > 37°C. A blood administration set with an in-line, 18-mm, micropore filter is used when plasma is infused intravenously.

**Table 8-9. Colloid Solutions and Indications for Use**

| Type of Colloid | Uses |
|---|---|
| **SYNTHETIC** | |
| Oxypolygelatin | Rapid, short-term intravascular volume resuscitation from hypovolemic shock |
| Dextran 40 | Rapid short-term intravascular volume resuscitation from hypovolemic shock; rapid improvement of microcirculatory flow; prophylaxis of deep vein thrombosis or pulmonary emboli |
| Dextran 70 | Rapid intravascular volume resuscitation from hypovolemic, traumatic, or hemorrhagic shock |
| Hetastarch | Rapid intravascular volume resuscitation from all forms of shock; volume replacement and maintenance of colloid oncotic pressure for patients with systemic inflammatory response syndrome (increased capillary permeability and albumin leakage); small-volume resuscitation |
| **NATURAL** | |
| Fresh whole blood | Rapid volume resuscitation during or after acute hemorrhage; anemia with hypoalbuminemia; significant bleeding from coagulopathy or thrombocytopenia |
| Stored whole blood | Rapid volume resuscitation during or after acute hemorrhage; anemia with hypoalbuminemia; significant bleeding other than in cases of thrombocytopenia; deficiency of factor V or VIII |
| Plasma | Coagulopathies (fresh frozen for factor V or VIII deficiency); low antithrombin; acute hypoalbuminemia, disseminated intravascular coagulation |

Modified from Rudloff E, Kirby R. The critical need for colloids: administering colloids effectively. Compend Contin Ed 1998;20:27–43.

    b.    It has been recommended that for dogs, the recipient should receive 28 to 33 mL/kg of plasma to administer 1 g/kg of albumin when the plasma protein concentration of the donor is 30 to 35 g/L.

    c.    Alternatively, the total protein deficit may be estimated as follows:

$$\text{donor plasma required (mL)} = \left[\frac{(\text{desired TP} - \text{actual TP})}{\text{donor plasma TP}}\right] \bullet \text{recipient plasma volume (mL)}$$

2.    Patients who are severely anemic or who have a significantly decreased packed cell volume are candidates for **whole blood** transfusion, **packed red cells,** or the hemoglobin substitute **oxyglobin.**

    a.    **Acute blood loss** in the perioperative period in excess of 10 to 15% of the patient's blood volume should be replaced with whole blood. **Chronic reductions** in hematocrit to 15% in a healthy nonexercising animal does not necessarily result in clinical signs of oxygen debt. When the cardiopulmonary effects of most anesthetic agents are considered, however, it is advisable to maintain a hematocrit of at least 25%, or a hemoglobin concentration of 70 g/L in the surgical patient.

    b.    Whole blood or packed cells that are properly stored in ACD may be used up to 21 days after collection, whereas CPD and CPAA-1 maintain adequate red cell viability for to 30 and 35 days, respectively.

        Storage of red blood cells results in dramatic reductions in 2,3-diphosphoglycerate (2,3-DPG), which shifts the oxyhemoglobin dissociation curve to the left in dogs. The left shift of the oxyhemoglobin dissociation curve results in a decrease in oxygen available to the peripheral tissues.

    c.    When possible, all donors should be typed and all potential transfusion recipients should be typed and cross-matched with the donor (Table 8-10). If donors are not typed, then a cross-match should be carried out on fresh blood collected from the donor and recipient.

| Table 8-10. Major Blood Groups of Domestic Animals | | |
|---|---|---|
| Species | Number of Major Groups | Clinically Significant Groups |
| Bovine | 12 | B, J |
| Canine | 7 | DEA 1.1, 1.2, 7 |
| Caprine | 5 | ? |
| Equine | 9 | A, C, Q |
| Feline | 2 | A, B |
| Ovine | 7 | B, R |
| Porcine | 16 | ? |

d. Whole blood and packed red cells, like plasma, must be rewarmed slowly to 37°C before being transfused into the patient. Temperatures in excess of 37°C should not be used to rewarm whole blood or blood products.

    i. Packed red cells may be diluted with 0.9% saline to facilitate the transfusion process by reducing the viscosity of the suspension.

    ii. Intravenous administration sets used for transfusion purposes should contain in-line filters with a pore size of 80 υ so that cellular debris and blood clots are not transfused into the patient.

    iii. In cats, from which blood is often collected into a syringe, syringe filters (e.g., Hemo-nate; Gesco, San Antonio, TX) may be used to accomplish the same purpose.

    iv. All blood transfusions should be administered through a separate intravenous access.

    v. The **volume** of blood to be **administered** may be set empirically at 10 to 40 mL/kg in dogs and 5 to 20 mL/kg in cats. Or the volume can be calculated using the following formulas. For cats:

$$\text{blood required (mL)} = BW_{kg} \times 70 \left[ \frac{(\text{desired PCV} - \text{patient PCV})}{\text{donor PCV}} \right]$$

For dogs:

$$\text{blood required (mL)} = \\ BW_{kg} \times 90 \left[ \frac{(\text{desired PCV} - \text{patient PCV})}{\text{donor PCV}} \right]$$

vi.   Whole blood or suspensions of packed red cells may be administered at rates of 5 to 10 mL/h. In critical situations, when rapid restoration of blood volume is of concern, administration rates of 22 mL/kg/h for dogs and 40 mL/kg/h for cats may be used. Transfusions should be completed within 4 h to avoid bacterial contamination and functional loss of the blood's components. When blood products are unavailable, the hemoglobin substitute product oxyglobin can be administered to improve the oxygen carrying capacity of blood. The recommended dose of oxyglobin is 30 mL/kg IV at a rate not to exceed 10 mL/kg/h. Duration of efficacy is approximately 24 h.

vii.  The patient must be continuously monitored for clinical signs that suggest that there is an adverse reaction to the transfusion. Adverse reactions may occur owing to prior bacterial contamination of the donor's blood, allergic or immunologic reactions to the transfusion itself, circulatory overload, or citrate-induced hypocalcemia.

3.  **Dextrans** are low to average molecular weight polysaccharides that are produced as a result of bacterial enzymatic action on sucrose. Dextran 40 is a low molecular weight polysaccharide with an average molecular weight of 40,000 and a molecular weight range of 10,000 to 70,000. Dextran 70 and 75 consist of glucose polymers with an average molecular weight of 70,000 and 75,000, respectively. Both preparations have a molecular weight range of 20,000 to 200,000; thus their clinical effects are similar. Polymers with a molecular weight < 50,000 are eliminated from the circulation by glomerular filtration and renal excretion. Polysaccharides with a molecular weight > 50,000 are

eventually stored in the reticuloendothelial system and subsequently metabolized.

a. Dextran solutions are used for **plasma volume expansion** when hematogenous products are not available. They are not a substitute for whole blood and possess no oxygen carrying capacity. Therefore, care should be exercised when dextrans are used in the treatment of severe hemorrhage so that the patient's hematocrit is not reduced to critical levels.

b. **Dextran 70 and 75** are slightly hyperoncotic compared to plasma and induce a water shift from the interstitial fluid space into the vascular system of 20 to 25 mL/g. Dextran 70 and 75 increase the plasma volume by an amount that is slightly in excess of the colloidal volume administered. The maximum increase in plasma volume occurs within 1 h of the termination of the infusion and lasts for up to 6 h.

c. The primary concerns with respect to the use of dextran solutions relates to the potential for allergic reactions or interference with the normal hemostatic mechanisms of blood.

d. The recommended dose for dextran 40, 70, or 75 is 10 to 20 mL/kg/day or 1.5 g /kg/day to reduce the possibility of an adverse or allergic reaction in the patient.

e. Infusion rates of 5 mL/kg may be used in noncritical situations.

f. Administration rates of up to 20 mL/kg/h have been recommended for **emergency** situations (Table 8-11).

4. **Hydroxyethyl starch,** or hetastarch, is a synthetic polymer that is synthesized from a waxy starch composed primarily of amylopectin. Commercially available preparations are sterile, nonpyogenic solutions of 6% hetastarch in 0.9% saline. The average molecular weight of hetastarch is 69,000. Approximately 40% of the hetastarch is excreted in the urine within 24 h in patients with normal renal function. The larger molecules are slowly degraded by serum amylase, resulting in a sustained ability of hetastarch to

| Table 8-11. Colloid Dosage and Administration Guidelines |
| --- |

| Type of Colloid | Dosage | Administration Guidelines |
| --- | --- | --- |
| **NATURAL** | | |
| Whole blood | *Felines:* 10 mL/kg or until PCV can support tissue oxygenation (25–30%)<br>*Canines:* 20 mL/kg or until PCV can support tissue oxygenation (25–30%) | In cases of acute, life-threatening hemorrhagic shock, whole blood is administered as rapidly as possible to sustain a MAP of 80 mmHg; whole blood is given over 4–6 h to hemodynamically stable patient<br>For dogs and cats in distributive shock owing to SIRS, once the PCV is > 25%, the initial infusion of blood can be followed by a CRI of hetastarch (10–20 mL/kg/day) |
| Plasma | *Felines:* 10 mL/kg over 4–6 h or until plasma Alb is > 2.0 g/dL<br>*Canines:* 250 mL/10–20 kg over 4 to 6 h or until plasma Alb is > 2.0 g/dL | 6–10 U frozen plasma may be required to raise the plasma Alb level to 2.0 g/dL in large dogs with SIRS<br>For dogs and cats in distributive shock owing to SIRS, once the plasma Alb is > 2.0 g/dL, a CRI of hetastarch can be instituted: 10–20 mL/kg/day (canines); 10–40 mL/kg/day (felines) |
| **SYNTHETIC** | | |
| Oxypolygelatin | 5 mL/kg over 15 min; titrate to effect; do not exceed 15 mL/kg total dose | If further volume is required for volume resuscitation, another synthetic colloid can be administered<br>For dogs and cats in distributive shock owing to SIRS, the initial resuscitation can be followed by a CRI of hetastarch |
| Dextran | *Felines:* 5 mL/kg increments given over 5 to 10 min; repeat to effect; up to 20 mL/kg<br>*Canines:* 10–20 mL/kg/day; IV bolus to effect | For dogs and cats in distributive shock owing to SIRS, the initial bolus of dextran can be followed by a CRI of hetastarch |

*Continued*

| Type of Colloid | Dosage | Administration Guidelines |
|---|---|---|
| Hetastarch | *Felines:* 5-mL/kg increments given over 5 to 10 min; repeat to effect; up to 40 mL/kg<br>*Canines:* 10–40 mL/kg/day; IV bolus to effect | For dogs and cats in hypovolemic cardiogenic shock, with pulmonary contusions, or with head injury, 5-mL/kg boluses are administered to effect, using the smallest volume possible to maintain the MAP at least 80 mm Hg<br>For dogs and cats in distributive shock owing to SIRS, the initial bolus of colloid is followed by a CRI of hetastarch to maintain a MAP of at least 80 mm Hg and a COP > 14 mm Hg |

Modified from Rudloff E, Kirby R. The critical need for colloids: administering colloids effectively. Compend Contin Ed 1998;20:27.
*PCV,* packed cell volume; *MAP,* mean arterial pressure; *SIRS,* systemic inflammatory response; *CRI,* constant rate of infusion; *COP,* colloid osmotic pressure.

maintain vascular volume expansion compared to dextran preparations.

a. The colloidal properties of hetastarch are similar to that of albumin.

b. The infusion of hetastarch results in a plasma volume expansion only slightly in excess of the volume infused. The volume expansion effect lasts < 12 h. As a result, multiple doses may be required for patients with ongoing protein losses.

c. Hetastarch should not be used in normovolemic patients owing to the potential for volume overload.

d. Other complications associated with the infusion of hetastarch solutions include anaphylactoid reactions and coagulopathies.

e. A dose of 10 to 20 mL/kg/day of 6% hetastarch has been recommended. Rapid infusion of hetastarch in cats may provoke moderate reactions, such as nausea with occasional vomiting. Table 8-11 lists recommended dosages of several colloid solutions and administration guidelines for dogs and cats.

### F. Considerations for Fluid Therapy

The degree of **dehydration** can be estimated by assessing the patient's **skin turgor** and correlating that information with the other clinical findings. Age, nutritional status of the animal, and individual variations make assessment of skin turgor difficult. In small animals, skin turgor is tested by pinching a skin fold over the torso and twisting it while the animal is in lateral recumbency. Skin turgor can also be used to determine the hydration status of avian patients.

1. **Total body water deficit** in liters is calculated in terms of percentage of body weight measured in kilograms. A patient that is estimated to be 10% dehydrated has lost a volume of water in liters equivalent to 10% of the animal's weight.

   a. Patients with a history of water loss but that have no obvious clinical signs associated with dehydration are assumed to be < 5% dehydrated. The skin tent persists for less than 2 s in these animals.

   b. An animal is assumed to be 6 to 8% dehydrated if on clinical examination the eyes are mildly sunken in their orbits, the mucous membranes are sticky to dry, and the skin tent persists for more than 3 s.

   c. Clinical signs are very pronounced when the animal is 10 to 12% dehydrated. The eyes will be deeply sunken into the orbits, with as much as a 2- to 4-mm gap between the eyeball and bony orbit. The mucous membranes are dry and possibly cold to the touch. The skin tent and twist will persist indefinitely.

2. **Hematocrit** and **total protein** values are commonly used to determine the degree of hemoconcentration or hemodilution that exists in the patient.

   a. The hematocrit should not be permitted to decrease below a value of 21% in the anesthesia candidate. In dogs, normovolemic reductions in packed cell volume to 25% results in optimal delivery of oxygen to peripheral tissues.

      b.    Stable, healthy surgical patients will tolerate normo-volemic reductions in hematocrit to 21% or hemo-globin levels of 70 g/L, if cardiac output is maintained and arterial oxygenation is ensured in the perioperative period. Further reductions in hematocrit increases the potential for inadequate oxygen delivery to peripheral tissues of the anesthetized patient. This is of particular importance to the patient with hemodynamic instability or pulmonary disease.

      c.    **Polycythemia,** on the other hand, increases blood viscosity and reduces capillary flow, which can result in a reduced oxygen delivery capacity of blood with respect to peripheral tissues.

      d.    **Serum protein levels** should be maintained above 35 g/L (3.5 g/dL) and albumin levels above 15 g/L (1.5 g/dL) to ensure that there is no net loss of water from the vascular space, resulting in interstitial edema.

3.    Urine should be collected; and its specific gravity, osmolality, and pH should be determined. In addition, the sample should be tested for the presence of protein, red blood cells, and glucose.

## G.   Fluid Replacement

Selection of the appropriate fluid for replacement purposes depends on the nature of the disease process and the composition of the fluid lost from the patient.

1.    The following **criteria** have been used for determining the appropriate therapeutic intervention: volume deficit; packed cell volume and total serum protein concentration; plasma osmolality; electrolyte concentrations; acid–base status; calorie, water-soluble vitamin, carbohydrate, and amino acid requirements; and trace element concentrations.

2.    It is preferable to replenish total body water and correct electrolyte deficits over a 24- to 48-h period. The patient may be stabilized over the first 4 to 6 h, and 50% of the estimated deficit should be corrected during that time period.

3. In **critically ill** or **moribund** patients, vascular and interstitial volume deficits must be corrected as rapidly as is necessary to ensure the survival of the patient. In the treatment of shock, fluid administration rates of 90 mL/kg/h for dogs and 50 to 60 mL/kg/h for cats have been recommended for the first hour. In subsequent hours, when appropriate, reductions in fluid administration rates to 10 to 12 mL/kg/h for dogs and 5 to 6 mL/kg/h for cats have been suggested.

4. Fluids may be administered orally, subcutaneously, or directly into the vascular space by the intravenous or intraosseous routes.

   a. **Oral administration** of fluids is recommended unless the animal is in critical condition or has severe gastrointestinal disease. Isotonic, nonirritating maintenance solutions may be administered subcutaneously if time and the clinical condition of the patient permit.

   b. The **intraosseous space** provides an alternative route for the parenteral administration of fluids and therapeutic agents into the vascular space.

      i. In **small animals,** the intraosseous space may be accessed through the tibial tuberosity, the trochanteric fossa of the femur or the flat medial surface of the proximal tibia just distal to the tibial tuberosity.

      ii. In **avian species,** the distal end of the ulna is cannulated, because pneumatic bone must be avoided.

## H. Interoperative Period

The most common changes that occur during the **intraoperative period** are alterations to the volume or composition of the extracellular fluid. These changes occur as the result of evaporative losses of free water, sequestration of intracellular and plasma water into traumatized tissues (third space), and hemorrhage.

1.  **Third space losses** occur as the result of translocation of plasma and intracellular water into surgically traumatized tissues. The degree to which the vascular volume is reduced is directly related to the extent of the surgical trauma to the patient.

    a.  Third space losses are replaced with a balanced electrolyte solution using an administration rate of up to 2 mL/kg/h for superficial procedures, 3 to 5 mL/kg/h for mildly traumatic procedures, 5 to 10 mL/kg/h for moderately traumatic surgeries, and up to 15 mL/kg/h for severely traumatic procedures.
    b.  In the avian species intraoperative fluid administration rates of 10 mL/kg/h for the first 2 h and 5 to 8 mL/kg/h for subsequent hours have been recommended.
    c.  This volume of fluid is administered in addition to that which is being administered for maintenance purposes to the surgical patient.

2.  Acute, **intraoperative losses of blood** in excess of 15% of total blood volume in the normal patient or 10% in the critically ill patient should be replaced with whole blood or packed red cells. Oxygen-carrying acellular fluids (oxyglobin), although costly, may be of value when whole blood or packed red cells are not available. Losses that do not exceed these limits may be replaced with balanced electrolyte or replacement solutions.

3.  Consideration must also be given to the administration of fluids to maintain **cardiovascular stability** and organ perfusion, which might be altered owing to the hemodynamic effects of the anesthetic protocol.

    a.  The total volume of fluid that is administered to the patient in the perioperative period should be adjusted to ensure that vital signs, such as blood pressure and urine production, are maintained above critical levels. It is important to remember that perioperative antidiuretic hormone (ADH) release can reduce the volume of urine production. This will complicate the use of urine production as a prognostic tool with respect to vascular volume expansion.

    b.    The administration of large volumes of replacement fluids can lead to **hemodilution** and the interstitial accumulation of fluids. Although some degree of hemodilution can be beneficial, the hematocrit should be maintained at approximately 21 to 25%, hemoglobin in excess of 70 g/L, and total serum protein levels should not be permitted to decrease below 35 g/L (3.5 g/dL).

  4.    Postsurgical **alterations in aldosterone and ADH** activity result in reduced free water clearance in the postoperative period. Once the neurohormonal responses to the surgical procedure abates, third space fluid and the excess fluid in the interstitial space is mobilized and returned to the vascular space. This can result in a volume overload that might be detrimental to the critically ill patient (e.g., pulmonary edema).

## I.   Sodium Balance

**Alterations in sodium balance** may occur as the result of depletion or retention of water or sodium or both. Sodium is the osmolar skeleton of extracellular fluid. Compositional changes in the extracellular fluid during the perioperative period may result from previous or ongoing disease processes or they may be iatrogenic in origin. Plasma electrolyte and osmolality values for dogs and cats are listed in Table 8-12.

  1.    **Hyponatremia** exists when serum sodium concentrations are < 136 mEq/L.

    a.    **Clinical signs** relating to neurologic dysfunction occur when sodium concentrations are < 120 mEq/L and become marked when serum sodium is < 110 mEq/L. Clinical signs that might be observed include anorexia, lethargy, weakness, vomiting, muscle cramping, myoclonus, seizures, tachycardia, shock, and coma.

    b.    The **ECG** may reveal a widened QRS complex with an elevated ST segment and a nonrespiratory dilutional acidosis may develop. Ventricular tachycardia or fibrillation can occur when serum sodium levels are < 100 mEq/L.

c. Severe hyponatremia may be corrected with the careful administration of 3% saline over 24 h.

2. **Hypernatremia** occurs most commonly owing to water loss in excess of the loss of sodium in small animal patients. Those animals that do not have free access to water are prone to develop hypernatremia if they have increased water losses such as would occur from heat prostration or burns. Serum sodium concentrations > 156 mEq/L in dogs and > 160 mEq/L in cats constitute hypernatremia.

**Table 8-12. Normal Fluid and Electrolyte Values**

| Factor/Units | Canine | Feline |
| --- | --- | --- |
| Sodium, mmol/L | 144–162 | 150–160 |
| Potassium, mmol/L | 3.6–6.0 | 4.0–5.8 |
| Chloride, mmol/L | 106–126 | 118–128 |
| Calcium, mmol/L | 2.24–3.04 | 2.23–2.80 |
| Phosphorus, mmol/L | 0.82–1.87 | 1.03–1.92 |
| Magnesium, mmol/L | 0.70–1.16 | 0.74–1.12 |
| Urea, mmol/L | 3.0–10.5 | 5.0–11.0 |
| Creatinine, µmol/L | 60–140 | 90–180 |
| Glucose, mmol/L | 3.3–5.6 | 3.3–5.6 |
| Total protein, g/L | 51–72 | 68–80 |
| Albumin, g/L | 22–38 | 22–38 |
| A:G ratio | 0.60–1.50 | 0.60–1.50 |
| Hemoglobin, g/L | 120–180 | 80–150 |
| Hematocrit, L/L | 0.37–0.55 | 0.24–0.45 |
| RBC, ×$10^{12}$/L | 5.5–8.5 | 5.0–10.0 |
| Reticulocytes, % | 0–1.5% | 0–1% |
| Platelets, ×$10^9$/L | 200–900 | 300–700 |
| Calculated osmolality, mOsm/kg | 280–320 | 280–320 |
| Anion gap, mmol/L | 14–26 | 13–26 |

    a.    **Clinical signs** include lethargy, confusion, muscle weakness, myoclonus, seizures, and coma.

    b.    **Treatment** depends on the initial cause of the hypernatremia and the chronicity of the electrolyte imbalance.

**J.   Calcium Balance**

**Calcium** plays a major role in the physiology of neuromuscular function, cell membrane permeability, muscle contraction, and hemostasis. Total serum calcium consists of an ionized portion, a protein-bound portion, and a portion that is bound to divalent anions such as phosphate and bicarbonate. Close to 50% of total serum calcium is bound to proteins, primarily albumin. Serum ionized calcium levels are pH dependent: Alkalemia reduces and acidemia increases ionized serum calcium levels.

   1.   Symptomatic **hypocalcemia** can occur as a result of hypoparathyroidism or eclampsia. **Intraoperative hypocalcemia,** induced by the administration of large volumes of citrated whole blood, reduces ventricular function and systemic blood pressure.

       a.    Hypocalcemia exists when serum calcium levels are < 7 mg/dL. Hypoalbuminemia may induce a hypocalcemia in small animals of 7 to 8 mg/dL. Serum calcium concentrations < 6.5 mg/dL are generally the result of a metabolic disorder.

       b.    **Clinical signs** include restlessness, muscle fasciculations, tetany, or convulsions. The **ECG** may show prolonged QT and ST segments owing to prolonged myocardial action potentials.

       c.    Acute, **intraoperative hypocalcemic** episodes that are iatrogenic in origin may be treated with 10% calcium chloride or gluconate.

          i.    The **dose** to be **administered** depends on the severity of the situation and ranges from 5 to 15 mg/kg administered over 1 h.

         ii.    If > 50 mL/kg blood or packed red cells are administered, calcium supplementation of the patient should be considered to counteract the effects of the citrate. Up to 6 mL of either calcium preparation per unit (450 to 500 mL) of blood may be administered via a separate intravenous route.

2. **Hypercalcemia** can result from hyperparathyroidism or malignancies in small animals. Hemoconcentration results in increased serum albumin levels. This may increase serum calcium levels to 13 mg/dL.

   a. Serum calcium concentrations in excess of 12 mg/dL in dogs and 11 mg/dL in cats indicate hypercalcemia.

   b. **Clinical** signs include anorexia, vomiting, and gastrointestinal dysfunction. Generalized locomotor weakness may also be evident. Bradycardia, a prolonged PR interval, and a shortened ST segment may be observed.

   c. Rapid increases in serum calcium levels in excess of 15 mg/dL may result in vagal stimulation and severe bradycardia, whereas severe but less acute increases may result in ventricular dysrhythmias.

## K. Potassium Balance

**Potassium** is the primary intracellular cation. Extracellular fluid potassium content represents approximately 2% of total body potassium. As a result, serum potassium concentration often does not accurately represent the extent or severity of a potassium disorder, particularly in chronic disease processes. Potassium is highly labile, and serum levels are altered significantly in the presence of acidemia, alkalemia, or extracellular fluid osmolality changes, or as the result of alterations in serum insulin, glucagon, or catecholamine concentration. Changes in extracellular fluid pH result in rapid and significant alteration in the potassium concentration of extracellular fluid. Acute reductions in $Paco_2$ of 10 mm Hg have been shown to increase plasma pH by 0.1 unit and decrease plasma potassium by 0.4 mEq/L in dogs. Similarly, in cats, serum potassium concentrations change on an order of 0.6 to 0.7 mEq/L per 0.1 unit change in pH.

1. **Hypokalemia** results from reductions in dietary intake or increased losses through the urinary or gastrointestinal systems. Increased losses through the urinary system can be the result of osmotic diuresis, chronic steroid therapy, or the use of loop or thiazide diuretics. Alkalemia will result in a reduction of serum potassium levels as extracellular potassium moves intracellularly in exchange for hydrogen ions.

   a. The degree to which **clinical signs** become apparent depends on the rapidity by which the electrolyte alteration occurs and the chronicity of the disease process.

      i. An **acute** reduction in serum potassium levels to < 3 mEq/L results in clinical signs. These may include reduced gastrointestinal motility and generalized muscle weakness.

      ii. Rapid reductions in extracellular potassium levels disrupt the normal intracellular to extracellular potassium ratio and lead to hyperpolarization of myocardial cells. The **ECG** demonstrates evidence of prolonged repolarization times with a prolonged PR, QRS, and QT intervals, depression of the ST segment, and a flattened or inverted T wave. Severe cardiac manifestations of hypokalemia include sinus bradycardia, heart block, and AV dissociation.

      iii. Clinical signs may not be apparent until potassium concentration approaches 2.5 mEq/L in **chronic** conditions.

   b. Patients in which serum potassium levels have been acutely reduced to < 3 mEq/L should have their serum potassium levels corrected, if at all possible, before inducing anesthesia.

      i. Volume deficits and acid–base disturbances should be corrected early on to ensure adequate renal perfusion and to enable the clinician to determine plasma potassium levels in a more normalized situation with respect to the patient's acid–base status.

  ii. Potassium chloride may be infused at a rate of 0.5 mEq/kg to a maximum daily dose of 2 to 3 mEq/kg.

  iii. In addition to serial potassium determinations, the patient should be monitored with an ECG so the clinician can detect the early signs of potassium toxicity.

 c. When the potassium imbalance is the result of a chronic disease process, anesthesia and surgery should be delayed, if possible, and the imbalance corrected and medically managed over 3 to 5 days. In this situation, the goal is to replenish the total body potassium deficit without inducing clinical signs of potassium toxicity. This may be accomplished through the oral administration of potassium supplements or the parenteral administration of a maintenance solution in which the potassium level has been adjusted to at least 20 to 30 mEq/L.

 d. If the surgical procedure cannot be delayed, then it may be prudent not to correct serum potassium levels that have been reduced to values between 2.5 and 3.0 mEq/L as a result of a chronic process. Rapid corrections of plasma potassium concentration in this instance may acutely disturb the intracellular to extracellular potassium ratio and induce alterations in cell membrane stability.

2. **Hyperkalemia** exists when plasma potassium levels exceed 6.5 mEq/L. It may be iatrogenic in nature or occur as the result of renal failure, urethral obstruction, hypoadrenocorticism, or acidemia. Postoperatively, increased plasma potassium levels may occur owing to increased tissue catabolism or acidemia.

 a. **Clinical signs** become apparent once plasma potassium concentration exceeds 6.5 mEq/L. Myocardial contractility decreases and bradycardia develops. As the plasma potassium concentration approaches 8 mEq/L, the **ECG** will show peaked T waves and a decrease in the amplitude of the P wave. Plasma potassium concentrations in excess of 8 mEq/L have a significant effect on myocardial activity. There is a prolongation of the PR interval, and the P wave may be absent. As the potassium level increases, the QRS complex widens until it assumes a sine wave appearance and AV dissociation occurs. Eventually, asystole or ventricular fibrillation ensues.

b.    Patients with plasma potassium concentrations in excess of 6.5 mEq/L should not be anesthetized unless the patient's life is immediately threatened by some other process.

c.    Severe potassium-induced **cardiotoxicity** may be initially **antagonized** by the intravenous administration of **10% calcium chloride or gluconate** at a dose of 0.2 to 0.3 mEq/kg. If the dysrhythmias persist, the dose may be repeated in 5 min. Calcium helps restore cell membrane potentials; and although its effect will last only 10 to 20 min, it will provide enough time for the clinician to institute other therapeutic measures.

d.    Acute, intraoperative decreases in plasma potassium concentration may also be accomplished by instituting controlled ventilation of the patient to rapidly reverse respiratory acidosis. Correction of **acidemia** will result in an intracellular shift of potassium in exchange for hydrogen ions.

e.    **Dextrose solutions** not only provide free water for volume replacement purposes but also enhance the cellular uptake of potassium as part of the normal mechanisms of glucose metabolism. When plasma potassium levels are significantly increased, glucose may be administered at a dose of 0.5 to 1.0 g/kg to enhance the intracellular movement of potassium. The effect of glucose on serum potassium concentration may be facilitated by administering 1 U of regular insulin for every 2 g dextrose administered.

# Chapter 9

---

## Anesthesia and Immobilization of Dogs, Cats, Birds, Reptiles, and Amphibians

### Introductory Comments

*Anesthetic selection is based on the patient's physical status and temperament, the type of procedure for which anesthesia is being considered, the anesthetist's familiarity with the anesthetic drugs, the type of facility, and the available equipment and technical assistance. There is no single best method for **anesthetizing dogs and cats,** but familiarity with just one anesthetic technique limits the veterinarian's ability to perform the myriad surgical and diagnostic procedures commonly called for in a modern veterinary practice. A debilitated dog or cat undergoing extensive repair of a fractured limb will require a different anesthetic regimen from one undergoing routine neutering, one requiring short-term restraint for radiography or ultrasonography, one with gastric torsion, or one requiring extensive dental work. Some breeds respond atypically to routine administration of an anesthetic drug. For example, sighthounds are less tolerant to thiobarbiturate than comparably sized mixed-breed dogs. The one thing that should not vary among anesthetic procedures is the degree of monitoring vigilance. Early warning of an impending anesthetic emergency is the single most important factor for decreasing anesthetic related morbidity and mortality.*

*The principles and practices of **avian anesthesia** depend on an understanding of anatomy, physiology, and pharmacology. Data derived from mammalian studies are not applied to birds except for general physiologic, pharmacologic, and anesthetic principles that are applicable to avian species. **Reptiles and amphibians** are ectothermic animals, and their response to anesthetic drugs depends on their environmental temperature. Because many body functions are temperature dependent, a variable response of reptiles to anesthetic drugs will be seen if the patient is kept above or below the preferred temperature range. Drugs and dosages successfully used in one animal may prove to be inadequate in another.*

367

## Dogs and Cats
## Birds
## Reptiles
## Amphibians

---

## I.   DOGS AND CATS
*Richard M. Bednarski*

### A.   Preanesthetic Considerations

The history and physical examination are the most important components of the preanesthetic evaluation of mature animals; however, seemingly healthy young animals presented for routine neutering require a history and physical examination. These animals may have never been previously examined by a veterinarian; and congenital disorders, severe parasitism, or heartworm disease may be discovered.

1.   *Signalment*

a.   Most **breed-related** anesthesia problems are **anecdotally** reported. Veterinary anesthesiologists are often asked about the sensitivity to anesthesia of a variety of dog breeds, including, but not limited to, soft-coated wheaten terriers, the Chinese shar-pei, collies, and the Belgian breeds; and among cats, the Maine coon. All breeds have been successfully anesthetized using standard anesthetic regimens.

b.   **Sighthounds** are sensitive to barbiturates. **Brachycephalic breeds** have their associated airway problems and can present anesthetic challenges. **Toy breeds** require special attention to maintenance of body heat. Furthermore, a toy breed requires a relatively greater drug dose per kilogram than does a giant breed. Generally, there is no **sex-related** difference in the response to anesthesia.

c.   A history of the **estrous cycle** identifies recent estrus and its associated enlarged and **vascularized** uterus, which would cause concern for potential blood loss during an ovariohysterectomy. These patients should have an intravenous cannula inserted for crystalloid administration.

   d.   Age is an important anesthetic consideration. Generally the **very young** (< 11 weeks) and the **aged** (> 80% of the expected life span) do not metabolize anesthetic drugs as well as the young, healthy patient does. Healthy geriatric patients should receive sedatives, hypnotics, and tranquilizers at 15 to 30% of the dose given to a comparable young healthy animal.

   e.   **Geriatric** dogs and cats should receive intravenous fluids perioperatively to maintain optimal perfusion of the vital organs.

2. *History*

In addition to questions concerning organ system function, the owner should be asked about any previous anesthetic episodes and past and current medication history, including heartworm prophylaxis. The time since the last feeding should be noted (see Table 2-1).

3. *Physical Examination*

The preanesthetic physical examination should be thorough, and all body systems should be considered (see Table 1-1). Any abnormality discovered or suggested by the medical history should be followed up with the appropriate laboratory test or other suitable diagnostic test. The assessment of the animal's temperament is critical. A vicious or aggressive dog requires a different approach to anesthesia than does the quiet relaxed individual.

4. *Laboratory Evaluation*

Young healthy dogs require minimal laboratory tests, **hematocrit** (packed cell volume; PCV), and **plasma protein.** These tests are inexpensive and easily and quickly performed. PCV indicates hemoglobin concentration. Hemoglobin (measured in grams per deciliter) can be approximated by dividing the PCV by 3. Middle-aged to older animals should have a blood dipstick test performed for **BUN**. If the results are out of the normal range, a more accurate test for BUN should be performed. Other laboratory tests should be performed if the history or physical examination suggests organ system disease.

5. *Physical Status*

Patients should be classified according to relative anesthetic risk. A system of classification has been adapted from suggestions by the American Society of Anesthesiologists (ASA). At physical stage I or II, patients are at less risk for anesthetic complications. At physical stage III through V, patients are at relatively greater anesthetic risk (see Chapter 1). This is not to imply, however, that stage I and II patients are at no risk of unanticipated anesthetic mishaps.

## B. Patient Preparation

1. *Fasting*

Healthy dogs and cats should receive no food for at least 6 h before being anesthetized. Water should be allowed free choice until just before anesthesia. Dogs and cats younger than 8 weeks of age and those weighing < 2 kg should not fast longer than 1 or 2 h. They should also receive intravenous fluids containing dextrose during any prolonged anesthesia (> 15 min).

2. *Patient Stabilization*

When possible, life-threatening disturbances should be corrected before administering anesthesia (Table 9-1).

---

**Table 9-1. A List of Conditions That Should Be Corrected before Administrating Anesthesia**

| | |
|---|---|
| I. Severe dehydration | IV. Pneumothorax |
| II. Anemia or hypoproteinemia | V. Cyanosis |
|    A. Packed cell volume < 20 with | VI. Oliguria or anuria |
|      acute blood loss | VII. Congestive heart failure |
|    B. Albumin < 2.0 g/dL | VIII. Severe, life-threatening cardiac |
| III. Acid–base and electrolyte disturbances |      arrhythmias |
|    A. pH < 7.2 | |
|    B. Potassium < 2.5–3.0 or > 6.0 | |

When impossible, anesthesia should never be delayed if immediate surgical or medical intervention is the only way to save the patient's life.

3.   *Venous Access*
Advantages of having an intravenous catheter in place include the following:

   a.   Tissue-toxic drugs, such as the thiobarbiturates, can be administered without perivascular administration.
   b.   **Intravenous fluid** administration is facilitated.
   c.   **The circulation** is immediately accessible for administration of emergency drugs.
   d.   The most common site for catheter insertion is the **cephalic vein.** The lateral and medial **saphenous veins** are also easily accessible.
   e.   The **jugular vein** can also be used.
   f.   An over-the-needle style of catheter, which is relatively inexpensive, is most suitable. A 20-gauge, 2-inch catheter is suitable for most dogs and cats weighing < 2 kg, and a 22-gauge, 1.25-inch catheter is suitable for those that are smaller. An 18-gauge catheter can be used in medium to large dogs if more rapid fluid administration is required.

4.   *Intravenous Fluids*

   a.   The purpose of perianesthetic administration of intravenous fluids is to maintain vascular volume, which is decreased as a result of anesthetic drugs, blood loss, and insensible fluid loss. For routine use, a balanced electrolyte solution such as lactated Ringer's solution is most suitable, because most fluid loss during anesthesia is isotonic. The patient's disease process may warrant the use of other fluids, such as normal saline, fluids containing dextrose, or a colloid solution (e.g., whole blood, plasma, or a plasma expander; see Chapter 8).
   b.   Several styles of fluid administration sets are available. An administration set with a 10 or 15 drop/mL

drip chamber is most convenient for patients weighing > 5 kg. For smaller patients, a 60 drop/mL drip chamber allows a more precise estimation of proper fluid rate. It is convenient to calculate the number of drops per minute necessary to deliver the calculated hourly fluid amount.

c. A danger of perioperative fluid administration to very small animals is inadvertently administering too much fluid by improperly adjusting the drip rate. This problem can be minimized by attaching a measured volume administration set to the fluid line.

## C. The Anesthetic Plan

The anesthetic technique chosen depends upon a variety of considerations (see Table 1-6). Some of the more commonly used techniques include the following:

1. **Local anesthesia** is usually accompanied by mild to strong sedation and is used more frequently in dogs than in cats. The techniques most commonly used are lumbosacral epidural block, local infiltration or line block, and Bier block.

2. **Injectable anesthesia** may be induced by either the intramuscular or intravenous routes. The intramuscular route is often used with opioids, ketamine, and benzodiazepines. The thiobarbiturates and propofol are always given intravenously.

3. **Inhalation anesthesia** is usually initiated after induction of injectable anesthetics but may be administered from an induction chamber or by use of a face mask. The injectable and inhalation techniques commonly overlap.

4. **For procedures < 15 min in duration,** the following methods can be used:

   a. The **thiobarbiturates** are relatively inexpensive and are suitable for short-term restraint of most healthy dogs and cats. The disadvantage of their use is that full recovery usually takes up to 1 h and can be associated with ataxia and disorientation. These effects are reduced when the thiobarbiturate is preceded by a tranquilizer, such as **acepromazine.** Another disadvantage is that they must be administered intravenously, a problem with fractious or uncooperative animals (Table 9-2).

b.   Alternatives to the thiobarbiturates include **propofol, etomidate,** and the combination of **diazepam** and **ketamine.** These drugs are more expensive than the thiobarbiturates; and the duration after one bolus dose is shorter, generally < 10 min. Preceding these drugs with a sedative or tranquilizer such as **acepromazine, xylazine,** or **diazepam** decreases the dose and improves the quality of recovery (Tables 9-2 and 9-3).

c.   **Neuroleptanalgesic combinations** are suitable for short-term restraint for mildly invasive procedures or for procedures not requiring general anesthesia (Table 9-4). An advantage is that one or both components of neuroleptanalgesia are reversible, allowing rapid return to preanesthetic mentation.

d.   The relatively cumbersome nature of **inhalation anesthesia** makes it less suitable for very short proce-

| Table 9-2. Injectable Anesthetic Drugs | | |
|---|---|---|
| **Drug** | **Dosage, mg/kg** | **Comments** |
| Thiamylal | 6.0–15.0 IV | Use lower dosage after premedication |
| Thiopental | 8.0–20.0 IV | Use lower dosage after premedication |
| Methohexital | 3.0–8.0 IV | Muscle rigidity; best if preceded by a tranquilizer sedative; 3–5 min duration |
| Etomidate | 0.5–2.0 IV | Duration 5–10 min; myoclonus, gagging/retching |
| Propofol | 4.0–6.0 IV | Duration 5–10 min after single bolus dose; |
| | 0.4–0.8 mg/kg/min | apnea several minutes with rapid injection |

dures. The rapid induction and recovery associated with isoflurane, however, make it the most suitable of the approved inhalants for short-term restraint.

5. **For procedures between 15 and 60 min (intermediate duration),** the drugs described above can be used and re-dosed to effect. Typically, one-third to one-half the original dose is administered to prolong the anesthetic effect. The thiobarbiturates should not be repeatedly re-dosed, however. Although their initial duration of action primarily depends on redistribution away from the brain to other tissues, such as muscle, when the tissue are saturated, metabolism is ultimately responsible for awakening. Again, inhalation anesthesia is also appropriate for procedures of intermediate duration.

6. **Procedures > 1h (long duration)** are best managed with inhalation anesthesia. Awakening from halothane and isoflurane anesthesia is predictably rapid. Even sick and debilitated patients recover from prolonged periods of inhalational anesthesia relatively quickly.

| Table 9-3. Cyclohexamines and Cyclohexamine Combinations | | |
|---|---|---|
| **Drugs** | **Dosage, mg/kg** | **Comments** |
| Ketamine | 2.0–10.0 IV, IM | Not useful alone in dogs; useful restraint in cats; lasts 5–30 min |
| Ketamine-diazepam and ketamine/midazolam | 5.5/0.20 IV | Diazepam and midazolam are equally effective in this combination; useful restraint; lasts 5–10 min; poor muscle relaxation and analgesia |
| Ketamine-xylazine | 10.0/0.7–1.0 | Useful restraint; lasts 20–40 min |
| Ketamine-acepromazine | 10.0/0.2 | Useful restraint; lasts 20–30 min |
| Tiletamine-zolazepam (Telazol) | 2.0–8.0 IV, IM | Limited shelf-life after reconstitution; useful restraint for 20–60 min |

**Table 9-4. Opioids and Neuroleptanalgesic Combinations**

| Drugs | Dosage,[a] mg/kg | Comments |
|---|---|---|
| Oxymorphone | 0.05–0.1 IV, IM, SC | Excitement when used alone in young healthy dogs; duration 1–4 h |
| Morphine | 0.2–0.6 IV, SC | Mild sedation when used alone; duration 1–4 h |
| Butorphanol | 0.2–0.4 IV, IM, SC | Minimal sedation when used alone; duration 1–3 h |
| Fentanyl-droperidol (Innovar-Vet) | 1 mL/10–30 kg IV, IM | Excellent for aggressive dogs; dose-dependent sedation; duration 30–60 min |
| Acepromazine-oxymorphone | 0.05/0.05–0.1 IV, IM | Can be combined in same syringe; duration 15–60 min |
| Acepromazine-butorphanol | 0.05/0.2 IV, IM | Can be combined in same syringe; duration 15–60 min |
| Acepromazine-buprenorphine | 0.03/0.01 IV | Moderate sedation; duration 2–3 h |
| Midazolam-oxymorphone | 0.1–0.2/0.05–0.1 IV, IM | Can be combined in same syringe; duration 15–40 min |
| Midazolam-butorphanol | 0.1–0.2/0.2 IV, IM | Can be combined in same syringe; duration 15–40 min |
| Xylazine-oxymorphone | 0.4–0.6/0.05–0.1 IV, IM | Both drugs are reversible; duration 30–40 min |
| Xylazine-butorphanol | 0.4–0.6/0.2–0.4 IV, IM | Both drugs are reversible; duration 30–40 min |

[a]Use low end of opioid dosage for cats.

## D. Premedication

Inhalation anesthesia can be initiated without premedication; however, premedication with a **sedative, tranquilizer,** or other injectable drug is recommended (Tables 9-5 and 9-6). Preanesthetic drugs aid in restraint, reduce apprehension, decrease the quantity of potentially more dangerous drugs used to produce general anesthesia, facilitate induction, enhance analgesia, and reduce autonomic reflex activity. Drugs for premedication are usually administered intramuscularly or subcutaneously 15 to 20 min before induction. The choice of premedication depends on species, temperament, physical stage, the procedure to be performed, and clinician's preference. For procedures associated with significant postoperative pain, premedication should include an analgesic such as an opioid or $\alpha_2$-agonist. When analgesia is provided before initiation of a painful stimulus (pre-emptive analgesia), need for postoperative analgesics is lessened. See Chapter 2 for further discussion on perioperative pain management.

### E. Induction

Induction is most easily accomplished with an ultra-short-acting barbiturate or other equally short-acting drug(s) (Tables 9-2

| Table 9-5. Suggestions for Premedication in Canines and Felines[a] | |
|---|---|
| **Species** | **Drugs** |
| Canines | |
| Young, normal healthy | Acepromazine |
| | Xylazine |
| | Acepromazine-oxymorphone |
| | Acepromazine-butorphanol |
| Aggressive/vicious | Fentanyl-droperidol |
| | Acepromazine-oxymorphone |
| | Tiletamine-zolazepam |
| Geriatric | Acepromazine |
| | Diazepam |
| | Midazolam-oxymorphone |
| | Midazolam-butorphanol |
| Painful procedures | Acepromazine-oxymorphone |
| | Acepromazine-butorphanol |
| | Midazolam-oxymorphone |
| | Midazolam-butorphanol |
| Felines | Acepromazine-oxymorphone |
| | Ketamine |
| | Ketamine-acepromazine |
| | Xylazine |

[a]All can be given intramuscularly or subcutaneously, except diazepam, which should be given intravenously immediately before administering the induction drug.

**Table 9-6. Sedatives and Tranquilizers**

| Drug | Dosage,[a] mg/kg | Comments |
|------|------------------|----------|
| Acepromazine | 0.025–0.2 IV, IM, SC (3–4 mg maximum) | Mild to moderate sedation; duration 1–2 h |
| Xylazine | 0.3–2.2 IV, IM | Moderate to deep sedation, analgesia; duration 20–60 min |
| Medetomidine | 0.01–0.02 IV, IM (canines) 0.02–0.03 IV, IM (felines) | Similar effects to xylazine; duration 1–3 h |
| Diazepam | 0.2–0.4 IV, IM | Most useful when combined with other sedatives, opioids, or ketamine; avoid IM in cats and small dogs |
| Midazolam | 0.1–0.3 IV, IM, SC | Similar to diazepam, but also useful IM or SC |

[a]Generally, the low end of the dosage range is used intravenously and in sick and debilitated patients.

and 9-3). Advantages to this method of induction include rapid loss of consciousness and ability to quickly intubate. Alternatives to rapid induction are chamber or mask induction and opioid induction. These techniques can be useful in special circumstances; but for routine use, their disadvantages outweigh their advantages.

1. *Chamber and Mask Induction*

   A disadvantage to chamber and mask induction is the associated waste gas pollution. Another disadvantage in nonpremedicated healthy animals is the struggling and associated stress during the induction phase. Mask induction is most easily accomplished in moribund animals, tractable dogs, and those that have been adequately sedated. **Chamber induction** is most useful in cats or tiny dogs. Isoflurane and halothane are suitable drugs, because they produce a fairly rapid induction. Relatively high oxygen flow rates (4 L/min for chamber; 3 L/min for mask) and vaporizer settings (4% halothane or isoflurane in healthy animals) are used. The use of nitrous oxide is not necessary during chamber and mask induction. During chamber induction, once the animal loses its righting reflex and is unresponsive when the chamber is tilted from side to side, the animal is removed from the chamber and induction is continued using an appropriately sized mask. **Mask induction** is begun by exposing the animal to the mask and oxygen. The inhalation concentration is slowly increased to 4%. This is accomplished with a nonrebreathing circuit by gradually increasing the vaporizer setting from 0 to 4% over 2 to 3 min. The vaporizer can be initially set to 4% if a circle system is used, because the concentration within the circle gradually increases.

2. *Opioid Induction*

A disadvantage to opioid induction is the attendant relatively slow loss of consciousness. Advantages include good cardiovascular stability and the attenuation of the stress response associated with anesthesia and surgery. Opioid induction works best in debilitated dogs and is not recommended in cats or young healthy dogs that are not well sedated. Low doses of oxymorphone or fentanyl are alternated with low doses of diazepam or midazolam until the dog can be intubated (Tables 9-3 and 9-4).

## F. Maintenance

The maintenance phase of anesthesia begins when unconsciousness is induced and continues through the time the patient is disconnected from the anesthesia breathing circuit. After the loss of consciousness, a properly sized cuffed endotracheal tube or alternative airway is inserted. Adequate cardiovascular function is verified, and the anesthetic vaporizer is turned on. The initial and subsequent anesthetic **vaporizer settings** vary with the condition of the patient, the type of vaporizer, the type of breathing circuit, and the fresh gas flow rate (Table 9-7). The relatively high fresh gas flow rate and vaporizer setting that are initially used after induction are decreased to maintenance settings when the **palpebral reflex** disappears and the heart rate begins to decrease. The vaporizer setting is adjusted according to signs of anesthetic depth, which include muscle tone (assessed by opening the mouth to its full extent), **heart** and **respiratory rates,** and **systemic blood pressure.** All but the

| Table 9-7. Vaporizer Settings[a] | | |
|---|---|---|
| **Drug** | **Induction Phase (%)** | **Maintenance Phase (%)** |
| **VAPORIZER OUT OF CIRCLE**[b] | | |
| Isoflurane | 3–4 | 1.5–3.0 |
| Halothane | 3 | 1.0–2.0 |
| Methoxyflurane | 3 | 0.5–1.5 |
| Enflurane | 4–5 | 2.5–4.0 |
| **VAPORIZER IN CIRCLE**[c] | | |
| Isoflurane | 2/3 open | 1/8–1/2 open |
| Halothane | 2/3 open | 1/8–1/2 open |
| Methoxyflurane | 2/3 to full open | 1/8–1/2 open |

[a]Assuming a fresh gas flow of 1–2 L/min during the induction phase and a fresh gas flow of 10 mL/kg/min during the maintenance phase. Low-flow system vaporizer settings are typically 1 to 2% higher.
[b]Induction phase listed as percent.
[c]For example, the Stephens vaporizer or the Ohio 8 vaporizer. The wick in these vaporizers is used only for methoxyflurane.

systemic blood pressure are easily and inexpensively monitored and should be performed routinely.

An anesthetic record should be maintained and should include patient status, the anesthetic drugs used (including dose and effect), the duration of the surgery, and any significant perioperative events. Ideally, heart rate, respiratory rate, blood pressure, and any other monitored variables should be recorded at regular intervals, which creates a visual aid that assists in determining the change in patient status over the course of the anesthetic episode. For example, a decrease in heart rate and blood pressure during a 15-min interval could signal increasing anesthetic depth and should alert the clinician to decrease the vaporizer setting. This change over time is easily observed on the anesthetic record but may not be noticed without the visual prompt of the record.

## G.   Recovery

1.   Recovery begins when the procedure for which the patient has been anesthetized is finished and the anesthetic drugs have been discontinued.

2. Patient monitoring should occur regularly during the recovery period until the patient is **alert and extubated** and the heart rate, respiratory rate, and body temperature have returned to normal.

3. Young, healthy animals undergoing routine procedures need not receive supplemental oxygen during recovery unless nitrous oxide was used. If nitrous oxide was used, the breathing circuit should be repeatedly flushed with oxygen, and the patient should be allowed to breathe an oxygen-enriched gas mixture for the first 5 to 10 min to help prevent **diffusion hypoxia.**

4. Sick or debilitated dogs and cats benefit from supplemental oxygen during recovery. **Shivering** signifies increased oxygen consumption. Some loss of body heat is unavoidable during anesthesia and surgery, and the patient should be warmed during recovery. Devices are available for patient warming, including circulating warm water heating blankets, infrared heat lamps, incubators, and circulating warm air blankets. Electric heating pads should never be used, because they have been associated with severe burns, which are usually manifest several days to a week after contact. Care must be used with heat lamps, because they also have produced thermal burns by being placed too close to unprotected skin. An advantage of using warm water heating blankets is that the temperature is uniform over the entire surface; furthermore, their maximum temperature is well below 40.5°C (105°F), the maximum safe level. Warming is hastened if the patient is cocooned within the warm water heating blanket. Incubators are convenient for warming small dogs and cats; and if needed, supplemental oxygen can be introduced during the warming period. Circulating warm air blankets that cocoon the patient are the most effective devices for postoperative warming.

5. The endotracheal tube cuff should be deflated and the gauze securing the tube should be untied when the patient is disconnected from the anesthetic machine. This permits extubation in the event that the patient rapidly awakens

and begins chewing. Similarly, if an esophageal stethoscope was used, it should be removed at this time. Dogs and cats should be extubated as soon as the swallowing reflex returns, unless there is some specific contraindication to removing the endotracheal tube. Dogs and cats should be constantly observed when the endotracheal tube is still in place.

6. Occasionally, a dog or cat will be disoriented when it awakens from anesthesia and will vocalize, paddle, and appear incoherent. This is most often caused by emergence delirium or pain. Emergence delirium occurs most frequently in nonpremedicated animals and, in particular, patients awakening rapidly from anesthesia. Dogs and cats suffering from emergence delirium will usually become quiet and more comfortable within a short time, ~ 10 min. A quiet, reassuring voice and restraint are all that is generally necessary to guide the animal through this period of excitement. Occasionally, a low dose of acepromazine (0.05 mg/kg IV) is needed to quiet the animal. If the apparent excitement is the result of postoperative pain, the animal should receive a systemic analgesic or some other analgesic technique. In rare instances, delirium may be associated with a drug effect that can be reversed with an antagonist (Table 9-8).

### Table 9-8. Antagonists of Various Classes of Sedative Drugs

| Drug | Dosage, mg/kg |
|---|---|
| $\alpha_2$ | |
| Yohimbine | 0.1 IV, IM |
| Atipamezole | 0.04–0.05 IM |
| Benzodiazepine | |
| Flumazenil | 0.2–5.0 IV |
| Opioid | |
| Naloxone | 0.003–0.01 IV, IM |

## II. BIRDS

*John W. Ludders and Nora Matthews*

### A. Form and Function

1. *Anatomy of the Pulmonary System*
   The avian respiratory system consists of two anatomically and functionally distinct components: one for ventilation (conducting airways, air sacs, thoracic skeleton, muscles of respiration) and one for gas exchange (the parabronchial lung).

   a. The **trachea** consists of four layers. The **mucous membrane** is made up of simple and pseudostratified, ciliated columnar epithelium with large numbers of simple alveolar mucous glands composed of typical mucus-secreting cells. The mucus glands give way to mucus goblet cells in the caudal portion of the trachea and within the lining of the syrinx. The other layers are the **submucosa, cartilage** (the tracheal cartilages form complete rings), and the **adventitia.**

   b. There are **species-related variations** in the tracheal anatomy.

      i. **Emus** have an inflatable saclike diverticulum (tracheal sac) arising from the ventral surface of the trachea approximately three-quarters of the way down the neck, where there is a slit-like opening in the tracheal rings. The caudal end of the sac may extend almost to the level of the sternum. This sac is present in both sexes.

      ii. The males of many **Anseriform species** (waterfowl such as ducks and mergansers) have a tracheal bulbous expansion, a bulb-like structure in the trachea.

      iii. **Double trachea** are found in some penguins and petrels. They consist of a median septum that divides part of the trachea into right and left channels. In both groups of birds, the septum extends cranially from the bronchial bifurcation; but its length is quite variable. For example, in the jackass penguin, the septum extends to within a few centimeters of the larynx; whereas in the rockhopper penguin, the septum is only 5 mm in length.

iv. Some species have **tracheal loops and coils** that, depending on the species, may be located in the caudal neck, within the keel, or within the thorax and the keel (Fig. 9-1).

c. Functionally, the **air sacs** serve as bellows to the lungs, because they provide tidal air flow to the relatively rigid avian lung. Based on their bronchial connections, air sacs are grouped into a cranial group (consisting of the cervical, clavicular, and cranial thoracic

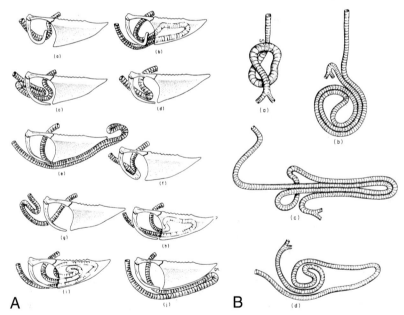

**Figure 9-1. A,** Different forms of tracheal loops found in birds. *a,* black swan (*Cygnus atratus*); *b,* whooper swan (*Cygnus cygnus*); *c,* white spoonbill (*Platalea leucorodia*); *d,* black curassow (*Crax alector*); *e,* helmeted curassow (*Crax pauxi*); *f,* crested guinea fowl (*Guttera edouardi*); *g,* capercaillie (*Tetrao urogallus*); *h,* crane (*Grus grus*); *i,* whooping crane (*Grus americana*); *j,* bird of paradise (*Manucodia* sp.). **B,** Extreme forms of tracheal loops found in birds. *a, Platalea* sp.; *b,* trumpet bird (*Phonygammus keradrenii*); *c,* magpie goose (*Anseranas semipalmata*); *d,* whooping crane (*Grus americana*). Reprinted with permission from McLelland J. Larynx and trachea. In: King AS, McLelland J, eds., Form and function in birds. Vol. 4. London: Academic Press, 1989:69–103.

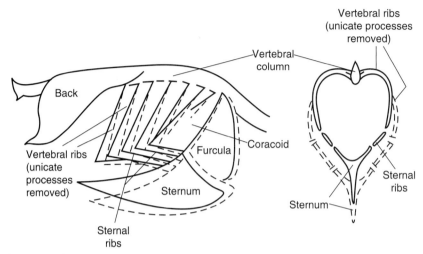

**Figure 9-2.** Changes in the position of the thoracic skeleton during breathing in a bird. *Solid lines,* thoracic position at the end of expiration; *dotted lines,* thoracic position at the end of inspiration. Reprinted with permission from Fedde MR. Respiration. In: Sturkie PD, ed., Avian physiology. 4th ed. New York: Springer-Verlag, 1986:191–220.

air sacs) and a caudal group (consisting of the caudal thoracic and abdominal air sacs). The volume is distributed approximately equally between the cranial and caudal groups of air sacs, and the ratio of ventilation to volume is similar for each air sac.

d.    In birds, inspiration and expiration are active processes that require muscular activity from the muscles of respiration and the thoracic skeleton. When the inspiratory muscles contract, the internal volume of the thoracoabdominal cavity increases; and because the air sacs are the only significant volume-compliant structures within the body cavity, the volume changes occur mainly in the air sacs (Fig. 9-2). Pressure within the air sacs becomes negative relative to the ambient atmospheric pressure; and air flows from the atmosphere into the pulmonary system, specifically into the air sacs and across the gas exchange surfaces of the lungs.

e.    A cross-current model of **gas exchange** describes the relationship between gas and blood flows within the avian lung. In birds, there is no equivalent of alveolar gas, because parabronchial gas continuously changes in composition as it flows along the length of the parabronchus. The degree to which capillary blood is oxygenated and carbon dioxide is eliminated depends on where along the length of the parabronchus the blood contacts the blood–gas interface. As a result, arterial blood is formed by the mixing of streams of end-capillary blood of widely varying gas composition.

2. *Control of Ventilation*
Birds have many of the same physiologic components for respiratory control as do mammals, such as a central respiratory pattern generator, central chemoreceptors that are sensitive to $P_{CO_2}$, and many similar peripheral chemoreceptors. Birds do have a unique group of peripheral receptors located in the lung, called **intrapulmonary chemoreceptors (IPC),** that are not mechanoreceptors and are acutely sensitive to $CO_2$ and insensitive to hypoxia.

3. *Implications for Anesthesia*
An overly inflated endotracheal tube cuff can traumatize and even rupture the tracheal mucosa and rings. For this reason, an endotracheal tube cuff either should not be inflated or should be inflated only sufficiently to form an effective seal when ventilation is assisted. During anesthesia, mucus production can be copious; and with the drying effects of the inspired gases, the mucus becomes thick and tenacious. Endotracheal tubes with small internal diameters can impose significant resistance to air flow, which that will be exacerbated by mucus accumulation in the tube. Signs of endotracheal tube obstruction can be detected by monitoring the bird's pattern of ventilation. An anticholinergic, such as atropine or glycopyrrolate, reduces mucus production and decreases mucus plug formation but may also increase mucus viscosity, making it harder to clear.

a. As noted, the vessel-poor **air sacs** do not significantly participate in gas exchange. For this same reason they do not play a major role in the uptake of inhalant anesthetics; nor, as has been suggested, do they accumulate or concentrate **anesthetic gases.**

b.   During **positive pressure ventilation** it is possible that the direction of gas flow within the avian lung may be reversed; but such a reversal does not affect gas exchange, because the efficiency of the crosscurrent model does not depend on the direction of flow.

c.   The follow-through (**unidirectional**) nature of the avian respiratory system makes it possible to ventilate birds by flowing a continuous stream of gas through the trachea and lungs, and out through a ruptured or cannulated air sac. This same technique can be used to induce and maintain anesthesia in birds. This technique also offers an effective means by which to ventilate and resuscitate an apneic bird or a bird with an obstructed airway.

d.   Because inspiratory and expiratory **muscle activity** is essential for ventilation in birds, any depression of muscle activity affects ventilatory efficiency.

e.   The **body position** of the bird during anesthesia can significantly affect ventilation. A number of factors contribute to this phenomenon, not the least of which is the weight of the abdominal viscera compressing the abdominal air sacs and thus reducing their effective volume.

f.   Because birds have many of the same mechanisms for controlling ventilation as mammals it seems reasonable to assume that anesthetics will similarly depress avian **ventilatory control mechanisms.**

g.   During anesthesia, the lack of a significant functional residual volume in birds limits the period of time that a bird can remain apneic. During induction of anesthesia in birds, especially waterfowl, apnea and bradycardia can occur and last for 3 to 5 min. Anesthetic gases are not required to elicit this response, as it can occur by placing a mask snugly over a bird's beak and face. This response has been referred to as the **dive response,** but it is actually a stress response that appears to be mediated by stimulation of trigeminal receptors in the beak and nares of diving ducks. During the stress response, blood flow is preferentially distributed to the kidneys, heart, and brain. This stress response makes safe induction of anesthesia in these birds a challenge. This response may be ameliorated by the use of premedicants such as diazepam or midazolam.

4.  *Anatomy of the Cardiovascular System*
    Birds have larger hearts, larger stroke volumes, lower heart rates, and higher cardiac output than do mammals of comparable body mass. Birds also have higher blood pressures than do mammals. The atria and ventricles are innervated by sympathetic and parasympathetic nerves. Norepinephrine and epinephrine are the principal sympathetic neurotransmitters in birds, and acetylcholine is the principal parasympathetic neurotransmitter.

5.  *Anatomy of the Renal Portal System*
    The avian kidney receives venous blood from the legs through the renal portal circulation and arterial blood through the arterial circulation. The flow of afferent venous blood, unlike in other nonmammalian vertebrates, is not obligatory, because blood can either perfuse the renal parenchyma or bypass it and enter the central circulation. A unique valve-like structure, containing smooth muscle and innervated by cholinergic and adrenergic nerves, is located within the external iliac vein at the point at which the efferent renal vein joins the external iliac vein. Epinephrine causes the valve to relax, whereas acetylcholine causes it to contract. When the valve contracts (closes), venous blood from the legs perfuses the kidney; but when the valve is relaxed (open), the venous blood is directed to the central circulation.

    a.  For walking birds, **intramuscular injections** are most commonly administered in the pectoral muscles; and in flying birds, they are generally injected in the leg muscles. Because birds possess a renal portal system, there has been some concern that injections in the leg muscles might result in excessive drug loss through the kidneys. Although the renal portal system may be an important variable in antimicrobial therapy, its effect on anesthetic drugs injected into the leg muscles is probably unimportant.

## B. General Considerations for Anesthesia

1. *Physical Examination*

   In general, quietly observing a bird in its cage provides a great deal of information. Awareness of and attention to its surrounding environment, body form and posture, feather condition, and respiratory rate all provide clues to a bird's physical condition. Birds should be removed from their cages and examined, with particular attention given to the nares and mouth. A stethoscope with a pediatric head for small species should be used to examine the heart and lungs. At the same time, the sharpness of the keel should be determined, because this is a good indicator of muscle mass and body fat.

2. *Acclimation*

   When possible a bird should be allowed to acclimate to the clinic or hospital environment before anesthesia. A bird brought into a new environment will be stressed.

3. *Fasting*

   In general, it has been recommended that birds either not be fasted or be fasted for no more than 2 to 3 h before anesthesia, because of their high metabolic rate and poor hepatic glycogen storage. Because of the hazards associated with regurgitation in minimally fasted birds, however, some practitioners recommend that avian species, regardless of size, be fasted overnight.

4. *Physical Restraint*

   Because birds cannot dissipate heat through the skin, they can become stressed and easily overheated with prolonged restraint. Psittacine owners often judge the expertise of a veterinarian by his or her ability to restrain their bird without bruising it around the face. In general, a bird must be restrained so that the wings and legs are controlled and not allowed to flap or kick about. For long-necked birds such as herons and cranes, the neck must also be controlled so that head, eye, and neck trauma is avoided.

Psittacines have very strong beaks that can cause severe soft tissue injury. Cranes and herons will use their long, pointed beaks in a spearing manner, and they seem to focus on handlers' eyes.

5. *Injectable Anesthetics*

There are many advantages associated with the use of injectable anesthetics, including their low cost and ease of use and the rapidity with which anesthesia can be induced. Furthermore, expensive equipment is not required for delivery or maintenance of anesthesia, and pollution of the work environment is not an issue. There are, however, inherent disadvantages associated with the use of injectables, including great interindividual and interspecies variation in terms of dose and response, difficulty in delivering safe volumes to small birds, ease in overdosing by any route, difficulty in maintaining surgical anesthesia without severe cardiopulmonary depression, and the potential for prolonged and violent recoveries.

## C.    Pharmacology

Pharmacologic principles that apply to mammals are applicable to birds.

1. *Injectable Drugs*

   a.    **Injection sites** for birds include subcutaneous, intramuscular, and intravenous sites.

      i.    **Subcutaneous:** the area over the back between the wings, the wing web, and the skin fold in the inguinal region.
      ii.   **Intramuscular:** pectoral and thigh muscles.
      iii.  **Intravenous:** ulnaris vein, dorsal metatarsal vein, and **jugular vein;** all can be used for intravenous injections as well as for catheterization. In general, the right jugular vein is larger and easier to visualize than the left jugular vein.

   b.    **Ketamine** is a cyclohexamine that produces a state of catalepsy and can be given by any parenteral route.

Doses range from 10 to 200 mg/kg, depending on species and route of administration. Drugs such as diazepam and xylazine have been combined with ketamine to prolong or improve the quality of anesthesia and provide muscle relaxation or additional analgesia. When used alone, ketamine is suitable for chemical restraint for minor surgical and diagnostic procedures, but it is not a suitable general anesthetic for major surgical manipulations. Higher doses of ketamine serve only to prolong its duration of action while decreasing its margin of safety.

  c.     The **benzodiazepines** include the following drugs.

       i.     **Diazepam** is a minor tranquilizer with excellent muscle relaxant properties, but it lacks analgesic properties. It should not be viewed as providing additional analgesia when combined with primary anesthetics, such as ketamine. Diazepam can be used to tranquilize birds before mask induction with inhalant anesthetics, thus reducing the stress and struggling associated with handling and anesthetic induction. Its duration of action is short, and recovery is not prolonged.

      ii.     **Midazolam** is a more potent, longer-acting benzodiazepine than diazepam. In Canada geese, midazolam (2 mg/kg IM) induced adequate sedation for radiography, and effective sedation lasted up to 20 min after injection. Mean arterial blood pressure remained stable; and arterial blood gases, which were measured in a select number of birds, were unchanged from baseline values. As with diazepam, midazolam can be given to facilitate induction of anesthesia. The effects of midazolam given to raptors and pigeons last for several hours after the termination of anesthesia. Although there have not been any complications associated with prolonged recoveries, they can be considered an undesirable feature of this drug.

      iii.     **Flumazenil** is a benzodiazepine antagonist. Flumazenil was administered to quail at a dosage of 0.1 mg/kg at the peak time of sedation with midazolam (6 mg IM). Flumazenil caused complete recovery from sedation induced with midazolam.

d. **Xylazine** has sedative and analgesic properties and has been used for minor surgical and diagnostic procedures. It has profound cardiopulmonary effects, including second-degree heart block, brady-arrhythmias, and increased sensitivity of the heart to catecholamine-induced arrhythmias. To enhance sedative and analgesic properties, xylazine is frequently combined with other anesthetic drugs, such as ketamine. When used alone in high doses, xylazine is associated with respiratory depression, excitement, and convulsions in some species.

e. To hasten recovery or to treat an $\alpha_2$-adrenergic agonist overdose, $\alpha_2$-**adrenergic antagonists,** such as **tolazoline** or **yohimbine,** can be used. **Atipamezole** is a very selective $\alpha_2$-antagonist and may be used to reverse the sedative effects of any $\alpha_2$-agonist drug.

f. **Propofol** is a substituted phenol derivative (2,6-diisopropylphenol) developed for intravenous induction and maintenance of general anesthesia. Its actions are characterized by rapid onset and recovery. In pigeons, propofol produced respiratory depression and apnea and was considered to have a narrow margin of safety. In chickens, propofol produced and maintained anesthesia when injected as a bolus intravenously (4.5 to 9.7 mg/kg) and infused at 0.5 to 1.2 mg/kg/min for 20 min. Arrhythmias were common, occurring in 13 of 14 birds. Induction and maintenance caused significant respiratory and cardiovascular depression; hypotension and hypoxemia were common.

g. With **barbiturates,** surgical anesthesia can be maintained for relatively long periods of time (1 to 12 h) by using intermediate- to long-acting barbiturates or combinations of drugs with intermediate duration of effect. **Pentobarbital** can be used to produce anesthesia of several hours' duration using doses of 25 to 30 mg/kg IV. Because it requires 10 to 15 min for full onset of action, the drug should be administered initially as a bolus consisting of half the total dose; the remainder should be titrated over several minutes until the desired plane of anesthesia is achieved.

h.    **α-chloralose** is a general depressant and tranquilizer that has been used to capture birds in the wild, such as cranes, crows, storks, wild turkeys, and Canada geese. The drug is usually mixed with a bait such as corn or bread that is attractive to the birds to be captured.

i.    **Local anesthetics** have been used in birds with unfortunate consequences, including seizures and cardiac arrest. The problem is the result of the small size of some avian species and inappropriate doses. For example, in a 30-g parakeet, 0.1 mL of 2% **lidocaine** administered intramuscularly or subcutaneously is equivalent to 67 mg/kg, a gross and toxic overdose for any animal! Lidocaine can be used in birds for local anesthesia if the dose does not exceed 4 mg/kg, a dose that is difficult to achieve in very small birds.

j.    The few studies evaluating the analgesic effects of **opioids** in birds are conflicting. Studies have shown that κ-opioid receptors account for 76% of the radiolabeling of pigeon forebrain tissues. Thus **butorphanol,** a κ-agonist, may be a better analgesic for birds than are **μ-opioid agonists.** This conclusion is supported by the fact that butorphanol produces an isoflurane-sparing effect in cockatoos.

2.    *Inhalant Anesthetics*

a.    The **advantages** of inhalant anesthetics are rapid induction and recovery, especially when inhalant anesthetics of low blood gas solubility are used (halothane and isoflurane), easier control of anesthetic depth, the concurrent use of oxygen thus providing respiratory support, and fast recovery that does not depend on metabolic or excretory pathways.

b.    **Nonrebreathing circuits** (Bain circuit or Norman elbow) are ideal for use in birds, because they offer minimal resistance to patient ventilation. The plastic Bain circuit is lightweight, which is an advantage when used in very small birds. When using a nonrebreathing circuit, **oxygen flows** should be 2 to 3 times minute ventilation, or 150 to 200 mL/kg/min.

c.   **Induction methods** include the following.

    i.    Induction can be accomplished with commercially available small animal **masks** or homemade masks fabricated from plastic bottles, syringe cases, syringes, and breathing hose connectors. Mask induction techniques can be used in a wide variety and sizes of birds, from the very small up to and including the emu. Mask inductions are unsatisfactory in adult ostriches.

    ii.    Birds can be induced by inserting their heads into **plastic bags** (preferably clear plastic) into which oxygen and anesthetic vapor are introduced via a nonrebreathing circuit. Plastic bags have been used to completely enclose a bird cage to induce anesthesia in a bird that is difficult to manage.

    iii.    Whatever technique is used for induction, the anesthetist must take precautions to control and eliminate anesthetic **gas pollution** in the work environment. If a mask is used, it should fit snugly over the bird's beak and face or over its entire head. If a plastic bag or chamber is used, it should be free of leaks.

    iv.    Any bird larger than a cockatiel or larger than 100 g can be **intubated.** Unique anatomic features, however, can interfere with intubation; and structures such as the median tracheal septum found in some penguins and the large bills of toucans and flamingos must be kept in mind as the clinician plans an intubation strategy. In most birds, the glottis is easy to visualize; and depending on the size of the bird, the larynx and trachea are easily intubated. Psittacine species, especially the smaller birds such as parakeets, can be difficult to intubate because of the awkward location of the glottis at the base of the humped, fleshy tongue.

   d.   **Halothane and isoflurane** are the two most commonly used inhalant anesthetics. Of these, isoflurane is the preferred choice for anesthesia in birds.

       i.   **Minimum anesthetic concentration** (MAC) values for halothane and isoflurane used in birds are similar to those reported for use in mammals (Table 9-9).

      ii.   Halothane and isoflurane, at all end-tidal anesthetic concentrations and in a dose-dependent manner, **depress ventilation.** Halothane and isoflurane appear to depress ventilation more in birds than in mammals. Hypoventilation makes it difficult to control the plane of anesthesia. Furthermore, the hypercapnia associated with anesthetic-induced ventilatory depression can have a variety of adverse effects on cardiopulmonary function through direct or indirect mechanisms. For these reasons, ventilation in birds should be assisted or controlled during general inhalant anesthesia.

     iii.   **Cardiac arrhythmias** frequently occur in birds anesthetized with halothane. Cardiac stability is one of the perceived advantages of isoflurane and is one of the reasons why it has so readily gained wide acceptance in clinical avian prac-

**Table 9-9. MAC Values for Halothane and Isoflurane in Selected Birds**

| Bird | Halothane | Isoflurane |
|------|-----------|------------|
| Cockatoo | | 1.44%[a] |
| Chicken | 0.85% | |
| Ducks | 1.05% | 1.32% |
| Sandhill cranes | | 1.35% |

[a]Personal communication, TG Curro, School of Veterinary Medicine, University of Wisconsin.

tice. In a study in which an electric fibrillation model was used to investigate the myocardial irritant effects of isoflurane and halothane, however, isoflurane was found to lower the threshold for electric fibrillation more than did halothane.

e. As with other anesthetic gases and vapors, **nitrous oxide** is not uniquely sequestered or concentrated in air sacs. The considerations for using nitrous oxide are the same as for its use in mammals: Pulmonary function should be adequate, and sufficient oxygen should be provided to meet the patient's metabolic demands ($\geq$ 30% oxygen). Diving birds, such as pelicans, have subcutaneous pockets of air that do not communicate with the respiratory system, and the use of $N_2O$ in these birds can result in subcutaneous gas accumulation.

3. *Muscle Paralytics*
   Muscle paralytics may be very useful in the anesthetic management of birds, especially during long surgical procedures that require adequate muscle relaxation and immobility. Atracurium (0.25 to 0.5 mg/kg) is a nondepolarizing muscle relaxant with a short duration that produces minimal cardiovascular effects. An anticholinesterase, such as edrophonium (0.5 mg/kg IV), can be given to reverse the effects of atracurium.

## D.   Monitoring the Avian Patient

1. **Physiologic variables to monitor** include respiratory rate and volume, heart rate and rhythm, body temperature, and muscle relaxation.

   a. **Respiratory frequency** can be misleading as a single indicator of the adequacy of ventilation and anesthetic depth. Ventilation should be monitored by watching the frequency and degree of motion of the sternum or movements of the reservoir bag on the breathing circuit. Respiratory pauses longer than 10 to 15 s should be treated by lightening the plane of anesthesia and, if possible, ventilating the bird by periodically squeezing the reservoir bag or by using a positive pressure mechanical ventilator. During positive pressure ventilation, airway pressure should not exceed 15 to 20 cm $H_2O$ to prevent **volotrauma** to the air sacs. Ventilation also can be assessed by noting the color and capillary refill time of mucous membranes. The color of the cere, beak, or bill, as well as coloration on the head can indicate the adequacy of cardiopulmonary function.

b.  The **heart function** can be assessed by monitoring mucous membrane color and refill time, ECG, and blood pressure and by palpating peripheral pulses. Standard bipolar and augmented limb leads can be used to monitor and record avian ECG. To ensure adequate skin contact for an interference-free signal, ECG clips can be attached to hypodermic needles inserted through the skin at the base of each wing and through the skin at the level of each stifle. **Pump function** can be assessed by monitoring the pulsations of blood through a peripheral artery or by monitoring blood pressure. It is possible to directly monitor arterial blood pressure in birds that weigh > 4 kg. The Doppler flow probe is an effective device for monitoring blood flow and blood pressure in any size bird. The probe can be placed over a digital artery, and a sphygmomanometer attached to a cuff placed around the leg can be used to indirectly measure systolic arterial blood pressure.

c.  During anesthesia, hypothermia is the most common problem. It decreases the requirement for anesthetic, causes cardiac instability, and prolongs recovery. In well-insulated birds (feathers, drapes, heating pads) hyperthermia can occur, which causes cardiac instability and an increased oxygen demand. **Body temperature** can be reliably monitored with an electronic thermometer and a long flexible thermistor probe inserted into the esophagus to the level of the heart. Temperature monitored from the cloaca can vary significantly owing to movements of the cloaca that affect the position of the thermometer or a thermistor probe. Body temperature can be adjusted by inserting or removing pads or blankets between the bird and cold surfaces, using circulating warm water blankets (not electric heating pads), maintaining a light plane of surgical anesthesia, raising or lowering the environmental temperature, or wetting the bird's legs with alcohol.

## E.    Recovery

Precautions should be taken to protect birds while they recover from anesthesia. Birds must be kept from flopping around, as this can lead to serious neck, wing, or leg injuries. Harmful activity can be prevented by lightly wrapping the bird in a towel, but wrapping poses its own hazards. If a bird is wrapped too tightly, sternal movements will be impeded and the bird may be unable to breathe. Wrapping can lead to excessive retention of body heat and cause hyperthermia.

## F.    Ratites

In general, young ratites (ostriches < 30 kg; emus < 18 kg) may be treated with the same methods and considerations as given to other birds. Hypoglycemia, hypothermia, hypotension, and hypoventilation tend to occur; and the equipment used is the same. Adult ostriches may average 114 kg and stand 6 feet tall. They can move rapidly and have very powerful feet, which they may use to strike forward. Techniques that facilitate handling include: **hooding** the bird (hood can be made with surgical stockinette), **herding** the bird using a solid object (e.g., large pad or plywood), or by **pushing** the bird by holding a wing at its base (Fig. 9-3). A **small bird** may be restrained by stepping over its back, grasping the legs below the hocks and folding the legs up to the body; an adult bird can be restrained in sternal recumbency, with the legs folded up under the body, by sitting on the bird.

1.    **Drug administration** can be via injection or catheter.

   a.    **Intramuscular injections** are best given into the large muscle mass of the thigh. Although ratites are reported to have a renal portal system, drugs are effective when given in this location.

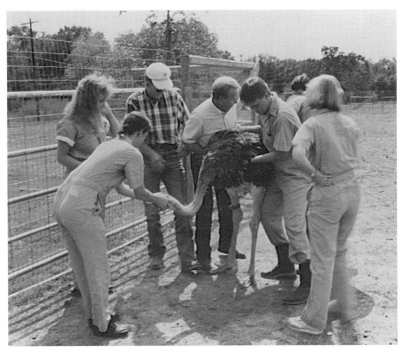

**Figure 9-3.** Manual restraint of a hooded ostrich.

b.  For **intravenous injections,** the jugular vein can be used—the right jugular is more prominent than the left. The branchial vein may be used in ostriches, but the wings are vestigial in emus. The metatarsal vein can be used in emus and rheas. Thick, cornified skin in ostriches makes this site difficult to use.

c.  For adult ostriches, a 14-gauge, 10-cm **catheter** can be used in the jugular vein, and smaller catheters are appropriate for immature birds. Branchial and metatarsal veins can also be catheterized.

2.  **Body weight** may be difficult or impossible to measure; and visual estimation is generally inaccurate, except by very experienced personnel. Feathers may conceal wasting. Food, but not water, should be withheld for 12 h in adult ratites. Regurgitation can occur.

3.  **Preanesthetics such as xylazine** (1 to 2 mg/kg IM) facilitates handling, placement of catheters, and induction of anesthesia in healthy birds. Preanesthetics are not necessary or indicated for sick birds. Anticholinergics should be used with intramuscular xylazine. Diazepam (0.4 to 1.0 mg/kg IM) is recommended for sick or debilitated ratites. Midazolam (0.4 mg/kg IM) is also an effective preanesthetic drug.

4.  **Induction of anesthesia** can be obtained with the following drugs.

    a.  **Ketamine** appears to be the most satisfactory drug for induction after various premedications (Tables 9-10 and 9-11). It can be administered intravenously to effect. Intramuscular injection, using a metabolically scaled dose at an intermediate value between passerine and nonpasserine birds.

    b.  **Tiletamine-zolazepam** can be given intramuscularly or intravenously. Inductions are smooth, but recoveries may be rough or prolonged.

    c.  **Carfentanyl** has been used, but induction and recovery are reported to be rough.

    d.  Mask induction with **isoflurane** is effective and smooth in smaller ratites. This technique is not recommended for adult ratites.

    e.  **Propofol** (4 to 6 mg/kg IV for induction; 0.2 to 0.4 mg/kg/min for maintenance) can be used for induction and maintenance. The clinician should be prepared to intubate and ventilate, because apnea is common after induction.

5.  **Intubation** is accomplished as follows.

    a.  Similar to many other avian species the **larynx** is readily accessible, the beak opens widely, and there is no epiglottis.

    b.  **Tracheal rings** are complete and portions of the trachea are collapsible. Careful inflation of the cuff is usually necessary to allow positive pressure ventilation. The **tracheal cleft** in emus, which is more highly developed in females but present in both

### Table 9-10. Data from Nine Anesthetized Ostriches[a]

| Induction | Procedure | Weight, kg | ASA Stage | Heart Rate, bpm | | | | Systolic/Diastolic (mean) Blood Pressure, mm Hg | | | | Respiratory Rate, breaths/min | | | | Complications |
|---|---|---|---|---|---|---|---|---|---|---|---|---|---|---|---|---|
| | | | | 15 | 30 | 45 | 60 | 15 | 30 | 45 | 60 | 15 | 30 | 45 | 60 | |
| Diazepam 0.35 mg/kg IM and IV Ketamine 6.3 mg/kg IV | Enterotomy | 79 | IVE | 45 | 45 | 45 | 40 | 100/75 (85) | 85/76 (78) | 90/65 (75) | 80/55 (65) | 10 | 10 | 10 | 10 | Cardiac arrest; hypovolemia; anemia |
| Diazepam 0.5 mg/kg IM Ketamine 6.6 mg/kg IV | Skin graft | 91 | II | 45 | 45 | 45 | 60 | N/A[b] | 165/125 (145) | 150/100 (130) | 165/120 (145) | 10 | 10 | 10 | 10 | None reported |
| Isoflurane mask | Proventriculotomy | 30 | III | 68 | 60 | 68 | 60 | 70/20 (30) | 60/20 (30) | 90/27 (45) | 115/30 (45) | 8 | 8 | 8 | 8 | Anemia, blood transfusion |
| Xylazine 3.6 mg/kg IM Ketamine 16.5 mg/kg IM | Tendon repair | 112 | II | 60 | 60 | 58 | 80 | N/A | 230/215 (225) | 225/205 (215) | 250/230 (240) | 15 | 6 | 8 | 8 | None reported |
| Diazepam 0.2 mg/kg IV Ketamine 16.4 mg/kg IV | Proventriculotomy | 95 | IVE | 35 | 35 | 38 | 35 | N/A | N/A | 205/175 (185) | 210/190 (200) | 8 | 8 | 8 | 8 | Bradycardia |
| Xylazine 3.2 mg/kg IM Ketamine 16.4 mg/kg IM | Phacofragmentation | 87 | I | 40 | 45 | 75 | 65 | N/A | N/A | 130/70 (88) | 130/60 (82) | 6 | 6 | 6 | 6 | None reported |
| Xylazine 1.9 mg/kg IM Diazepam 0.1 mg/kg IV Ketamine 7.1 mg/kg IV | Proventriculotomy | 106 | III | 60 | 95 | 90 | 85 | N/A | N/A | N/A | 110/95 (105) | 10 | 10 | 10 | 10 | Bradycardia in recovery |
| Xylazine 3.5 mg/kg IM Ketamine 17.7 mg/kg IM | Proventriculotomy | 85 | II | 70 | 70 | 68 | 68 | 65/45 (50) | 105/85 (95) | 115/95 (105) | N/A | 16 | 16 | 16 | 16 | None reported |
| Diazepam 0.1 mg/kg IV Ketamine 2.6 mg/kg IV Midazolam 0.57 mg/kg IM Ketamine 6.8 mg/kg IV | Cast application | 88 | II | 65 | 48 | 48 | 50 | N/A | 90/50 (65) | 120/72 (95) | 145/195 (120) | 10 | 10 | 10 | 10 | None reported |

[a]At the College of Veterinary Medicine, Texas A&M University, 1992. Data recorded at 15, 30, 45, and 60 min of anesthesia.
[b]Not available.

## Table 9-11. Data from 10 Anesthetized Emus[a]

| Induction | Procedure | Weight, kg | ASA Stage | Heart Rate, bpm | | | | Systolic/Diastolic (mean) Blood Pressure, mm Hg | | | | Respiratory Rate, breaths/min | | | | Complications |
|---|---|---|---|---|---|---|---|---|---|---|---|---|---|---|---|---|
| | | | | 15 | 30 | 45 | 60 | 15 | 30 | 45 | 60 | 15 | 30 | 45 | 60 | |
| Diazepam 0.37 mg/kg IM Ketamine 7.3 mg/kg IV | Egg bound | 41 | II | 155 | 150 | 145 | 125 | N/A[b] | 50/40 (45) | 75/45 (62) | 110/60 (95) | 12 | 12 | 12 | 12 | Hypotension |
| Diazepam 0.56 mg/kg IM Ketamine 14.8 mg/kg IV | Proventriculotomy | 27 | III | 58 | 60 | 72 | 58 | 135/60 (88) | 125/95 (108) | 115/90 (105) | 100/80 (90) | 15 | 15 | 15 | 15 | None reported |
| Midazolam 0.4 mg/kg IM Ketamine 1 mg/kg IV | Egg bound | 40 | II | 135 | 125 | 90 | 122 | N/A | N/A | 88/40 (52) | 100/55 (75) | 14 | 14 | 14 | 14 | None reported |
| Azaperone 2.7 mg/kg IM Ketamine 3.8 mg/kg IV | Skin graft | 26 | II | 50 | 30 | 30 | 40 | N/A | N/A | N/A | N/A | 8 | 8 | 8 | 8 | Bradycardia |
| Diazepam 1.0 mg/kg IM Ketamine 10 mg/kg IV | Wound débridement | 31 | II | 85 | 65 | 70 | 65 | N/A | N/A | N/A | N/A | 10 | 10 | 10 | 10 | None reported |
| Diazepam 1.0 mg/kg IV Ketamine 19 mg/kg IV | Tracheal endoscopy | 21 | IV | 105 | 110 | 140 | 142 | 175/105 (N/A) | 182/125 (N/A) | 200/130 (N/A) | 170/130 (N/A) | 15 | 17 | 17 | 15 | None reported |
| Diazepam 0.7 mg/kg IM Ketamine 6.7 mg/kg IV | Endoscopy | 45 | II | 92 | 92 | 80 | 70 | N/A | N/A | N/A | N/A | 6 | 6 | 10 | 8 | Regurgitation at recovery |
| Xylazine 4.5 mg/kg IM Xylazine 21 mg/kg IM | Papilloma removal | 35 | II | 20 | 30 | 40 | 40 | N/A | 128/100 (115) | 150/125 (135) | 140/130 (135) | 10 | 10 | 10 | 10 | Bradycardia |
| Diazepam 0.5 mg/kg IV Ketamine 7.0 mg/kg IV | Endoscopy | N/A | II | 100 | 130 | 90 | 125 | 120/155 (175) | 195/140 (160) | 170/115 (135) | 155/100 (120) | 25 | 25 | 32 | 32 | None reported |
| Xylazine 4.7 mg/kg IM Ketamine 25 mg/kg IM | Osteotomy | 17 | 2 | 40 | 35 | 35 | 32 | 128/70 (95) | 100/50 (65) | 100/40 (48) | 80/40 (50) | 12 | 12 | 12 | 12 | None reported |

[a] At the College of Veterinary Medicine, Texas A&M University, 1992. Data recorded at 15, 30, 45, and 60 minutes of anesthesia.
[b] Not available.

sexes, does not complicate intubation; however, it does make positive pressure ventilation difficult. Expansion of the cleft can be overcome by wrapping the neck with Vetrap.

6. **Maintenance** of anesthesia for ratites is as follows.

    a.    **Isoflurane** is recommended for maintenance. Emus and ostriches < 130 kg can be maintained on a small animal breathing circuit. Larger ostriches should be maintained on a large animal breathing circuit.

    b.    **Positive pressure** ventilation is recommended for adult ostriches. Ventilation appears to be depressed by anesthetic drugs. Ventilation facilitates uptake of the inhalant anesthetic, thereby helping maintain a stable plane of anesthesia. Adult ostriches have a large respiratory volume (~ 15 L). The ostrich may have a functional shunting system, which appears to affect uptake of inhalant.

    c.    **Muscle relaxants** appear to be effective in ratites. Duration of effect seems to be similar to mammalian species. The dose of atracurium is 0.3 mg/kg IV; the dose of vecuronium is 0.08 mg/kg IV. Peripheral nerve stimulator can be used to assess the block; the electrodes are placed on the proximal and distal ends of the wing.

7. **Monitoring** guidelines are as follows.

    a.    **Electrocardiogram** leads can be positioned with one electrode in the neck region, one in the wing fold, and the third near the keel or opposite wing. Standardization of lead placement is complicated by tight skin and surgical incision sites.

    b.    **Blood pressure** can be measured directly or indirectly. Indirect measurement can be made with a Doppler flow probe placed over the tibial artery. An oscillometric technique can be used by placing the cuff on the leg above the tarsus. Direct measurement can be taken by placing an arterial catheter in the brachialis or ulnaris artery of the ostrich wing or in the metatarsal artery of a pelvic limb (Fig. 9-4). In the **emu,** the brachialis artery is small, so the pedal artery is preferred. Tourniquet-induced hypertension has been reported and may cause high blood pressure recordings.

c.   **Oxygen saturation** can be measured with a pulse oximeter probe placed on the upper or lower beak. The accuracy of the readings is unknown because there are quantitative differences in the oxyhemoglobin dissociation curve between birds and mammals.

d.   **Positive pressure ventilation** appears to be effective with tidal volume settings of 10 to 13 mL/kg, respiratory rates of 8 to 16 breaths per minute, and inspiratory pressures of 10 to 15 cm $H_2O$.

8.   Clinical experience shows that **complications** involve a high incidence of cardiac arrhythmias in adult ratites. Bradycardia (heart rate < 30 bpm) is usually associated with the use of xylazine as a preanesthetic, especially when a large dose is used. Bradycardia responds to glycopyrrolate (0.01 mg/kg IV) or reversal of xylazine with yohimbine (dosed slowly intravenously to effect).

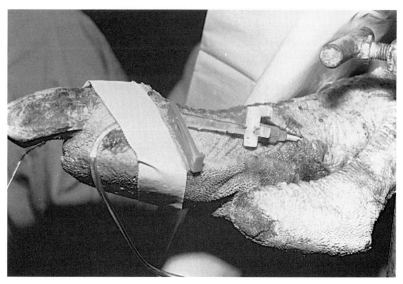

**Figure 9-4.** A catheter in the digital artery of an ostrich is used for measuring arterial blood pressure and collecting arterial blood samples for analysis of pH, $Pa_{CO_2}$, and $Pa_{O_2}$.

9. **Recovery** from inhalant anesthesia can be quite slow. Adult ratites recover best if moved to a darkened, padded area or well-bedded stall. Manual restraint is dangerous, but protection of the head and neck are desirable. Ratite-Rap (Jorgensen, Loveland, CO) can be used to restrain an adult ratite during the recovery period.

# III. REPTILES

*Juergen Schumacher*

## A. Physical Restraint

1. Turtles (***Chelonia*** sp.) should be observed undisturbed in their tank or cage. Level of activity, respiratory efforts, normal signs, and signs of illness should be noted. The legs should be examined as well as the cloacal region. The head should be examined, with particular focus on the eyes, tympanic membranes, and nares. **Aquatic turtles** are often very agile and can inflict a painful bite. Snapping turtles and adult marine turtles are capable of crushing the examiner's hand; and in some cases it is advisable to perform the physical examination and collect the diagnostic samples after the animal has been sedated or anesthetized. Often it is a major challenge to secure the head for examination. Pressure on the hind limbs may encourage tortoises to protrude their head from the shell so that it can be grasped quickly. Care should be taken to avoid injury to the animal; and excessive force should not be applied to pull out the legs or the head. In some cases, placing the tortoise in dorsal recumbency will encourage it to protrude its legs and head.

2. **Crocodilians** can be dangerous to restrain. In general, alligators are more docile and easier to work with than crocodiles. Members of both species ≤ 3 feet long may be manually restrained by an experienced person. The greatest potential for injury are from the teeth and tail, which will be violently thrashed around for defense and attack purposes. The first step should be to secure the mouth. When transporting the animal, it should be supported along the entire body axis, and the head and tail should be

secured. For ease of capturing, a pole with a loop at the end (snare) is suitable, especially for animals > 3 feet long. As soon as the snare is around the neck, the head and tail must be restrained to prevent the animal from twirling. Large crocodilians require the effort of several experienced people.

3. Restraint of lizards (*Sauria* sp.) is relatively easy to accomplish. The only exceptions are larger species, such as **Komodo dragons** (up to 100 kg) and some large monitors, which are potentially dangerous. They should be handled similarly to crocodiles. Most smaller species, although capable of inflicting serious and painful bites (**adult green iguanas** and **some lizards**), can be manually restrained if gloves are worn for protection. In all cases, a secure and firm grip should be placed around the head. Thumb and index finger should be placed around the neck, and one front leg should be placed between the other fingers to prevent the animal from spinning. The other hand can then, depending on the animal's size, be used either for manipulation of the animal or to support the rest of the body. Under no circumstances should iguanas and lizards be restrained by holding the tail alone. To support the body, the hand should be placed under the abdomen at the base of the tail to prevent it from hitting. As a rule, to visually examine an iguana, the clinician should let it sit on his or her hand and arm, with its whole body supported but not restrained. This is a stress-free situation for the animal, and visual examinations can be made this way. Gentle, manipulative examinations can be made by palpating the abdomen and the limbs and by examining the head. For poisonous species, such as the Gila monster and the beaded lizard, the head should be secured before examination begins.

4. Physical restraint of **nonpoisonous snakes** is, with the exception of large boid snakes, easy to accomplish. First, the head should be secured by placing the thumb and middle fingers on either side, with the index finger on the top of the head. The body should be supported by the other hand. Plexiglas tubes, which are available in different sizes, are useful. The snake can be manipulated to

crawl into the tube. This device allows easy access for injections or other procedures. They are especially useful when handling poisonous snakes. The most useful tool when working with poisonous or aggressive nonpoisonous snakes is a snake hook. It can be used for lifting the animal from its container, for manipulating it to crawl in a certain direction, or for pinning the head before manual restraint.

**Large boas and pythons** should always be restrained by several people. If possible, remove the snake from its cage or box, this allows more room to work in and may make the snake less territorial. To examine the head, the body of the snake can be left in a large pillow case with only the head exposed. As a rule, one person is responsible for the head and one person for each 3 feet of body length of a large snake. The head should be secured first. A plastic shield can be held in front of the snake to prevent it from striking.

**Poisonous snakes** can be handled with a snake hook or long forceps. They should be manipulated to crawl into a Plexiglas tube for further evaluation. For procedures in the oral cavity, such as abscess débridement, chemical restraint of the snake is advisable in most cases. When working with poisonous snakes on a regular basis, the clinician should contact local breeders, zoos, or research facilities that store antivenin for the most commonly kept species. Pinning the snake with a hook and holding the head between the fingers should be done only by experienced people.

## B.    Drug Administration Routes

In most cases, injectable anesthetic agents are administered by the intramuscular route. Oral administration is less reliable and clinically not practical, owing to variances in uptake and distribution of the drug. Subcutaneous administration will also result in prolonged induction times.

1.    In **reptiles,** a renal portal system has been described; therefore, drugs that are eliminated by the kidneys, such as ketamine, should be given in the forelimbs or the rostral half of the body.

2. In **snakes,** intramuscular injections are given in the front half of the body into the paravertebral muscles (Fig. 9-5). The right jugular vein in snakes is accessible for venous injection. A cutdown and dissection of the vein will allow the clinician to place a catheter for intravenous administration of drugs and fluids.

3. In **chelonians and lizards,** intramuscular injections are given into the muscles of the forelegs or the gluteal muscles of the hind leg (Fig. 9-5). Intravenous injection is more difficult and is often reserved for research purposes. An intravenous catheter can be inserted relatively easily and sutured or taped to the skin (Fig. 9-6).

4. In **lizards** (especially in green iguanas), the presence of a large abdominal vein allows for easy collection of blood, intravenous injection, and placement of an intravenous catheter (Fig. 9-7). The vein can easily be visualized within the connective tissue underneath the skin.

5. In **tortoises, crocodilians,** and **lizards** an intraosseous catheter may be placed in the ulna or tibia for administration of fluids. Depending on the size of the patient, a spinal or hypodermic needle is suitable.

## C.   Preanesthetic Evaluation

1. Ideally, the reptilian patient should be maintained at and acclimated to its optimum **body temperature** for several days before anesthesia.

2. Supportive care, initiated before anesthesia—including administration of a **balanced electrolyte solution,** heat, nutritional support, and antimicrobial therapy—will decrease anesthetic and surgical risks. **Lactated Ringer's** solution may be given intravenously, subcutaneously, or intracelomically. Although guidelines for reptilian fluid requirements have not been established, administration volume may be calculated on the basis of that required for mammals, with the exception of large turtles.

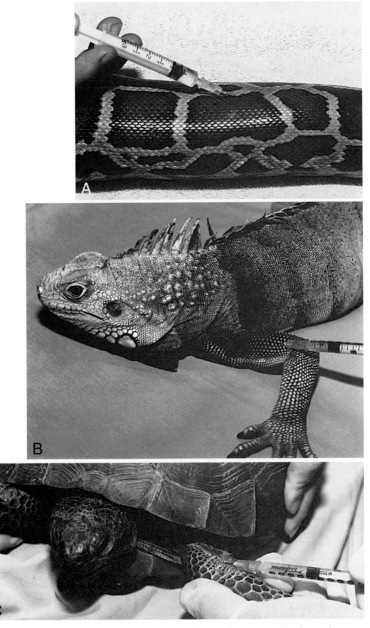

**Figure 9-5.** Intramuscular injection of ketamine HCl in (*A*) the paravertebral muscle group of a Burmese python (*Python molurus bivittatus*), (*B*) the front leg of a green iguana (*Iguana iguana*), and (*C*) a gopher tortoise (*Gopherus polypherus*).

### D.  Injectable Sedation and Anesthesia

Reptiles are most commonly anesthetized with injectable anesthetics that offer the advantages of ease of administration and a relatively low cost. A major disadvantage after injectable anesthesia is prolonged recovery, which may take several days. Recovery depends on the drug and the species anesthetized. Injectable drugs are more commonly given by the intramuscular route, often requiring higher doses than would be required by the intravenous administration.

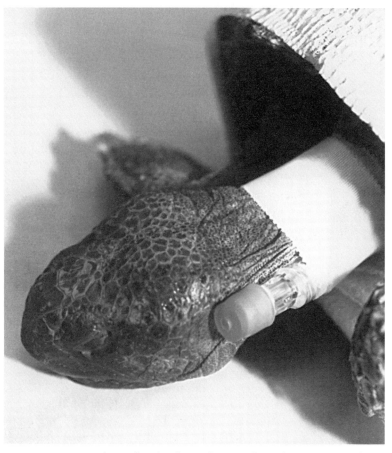

**Figure 9-6.** Intravenous catheter placed in the jugular vein of a gopher tortoise (*Gopherus polyphemus*).

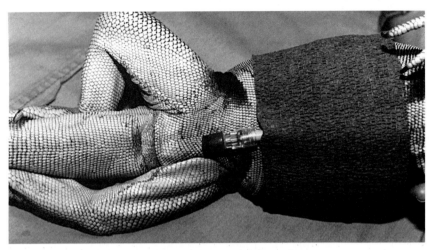

**Figure 9-7.** Intravenous catheter placed in the ventral abdominal vein in a green iguana (*Iguana iguana*).

1.  *Chelonians*

    a.  **Ketamine** alone or in combination with diazepam or midazolam has been used to produce sedation and anesthesia in tortoises and turtles. Ketamine (22 to 44 mg/kg IM or SC) induces good sedation. A dose of 55 to 88 mg/kg is recommended for a surgical plane of anesthesia. Induction time is between 10 and 30 min; but recovery may be prolonged, ranging up to 96 h. As a rule for inducing anesthesia, smaller tortoises and turtles require less ketamine per unit of body weight than do larger species. It is recommended that ketamine be used in combination with diazepam (0.2 to 1 mg/kg IM) or midazolam (up to 2 mg/kg IM) to enhance muscle relaxation. Ketamine (10 to 30 mg/kg IM) is routinely administered in combination with butorphanol (0.5 to 1.5 mg/kg IM) for minor surgical procedures, such as shell repairs and limb trauma.

    b.  Large tortoises may be given tiletamine-zolazepam (**Telazol**) at a dose of 5 to 10 mg/kg IM or IV to facilitate tracheal intubation. If sedation of the animal is too light for tracheal intubation after tiletamine-zolazepam administration, mask induction with isoflurane or sevoflurane is preferred instead of repetitive dosing.

c.    **Alphaxalone-alphadolone** (Althesin) has been recommended as a preanesthetic before inhalation anesthesia in reptiles. If administered intravenously, induction time is between 2 and 4 min, allowing for rapid tracheal intubation and administration of an inhalant anesthetic. In contrast, after intramuscular administration, induction may take up to 30 min. The optimum dose in lizards and chelonians is 15 mg/kg IM, which allows 15 to 30 min of anesthesia. Its action in snakes is more variable. Because relatively large volumes are required, multiple intramuscular injection sites should be used. Complete recovery after alphaxalone-alphadolone may require 2 to 4 h.

d.    **Propofol** is an ultra-short-acting hypnotic commonly used in dogs. Its use is followed by rapid induction, minimal accumulation after repeated administrations, and rapid excitement-free recovery. Propofol appears to be the induction agent of choice in chelonians and in any species in which a vein can be catheterized. A propofol dosage of 5 of 10 mg/kg IV will induce anesthesia in most chelonians. Further doses of propofol may be given to extend anesthesia.

2.   *Alligators and Crocodiles*
     Alligators and crocodiles detoxify drugs slowly, predisposing these species to prolonged recovery when injectable drugs are used.

a.    **Pentobarbital** has been given both orally and intraperitoneally to anesthetize alligators and crocodiles. Alligators given tricaine methanesulfonate (MS-222) (80.0 to 90.0 mg/kg IM) are completely relaxed in 10 min. Recovery does not occur for 9 to 10 h.

b.    In large crocodilians, either **ketamine** (12 to 15 mg/kg IM) or **tiletamine-zolazepam** (2 to 10 mg/kg IM) can be given, followed by tracheal intubation and maintenance of anesthesia with an inhalant. This regimen provides safe inductions and recoveries. Tracheal intubation in the adequately sedated animal is achieved by using a mouth gag and manual placement of the endotracheal tube.

c.   **Etorphine** has been used in reptiles with variable success. Most often, it has been used for capture and restraint of large crocodilians. Major disadvantages for its use include potential danger for the veterinarian and its relatively high cost.

d.   The **immobility reflex** can be used to induce a hypnotic state in young alligators. They are turned on their backs, and their abdomen is stroked.

3.   *Green Iguanas*
Green iguanas may hold their breath for long periods of time when stressed. Low doses of ketamine (5 to 10 mg/kg IM) decrease the breath holding. Clinical experience has shown that butorphanol (1 to 1.5 mg/kg IM) 30 min before induction with isoflurane provides smoother and shorter inductions and improves analgesia during surgery.

4.   *Serpentes*

a.   Many injectables have been used in snakes; but **ketamine,** either alone or in combination with diazepam, is preferred for sedation. Although the use of a variety of drugs may provide satisfactory sedation for diagnostic procedures, it is recommended that an inhalant be used for prolonged procedures or if a surgical plane of anesthesia is required. For sedation, a ketamine dose of 22 to 44 mg/kg has been reported. It is recommended that diazepam (0.2 to 0.8 mg/kg IM) or butorphanol (up to 1.5 mg/kg IM) be given to improve muscle relaxation. Induction times after ketamine administration may be up to 30 min.

b.   **Metomidate** is a nonbarbiturate that has been used for anesthesia in birds of prey and in domestic and nondomestic mammals. It reportedly is useful as a sedative in snakes to facilitate noninvasive diagnostic procedures. It has a rapid onset of action, even after intramuscular injection, and results in profound sedation within 10 to 20 min. Metomidate has no analgesic properties, and should be used only for sedation or as a preanesthetic before inhalation anesthesia.

### E.  Inhalational Anesthesia

The advantages of using inhalants include better controllability of anesthetic depth and a more rapid induction and recovery than are possible with injectable agents. Establishment of an airway allows for positive pressure ventilation and administration of oxygen. In most reptiles, **endotracheal intubation** is easily achieved, because the glottis can be visualized. Intubation can be performed either after a sedative dose of an injectable agent or after mask induction (Fig. 9-8). In chelonians and crocodilians, the tracheal rings are complete; and care should be taken not to overinflate the cuff, which may cause damage to the tracheal mucosa. A tight-fitting uncuffed tube may be more beneficial and safer. When intubating chelonians, care should be taken not to intubate one bronchus, because these species

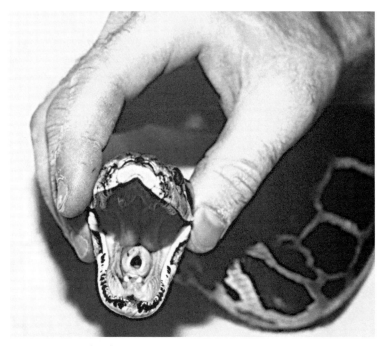

**Figure 9-8.** The glottis in a Burmese python (*Python molurus bivitattus*).

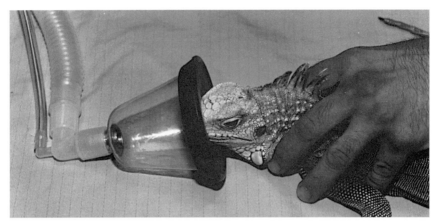

**Figure 9-9.** Mask induction of a green iguana (*Iguana iguana*). A suitable face mask may also be constructed from an empty syringe case.

have relatively short tracheas. If endotracheal intubation is not performed and anesthesia is maintained via face mask, a clear plastic mask available for dogs and cats or syringe cases are recommended (Figs. 9-9).

1. The use of a **precision vaporizer** is recommended. For reptiles weighing < 10 kg, the use of a nonrebreathing system has the advantage of little resistance and minimal dead space. Because the normal respiratory rate of anesthetized reptiles is 2 to 4 breaths per minute, it is recommended that positive pressure ventilation also be set at a rate of 2 to 4 breaths per minute. **Breath holding** is a common problem in reptiles, especially in turtles and crocodiles. Increasing the anesthetic concentration in increments will tend to decrease breath holding, and the addition of nitrous oxide to the volatile anesthetic will often decrease induction times. Generally, when using a glass aquarium or chamber for inducing anesthesia in small or poisonous reptiles, the animal can be carefully removed from the chamber and intubated when it no longer is capable of righting itself when tipped onto its back.

2. For **induction of anesthesia** of most reptiles, a concentration of 3 to 5% isoflurane is used, which may require 20 to 30 min. Maintenance of anesthesia is usually accomplished

with a concentration of 1.5 to 2.5% halothane or isoflurane. In debilitated metabolically compromised reptiles, isoflurane is the anesthetic agent of choice.

### F. Deliberate Cooling

Rapid cooling to a hypothermic temperature will not provide analgesia and may be painful and stressful. Because reptiles are poikilothermic animals, cooling reduces the patient's metabolism. Lower temperatures have been associated with necrotic changes in the brain of snakes and tortoises. The use of body cooling as a substitute for anesthesia in reptiles is inappropriate. Placing an animal on a heating blanket set at the reptile's optimal external temperature helps prevent rapid body cooling during and after anesthesia.

### G. Monitoring

Heart rate and rhythm and respiratory rate should be monitored. An esophageal stethoscope or a Doppler flow probe placed at the level of the heart will facilitate cardiac monitoring (Fig. 9-10). Monitoring respiratory rate may be difficult in some reptiles, especially in snakes. In most lizards, movement of the intercostal musculature is easier to observe. In turtles, the tonus of the head, neck, and limbs can be used to judge the depth of anesthesia. Respiratory movements can be observed as alternating concavity and convexity of the skin adjacent to the limbs and tail. ECG leads may be placed in reptiles in the conventional fashion (Fig. 9-11). Leads can be connected to hypodermic needles or alligator clips to improve lead contact. The heart is usually located after the first third to quarter of the body length in snakes.

The **righting reflex,** or the ability to turn over when placed in dorsal recumbency, is lost in relatively light planes of anesthesia. Its presence is most useful during the recovery period. In snakes not fully anesthetized, touching the muscles firmly along the vertebral column produces a spastic reaction. In snakes and some lizards, the **tongue withdrawal reflex** should still be present in a surgical plane of anesthesia. The patient is too deep if this reflex is absent. There is an obvious **dilation of the pupils** in deep surgical anesthesia. In chelonians, the **head withdrawal reflex** is helpful in determining level of anesthetic depth.

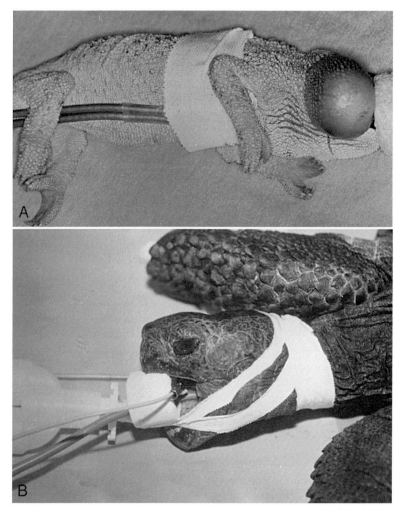

**Figure 9-10. A,** A Jackson's chameleon (*Chameleo jackson*) with a Doppler flow probe positioned at the level of the heart to monitor cardiac rate and rhythm. **B,** A Galapagos tortoise (*Geochelone elephantopus*) after tracheal intubation and placement of an esophageal ECG.

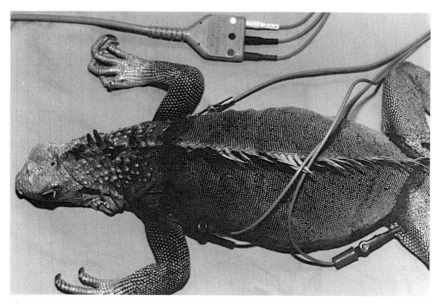

**Figure 9-11.** A green iguana (*Iguana iguana*) with ECG leads placed in a conventional configuration.

## H.   Analgesia

Information about the effects of analgesic agents in reptilians is scant. Every animal is capable of feeling pain. Although it is sometimes difficult to assess and evaluate pain in the reptilian patient, there is no reason to believe that the lack of more familiar responses to pain, such as vocalization, is equivalent to no pain sensation. Routine administration of analgesics to any reptile that undergoes invasive or painful surgery is recommended. Although no information is available on drugs and doses, the higher end of the dose range recommended for mammalian species is commonly used. A butorphanol dose of 0.4 to 1 mg/kg given intramuscularly appears beneficial.

## I.   Recovery

During the postoperative period, ectotherms should be placed in an incubator at a temperature and relative humidity within the optimal range for the species. Recovery times in reptiles tend to be longer than those of birds and mammals. Most reptiles will be in a state of respiratory depression during the recovery period. Respiration should be carefully monitored, especially after administration of ketamine or tiletamine-zolazepam. When using inhalants in snakes, recovery may be hastened by gentle evacuation of the lungs. This is accomplished by a milking action of the hand drawn from the cloacal end of the snake toward the head. Before extubation, spontaneous ventilation should be observed. The administration of **doxapram** (0.2 to 0.6 mL/kg IV or IM) will stimulate breathing in most reptiles. Return of the righting reflex is the most useful indicator of recovery. To prevent drowning, aquatic species, such as marine turtles, should be placed in deep water only after recovery is complete.

## IV.  AMPHIBIANS

*Juergen Schumacher*

### A.    Anatomy and Physiology

Amphibians are aquatic animals that spend at least the reproductive phase of their lives in an aquatic environment. One adaptation to their lives in the water is the development of glands to protect the skin. The secretions from these glands prevent the animal from desiccation and protect it from microorganisms. **Skin secretions** make it difficult for the veterinarian to handle these animals, because they make the body slippery. The secretions may irritate the handler's skin and damage of the film of secretions on the amphibian's skin may predispose the animal to infections. In addition, the skin of some amphibians serves as a supplemental respiratory organ. Amphibians are highly sensitive to changes in humidity and may rapidly dehydrate.

### B.    Physical Examination

The patient's **reflexes,** such as the righting reflex, and postural changes should be assessed. A sick amphibian often has changes in **skin color** and may appear congested. **Ascites,** indicating infectious disease processes, and osmotic imbalances are commonly seen. The general body condition should be critically assessed based on abdominal contents, visibility of the skeleton, and musculature. **Fecal examination** is recommended for assessing parasite infestation. Most amphibians can be handled manually for transfer and physical examination. To protect their sensitive skin, it is recommended that the clinician's **hands be moistened** when handling aquatic species. A wet paper towel also serves well. The restraint period should be kept as brief as possible. Almost all frogs and toads secrete a venom from their glands. Gloves should be worn, and contact with the eyes avoided. A few species **secrete a poison,** which in the case of the arrow-poison frog is highly toxic. Although smaller species rarely bite; larger individuals, especially large toads, are capable of inflicting a painful bite. In general, toads are less slippery than frogs and may be restrained by supporting the body and holding on to the hind limbs.

### C.   Anesthesia

**Depth of anesthesia** is evaluated by the loss of the righting reflex, by the loss of reflexes to pain (toe pinch), and by changes in the respiratory rate and pattern. Although at a surgical plane of anesthesia the ventilation rate will often be greatly depressed, cutaneous respiration will provide sufficient oxygenation. The clinician can take advantage of the amphibian's ability of cutaneous fluid absorption by immersion of the animal in a solution of anesthetic agent. Like reptiles, amphibians require an **optimum temperature** for proper metabolism and function of various organ systems. Before anesthetizing the amphibian patient, it should be kept in its optimum temperature range to reduce stress and metabolic compromise.

1.   **Local anesthesia** provides a safe and effective measure for certain procedures; 2% lidocaine in combination with ketamine for minor surgical procedures, such as removal of subcutaneous abscesses or amputation of digits, is effective. As an analgesic, butorphanol at a dosage of 0.2 to 0.4 mg/kg IM has been used with good success.

2.   **Injectable anesthesia** includes the following.

     a.   One of the more commonly used amphibian anesthetics is **tricaine methanesulfonate** (MS-222). This drug may be administered to frogs, salamanders, newts, and mudpuppies by bath or through injection. In frogs and toads, injections can be given in the dorsal lymph sac. The dorsal lymph sacs are paired organs located on either side of the last vertebra. Their location can be determined by observation of their rhythmic beating. In an adult leopard frog, 2 to 3 mL anesthetic can be injected at one time into these sacs. Anesthesia can be maintained by keeping the animal partially submerged in the bath and taking advantage of its capability of cutaneous uptake of the drug. When using a bath, a 0.1 to 0.3% solution should be prepared. Induction time may take up to 30 min and recovery up to 24 h.

b.  **Pentobarbital** has been used at a dose of 40 to 50 mg/kg administered into the dorsal lymph sac or intraperitoneally. Induction is prolonged (approximately 30 min), and anesthesia may last 9 h; recovery may require up to 24 h.

c.  The combination of **ketamine** (20 to 40 mg/kg IM) and **diazepam** (0.2 to 0.4 mg/kg IM) has been used with variable success. Although in some animals adequate anesthesia to perform surgical procedures was achieved, others required additional inhalant anesthetic.

d.  **Tiletamine-zolazepam** (10 to 20 mg/kg) given intramuscularly produces variable states of tranquilization or anesthesia in leopard frogs and bullfrogs. A dose of 50 mg/kg induces anesthesia consistently in bullfrogs but results in some mortalities. This same dose is uniformly fatal for leopard frogs. Sites for intramuscular injection of drugs are the muscles of the front and hind limbs. In frogs and toads, injections can be given into the dorsal lymph sac.

3.  **Inhalational anesthesia** includes the following.

a.  The inhalants of choice for amphibians are **isoflurane** and sevoflurane, because they provide a rapid induction and recovery. Induction of anesthesia is usually achieved with an induction chamber. With concentrations of 3 to 5%, loss of the righting reflex may take up to 30 min. Anesthesia is maintained with 1 to 2% isoflurane or 2 to 3% sevoflurane.

b.  **Tracheal intubation** is easily accomplished by the use of a 2-mm uncuffed endotracheal tube or, in smaller species, by the use of plastic catheters connected to the anesthetic circuit. In frogs and toads, the tracheal opening is positioned at the base of the tongue.

c.  During **recovery,** amphibians should be kept moist over their entire body and in a warm environment. As with aquatic species of reptiles, to prevent drowning, care must be taken that terrestrial species of amphibians do not become completely immersed in water until recovery is complete.

# Chapter 10

## Anesthesia Management of Patients with Disease

### Introductory Comments

*Management of anesthesia in patients with **cardiopulmonary dysfunction** or **systemic disease** of the major organ systems is increasingly common in modern veterinary practice. Appreciation for how pathophysiologic derangements associated with these conditions alter anesthetic actions is essential for the proper selection of anesthetic protocol and management of anesthesia in these patients. A brief review of selected disease entities of the major organ systems with suggestions for appropriate modifications of anesthetic management are presented in this chapter.*

**Cardiovascular Dysfunction**
**Pulmonary Dysfunction**
**Neurologic Disease**
**Renal Disease**
**Hepatic Disease**
**Gastrointestinal Disease**
**Endocrine Disease**

---

## I.  CARDIOVASCULAR DYSFUNCTION
*Robert R. Paddleford, Ralph C. Harvey*

The anesthetic management of the patient with cardiovascular dysfunction can be challenging, because most preanesthetic and anesthetic agents capable of CNS depression are also capable of producing cardiovascular depression. Patients with cardiovascular dysfunction may be more prone to fluid overload and dysrhythmias. Extremes in heart rate may cause severe problems, including heart failure. Patients with cardiovascular dysfunction may lack sufficient cardiac reserve to compensate for anesthetic-induced depression.

## A. Cardiovascular Physiology

The **function of the myocardial cell** is to rhythmically contract and relax with other myofibers so that the heart will act as a pump. The basic contractile unit of heart muscle is the sarcomere, which is composed of interdigitating protein filaments referred to as actin and myosin. The contraction of the heart muscle depends on the amount of free calcium ions available around the myofibril. Part of the contractile-dependent calcium originates from superficial sites on cell membranes that are in equilibrium with extracellular calcium and, therefore, can be affected by drugs that do not penetrate the myocardial cell.

1. Few clinically used drugs affect the actin–myosin proteins; however, many drugs can alter the availability of calcium for activation of the contractile process. Digitalis increases calcium movement to the troponin–tropomyosin protein unit and thus increases contractile strength. Barbiturates and inhalant anesthetic agents seem to disrupt calcium movements and thus cause a reduced contractile strength. Myocardial intracellular acidosis also inhibits the binding of calcium to the troponin–tropomyosin unit, causing decreased myocardial contractile strength.

2. **Blood pressure** is the product of peripheral vascular resistance and cardiac output. Cardiac output is the product of heart rate and stroke volume. Drugs that alter any or all of these parameters may greatly affect blood pressure and tissue blood flow. Preanesthetic and anesthetic agents can alter peripheral resistance (phenothiazine tranquilizers, $\alpha_2$-agonists, barbiturates, inhalant agents), heart rate (opioids, $\alpha_2$-agonists, dissociative agents, inhalants), and stroke volume (inhalant anesthetics). Patients that suffer from diseases causing impaired cardiac output (cardiomyopathies), patients with congenital heart disease, and those suffering from hypotension–hypovolemia, anemia, and/or heartworms are at a higher anesthetic risk.

3. The **primary goals in the anesthetic management** of patients with impaired cardiac output are to avoid tachycardia, decreased preload, and hypovolemia. These patients should be preoxygenated for 5 to 7 min before anesthetic induction. If pump function is adequate, the choice of anesthetic drugs is not specific for these patients; however, drugs that may produce tachycardia (anticholinergics, dissociative agents) are best avoided. The exception to this is dilated cardiomyopathy, in which an increased heart rate may help increase cardiac output.

4. **Opioids** are often used as preanesthetic medication because of their minimal effects on the myocardium, and they can be readily antagonized. They can be used in combination with acepromazine or a benzodiazepine tranquilizer for additional sedation. The fact that they slow the heart rate may be beneficial. If significant bradycardia occurs, however, atropine or glycopyrrolate should be given to effect. If only tranquilization is needed, a low dose of acepromazine (0.05 mg/kg IM to a maximum total dose of 1.5 mg) may be used. Acepromazine produces minimal direct myocardial depression; however, it can produce a decrease in peripheral vascular resistance, which can potentially lead to arterial hypotension. The $\alpha_2$-agonists should be avoided in patients with impaired cardiac output. These drugs can produce significant dysrhythmias including severe sinus bradycardia and SA and AV nodal blocks.

5. **Induction of anesthesia** can be accomplished by using thiopental, propofol, etomidate, or a neuroleptanalgesic. Isoflurane is the preferred inhalant, because of its preservation of a near normal cardiac index and its minimal dysrhythmic effects compared to halothane.

## B. Patients with Impaired Cardiac Output

1. **Cardiomyopathies** can be classified as hypertrophic or congestive. Hypertrophic cardiomyopathy is characterized by ventricular hypertrophy; decreased ventricular compliance; and impaired ventricular filling, which results in reduced cardiac output. Ventricular performance (pump

function) is usually not impaired. Dilated cardiomyopathy is characterized by marked ventricular dilation, increased ventricular diastolic volume, and poor ventricular performance. Often, congestive heart failure (CHF) is present. Commonly employed cardiovascular medications used for treatment of congestive heart failure are listed in Table 10-1.

2. **Pericardial tamponade** and **constrictive pericarditis** are associated with impaired cardiac output secondary to reduced preload. There is limited expansion of the cardiac chambers, resulting in decreased ventricular filling, stroke volume, and cardiac output. Pump function is not impaired.

3. **Valvular heart disease** is associated with impaired cardiac output and when severe can cause congestive heart failure. Mitral insufficiency is probably the most common valvular disease. Characterized by ventricular hypertrophy and dilation and pulmonary vascular engorgement, it may eventually cause right heart failure. Left ventricular pump function and systemic cardiac output are usually maintained until retrograde flow becomes severe. Preanesthetic and anesthetic drugs that increase afterload should be avoided.

## C. Patients with Congenital Heart Disease

When considering the anesthetic management of patients with congenital heart disease, the problems encountered are often similar to patients with congestive heart failure. The most common surgically correctable problems are patent ductus arteriosus (PDA) and persistent right aortic arch (PRAA).

1. **Patent ductus arteriosus** is usually recognized early in life before the patient deteriorates. If the patient is normal in other respects, the anesthetic protocol is designed for the pediatric patient undergoing a thoracotomy. There are no specific contraindications to any particular preanesthetic or anesthetic drug. Surgical manipulation around the heart may cause ventricular ectopic beats, which are usually transitory and do not require treatment. When the PDA is

**Table 10-1. Chronic Therapy for Congestive Heart Failure**

| Classes | Trade Name(s) | Mechanisms of Action | Effects on Contractility | Afterload | Maintenance Dose[a] |
|---|---|---|---|---|---|
| **INOTROPES** | | | | | |
| Digitalis | Cardoxin; Lanoxin | Inactivates $Na^+/K^+$ exchange, increasing $Ca^{2+}$ intracellularly | ↑ | ↑ | Canine: 0.005 mg/kg PO, BID Feline: 0.007 mg/kg PO, q 48 h |
| T3 | Triostat | Increases $Ca^{+2}$ adenosine ATPase activity; β-receptor up regulation | ↑ | — | NA[b] |
| **INODILATORS** | | | | | |
| Amrinone | Inocor | Class III phosphodiesterase inhibitors prevent breakdown of cAMP, which results from stimulation of β-adrenergic receptors; enoximome is more potent than older inodilators | ↑ | → | 3 mg/kg IV slowly to effect |
| Milrinone | | | ↑ | → | 0.5–1.0 mg/kg PO, BID |
| Enoximome | | | ↑ | → | NA[b] |
| **NITROVASODILATORS** | | | | | |
| Sodium nitroprusside | Nitropress | Activation of EDRF[c] or NO; act as substrates for the formation of NO; nitroprusside is an arterial dilator; nitroglycerin is a venodilator. | — | → | 1–10 mg/kg/min IV (monitor pressure) |
| Nitroglycerine | Nitrostat; Nitrolpaste | | — | → | 1–5 mg/kg/min IV; available in oral and transdermal paste formulations: Canine: ¼–½ in/20 kg QOD Feline: ⅛ in QOD |

| Generic | Trade | Mechanism | | | Dosage |
|---|---|---|---|---|---|
| Isosorbide dinitrate | | Formation of NO | — | → | 0.5 to 2.0 mg/kg PO, TID; also available as ointment |
| Hydralazine | Apresoline | Hydralazine interferes with $Ca^{2+}$ transport in smooth muscle | — | → | Canine: 1–3 mg/kg PO, BID; Feline: 2.5–5.0 mg/kg PO, BID |
| **ANGIOTENSIN-CONVERTING ENZYME INHIBITORS** | | | | | |
| Captopril | Capoten | Prevent conversion of $AI^a$ to AII, which decreases blood pressure and causes some venodilation; produce balanced vasodilation and prevent renal fluid retention | — | → | Canine and feline: 0.5 to 2.0 mg/kg PO, TID |
| Enalapril | Enacard | | — | → | Canine: 0.5 mg/kg PO, SID, BID; Feline: 0.25–0.5 mg/kg PO, SID, QOD |
| Benazepril | Lotensin | | — | → | Canine: 0.25–0.5 mg/kg PO, SID, BID; Feline: 0.25–0.5 mg/kg PO, SID, -QOD |
| **DIURETICS**[e] | | | | | |
| Acetazolamide | | Inhibit $Na^+$ from passing into proximal tubule; osmotic effect at glomerulus | — | → | Canine: 10 mg/kg q 6 h |
| Mannitol | | | — | → | Canine and Feline: 0.25–0.5 g/kg 5% solution IV |
| Aminophylline | | Increased vascular perfusion of glomerulus | ← | → | Canine: 11 mg/kg PO, TID; Feline: 5 mg/kg PO, BID, TID |

*Continued*

**Table 10-1. (continued)**

| Classes | Trade Name(s) | Mechanisms of Action | Effects on | | Maintenance Dose[a] |
|---------|---------------|----------------------|-------------|-----------|---------------------|
| | | | Contractility | Afterload | |
| Spironolactone | Aldactone | Inhibits aldosterone receptor in collecting tubule | — | ↓ | Canine and Feline: 1–2 mg/kg PO, BID |
| Furosemide | Lasix | Inhibits $Na^+$, $K^+$, and $Cl^{2-}$; cotransporter in thick ascending loop of Henle | — | ↓ | Canine: 1–4 mg/kg PO, SID, QOD Feline: 0.5–3.0 mg/kg PO 8–48 h |

[a]Patients usually are stabilized on congestive heart failure medications before undergoing anesthesia. Medications should *not* be discontinued when contemplating anesthesia and surgery.
[b]Dose is not available for canine or feline.
[c]Endothelium-dependent relaxant factor (= nitric oxide; NO). NO binds to a heme group in the enzyme guanylyl cyclase, activating the enzyme and resulting in the production of cGMP. cGMP produces relaxation as a second messenger in vascular smooth muscle.
[d]Angiotensin I and angiotensin II.
[e]If one diuretic does not produce increased urine flow, another class may be effective. Some diuretics result in salt wasting, so serum $[K^+]$ should be monitored to avoid complicating arrhythmias in the congestive patient.

ligated, increased blood pressure may cause a reflex slowing of the heart rate. In some instances, atropine may be
needed to counteract sinus bradycardia.

2. **Persistent right aortic arch** is also usually recognized early
in life and corrected at that time. If the patient is normal
in other respects, the anesthetic protocol is designed for
the pediatric patient undergoing a thoracotomy. It is
important to remember that a patient with PRAA may be
suffering from aspiration pneumonia. As with a PDA,
surgical manipulation around the heart may cause ventricular ectopic beats, and intraoperative hypothermia is of
concern.

### D. Patients with Hypotension–Hypovolemia: The Patient in Shock

Patients with hypotension–hypovolemia should be stabilized
with fluids and/or whole blood before anesthesia. Many preanesthetic and anesthetic drugs are potentially hypotensive; therefore, they can exacerbate pre-existing hypotension. **Shock** can
be defined as an acute clinical syndrome characterized by
progressive circulatory failure that leads to inadequate capillary
perfusion and cellular hypoxia. Shock is a complex, multisystem
disorder that may be caused by a variety of insults. Shock may be
classified as hypovolemic, cardiogenic, or vasculogenic.

1. **Hypovolemic shock** occurs when there is an inadequate
volume of fluid (blood) being pumped through the cardiovascular system. Hemorrhage (trauma, surgery), fluid
loss (vomiting, diarrhea, burns, diuresis), and trauma (sequestered fluid) can all cause hypovolemic shock.

2. **Cardiogenic shock** occurs when the heart is no longer an
effective pump. It can be caused by a failure in ventricular
filling (cardiac tamponade; tension pneumothorax; collapse of the vena cava caused by inadvertent closure of the
pop-off valve, resulting in airway and intrathoracic pressure buildup), or by a failure of ventricular ejection (ruptured chordae tendineae, cardiac dysrhythmias, severe
myocardial depression, severe and prolonged increase in
systemic vascular resistance).

3. **Vasculogenic shock** occurs when there are changes in the venous capacitance or peripheral resistance. Numerous causes can lead to vasculogenic shock, including sepsis (vasodilation occurs as a result of release of vasoactive substances, such as histamine, prostaglandins, and bradykinin), anaphylaxis (vasodilation occurs because of histamine release), neurogenic factors (loss of vasomotor tone caused by excessive general anesthesia, CNS trauma, spinal anesthesia), and a severe and prolonged increase in peripheral resistance.

4. **Always stabilize the patient in shock before anesthesia.** Once the patient has been treated and stabilized, there are no particular contraindications to any of the preanesthetic or anesthetics.

E. **Patients with Anemia–Hypoproteinemia**

1. **Anemic patients** are of concern from an anesthetic standpoint because the oxygen carrying capacity is diminished. These patients should be preoxygenated before anesthetic induction. Whole blood transfusion should be considered if the dog or cat has a packed cell volume (PCV) of < 25 to 30% before surgery or < 20% after surgery. Patients with chronic anemia seem to be able to better cope with the problem than those with acute anemia.

2. If there is less **plasma protein,** more drug is pharmacologically active and, therefore, will have an increased effect in the patient. Plasma protein is also required to maintain plasma oncotic pressure. Hypoproteinemic patients are less tolerant of fluid administration and more prone to fluid overload and pulmonary edema. Plasma proteins should be maintained above 3.5 g/dL. If the plasma proteins fall below this number, the administration of plasma proteins or other colloidal preparation should be considered.

3. **Supplemental oxygen** may be beneficial in the preanesthetic as well as the postoperative period in anemic patients. A high inspired oxygen tension allows more

oxygen to be dissolved into the plasma and thus helps counteract the decreased oxygen carrying capacity owing to low red blood cell numbers. A mask, nasal catheter, or oxygen cage can be used to deliver 40 to 100% oxygen to the patient.

### F.   Patients with Heartworm Disease

**Heartworm disease** in itself does not contraindicate any particular anesthetic regimen or protocol. If the patient is not exhibiting clinical signs, any standard anesthetic protocol is probably satisfactory. The clinician should be aware that patients with heartworms may be more prone to spontaneous cardiac dysrhythmias while under anesthesia. If a significant number of heartworms are present, cardiac output may also be decreased. Heartworms may also lead to pulmonary dysfunction, which could compromise the patient's ability to ventilate.

## II.   PULMONARY DYSFUNCTION
*Robert R. Paddleford*

Patients with **pulmonary dysfunction** are often difficult to safely anesthetize. Most preanesthetic and anesthetic drugs depress respiratory function, further compromising patients with pulmonary dysfunction.

### A.   Physiology of Ventilation

The **primary function of the lungs** is to exhale carbon dioxide generated by body metabolism and oxygenate venous blood. Alveolar ventilation can be assessed by measuring $Pa_{CO_2}$ or end-tidal carbon dioxide partial pressures. No conscious control is necessary to sustain ventilation. Many factors can alter the ventilatory pattern, including $Pa_{CO_2}$, arterial pH, $Pa_{O_2}$, pulmonary stretch and upper airway receptors, heat regulation, sensory input, and emotional factors.

1.   The **ventilatory control system** is a series of complex feedback loops made up of sensors, controllers, and effectors. The principal ventilatory receptors or sensors are the peripheral carotid-body chemoreceptors (located at the bifurcations of the carotid arteries); the central chemoreceptors (located near the surface on the ventro-

lateral aspect of the medulla oblongata); and the receptors sensing stretch, irritation, and proprioception in the lungs, airways, and muscles of respiration. The carotid-body chemoreceptors are responsive to oxygen and stimulate respiration when hypoxemia is present. The central chemoreceptors respond to carbon dioxide and stimulate ventilation when hypercarbia (respiratory acidosis) is present. Increased ventilation caused by metabolic acidosis may be mediated through either the central or peripheral chemoreceptors or the controllers of the ventilatory feedback loop located in the brain. The cortex controls voluntary and behavioral modifications of ventilation, and respiratory rhythm is controlled by the medulla. The effectors of ventilation are the muscles of respiration and include the intercostal muscles, the diaphragm, and the muscles of the upper airways.

2.  Many preanesthetic and anesthetic agents can alter the patient's ventilatory pattern. Most preanesthetic and anesthetic agents affect ventilation by altering the threshold of the respiratory centers to carbon dioxide, by changing the sensitivity of the respiratory centers to carbon dioxide, and/or by relaxing the muscles of ventilation.

**B.  Effects of Preanesthetic and Anesthetic Drugs**

Most preanesthetic and anesthetic drugs depress respiratory function, thereby further jeopardizing the patient with respiratory dysfunction. Drugs depress or stimulate ventilation by acting directly or indirectly on one or more of the elements of the ventilatory control system.

1.  **Atropine and glycopyrrolate** decrease airway resistance by causing direct dilation of the airways. Atropine also increases respiratory dead space by dilating the larger bronchi. Both drugs increase the viscosity of airway secretions.

2.  **Phenothiazine tranquilizers** have minimal effects on ventilation at therapeutic doses, although large doses can depress ventilation. They produce a decrease in respiratory

rate, but this is usually compensated for by an increase in tidal volume.

3. The $\alpha_2$-agonists (xylazine, detomidine, medetomidine) vary in their pulmonary depressant effects and are somewhat unpredictable. Their depressant effects range from mild to significant, depending on the dose and individual patient response.

4. The benzodiazepine tranquilizers (diazepam, midazolam) usually produce minimal respiratory depression at therapeutic doses.

5. Opioids are potentially potent respiratory depressants. The depression is drug and dose dependent and may occur at doses that do not produce marked CNS depression or analgesia. The opioids directly depress the pontine and medullary centers, causing a decrease in respiratory rate and tidal volume. The panting observed in some dogs after opioid administration may be caused by an initial stimulation of the respiratory centers and/or alteration of the thermoregulation center.

6. The barbiturates are potent respiratory depressants. At anesthetizing doses, the respiratory centers of the brain are depressed. Barbiturates can depress both the respiratory rate and tidal volume and thus minute ventilation.

7. The dissociative anesthetics (ketamine, tiletamine) may have a dual effect on ventilation. They may affect ventilation at two or more anatomic sites, causing stimulation at one and depression at another. Dissociatives produce apneustic ventilation but do not depress the pharyngeal or laryngeal reflexes; therefore, a patient may be more prone to laryngospasm, bronchospasm, and coughing. The dissociative agents increase salivation and respiratory secretions, sometimes resulting in aspiration and respiratory obstruction.

8. Propofol is a relatively new injectable anesthetic that produces respiratory depression in much the same manner as the barbiturates. The incidence of apnea with

propofol is comparable to the barbiturates, but the duration of apneic episodes may be slightly longer.

9. The **inhalant anesthetics** (methoxyflurane, halothane, isoflurane) depress ventilation by decreasing tidal volume. These anesthetics may produce an increase in respiratory rate, but it is not adequate to compensate for the decrease in tidal volume. Potent inhalation anesthetics increase the level of arterial carbon dioxide at which spontaneous ventilation ceases (i.e., the apneic threshold). Potent inhalation anesthetics depress the ventilatory response to hypoxemia. In addition, the interaction between hypoxemia and hypercarbia in stimulating ventilation is greatly attenuated or eliminated by moderate concentrations of these agents.

10. **Nitrous oxide** does possess some respiratory depressant properties, but they are minimal. Nitrous oxide should be used with care in patients with pulmonary dysfunction.

## C. Anesthetic Considerations in Patients with Respiratory Dysfunction

Patients with pulmonary dysfunction may lack the ability to properly expand the lungs (**extrapulmonary dysfunction**) and/or may have impairment of oxygen–carbon dioxide transfer across the alveolar membranes (**intrapulmonary dysfunction**). Examples of extrapulmonary dysfunction include diaphragmatic hernia, pneumothorax, hydrothorax, space-occupying lesions of the thorax, flail chest, and any condition that restricts chest wall expansion. Examples of intrapulmonary dysfunction include pneumonia; pulmonary edema; intrapulmonary hemorrhage (contusions); atelectasis; interstitial disease; and upper airway, tracheal, or bronchial obstruction. Patients with respiratory dysfunction are classified as follows:

Category I: dyspnea does not occur with exertion
Category II: dyspnea occurs with moderate exertion
Category III: dyspnea occurs with mild exertion
Category IV: dyspnea occurs at rest

Patients in categories III and IV are definitely at higher anesthetic risk.

1. **Thoracocentesis** should be done before anesthesia in patients who have moderate to severe pneumothorax or hydrothorax; and in some cases, a chest tube may be needed. Patients with respiratory dysfunction should be **preoxygenated** for 5 to 7 min before anesthetic induction. A mask, nasal catheter, or oxygen chamber may be used.

2. **Mild preanesthetic sedation** may be necessary to allow the patient to be handled without causing stress and exacerbating the respiratory dysfunction. Acetylpromazine produces minimal respiratory depression, especially in low doses. Butorphanol can produce a dose-related respiratory depression similar to that of morphine; however, butorphanol seems to reach a ceiling beyond which higher doses do not cause significantly more respiratory depression. The dose of acetylpromazine is 0.05 mg/kg IM to a maximum total dose of 1 mg. The recommended dose of butorphanol is 0.22 to 0.44 mg/kg IM to a maximum total dose of 20 mg. Because butorphanol can increase vagal tone, atropine at a dose of 0.044 mg/kg IM should be administered to the patient.

3. **Rapid anesthetic induction** may be accomplished using thiopental, propofol, etomidate, or ketamine intravenously. A rapid mask induction using halothane or isoflurane may be used; however, because of the patient's inability to ventilate properly, this technique may result in delayed anesthetic induction and struggling.

4. **Maintenance of anesthesia** is best achieved with an inhalant anesthetic and controlled or positive pressure ventilation.

## D. Controlled Ventilation

1. **Five components** can be adjusted in the ventilatory cycle during controlled ventilation: peak airway pressure, mean airway pressure, length of inspiratory phase, length of expiratory phase, and inspiratory to expiratory ratio.

   a. **Peak airway pressures** are measured by a pressure manometer in the anesthesia circuit. Peak airway pressures of 15 to 20 cm $H_2O$ are necessary to overcome lung resistance to expansion in dogs and larger species. In cats, slightly higher pressures may be needed.

b.    The **mean airway pressure** is the average pressure generated during the inspiratory and expiratory phases of positive pressure ventilation. Mean airway pressure should be kept low. It is kept low by not maintaining the positive airway pressure for longer than is necessary. Mean airway pressure correlates most closely with decreases in cardiac output.

c.    To produce minimal cardiovascular alteration, the **inspiratory phase** should be less than the **expiratory phase.** The inspiratory phase should last 1 to 1.5 s. Prolonged holding of the tidal volume at peak airway pressure will not increase tidal exchange but will increase mean airway pressure, thereby decreasing venous return and cardiac output.

d.    The **inspiratory to expiratory (I:E) ratio** is important during controlled or positive pressure ventilation. The inspiratory phase should be a third and no more than half of the total ventilatory cycle. An I:E ratio of 1:2 or 1:3 helps provide an adequate period for proper cardiac filling. Increased alveolar pressure also decreases pulmonary blood flow; thus maintaining proper peak and mean airway pressures and a proper I:E ratio is critical. **Lung damage** during positive pressure ventilation is always a possibility. Volotrauma can range from mild trauma, producing minimal alveolar hemorrhage, to severe trauma, producing airway rupture and a tension pneumothorax. If a major airway blowout occurs during positive pressure ventilation, it is owing to excessive peak airway pressures and/or pre-existing lung pathology.

2.    The **acid–base balance** will be changed with any change in alveolar ventilation. Hyperventilation causes a decreased arterial carbon dioxide level and an increased pH (alkalosis). Hyperventilation can also lead to cerebral vasoconstriction, which can be beneficial in cases of raised intracranial pressure owing to trauma or masses in the brain.

## III. NEUROLOGIC DISEASE

*Stephen A. Greene, Ralph C. Harvey, and Michael H. Sims*

For patients with **neurologic disease,** consideration of the dynamics of intracranial pressure (ICP), cerebral blood flow (CBF), and cerebrospinal fluid (CSF) production and flow is important to prevent neurologic morbidity or mortality. In normal awake animals, blood supply to the CNS is controlled by autoregulatory mechanisms. Alteration in the CBF can result from a variety of changes in arterial oxygenation, carbon dioxide accumulation, mean arterial pressure, and venous outflow. The brain and spinal cord are protected by the bony skull and vertebral column. Increases in the flow of blood within the noncompliant cranial vault cause an increase in the intracranial volume and pressure. Once increases in CBF cause the intracranial volume to exceed the limits of effective compliance, there is a sharp increase in intracranial pressure. When the ICP is already increased by intracranial masses, trauma, or derangement of autoregulation, slight changes in intracranial volume greatly increase ICP. Significant increases in the ICP may lead to cerebral ischemia and eventually brain herniation.

### A. Autoregulation of Cerebral Blood Flow

**Autoregulation of CBF** is usually effective for an arterial blood pressure range of 60 to 140 mm Hg. Within this range, several factors—including intracranial tumors, hypercapnia, severe hypoxia, and many anesthetics—interfere with autoregulation and cause changes in the ICP (Fig. 10-1). Blood vessels in the brain that supply diseased tissue or neoplasms may be fully dilated and unaffected by normal autoregulation mechanisms.

1. The CNS depression of general anesthesia is usually accompanied by a decrease in cerebral metabolic rate of oxygen ($CMR_{O_2}$). This decrease in oxygen requirement is thought to be protective in the possible event of relative ischemia during anesthesia and neurosurgery. There are conflicting reports on the efficacy of various anesthetics in reducing $CMR_{O_2}$, just as there are in regard to the relative effects of the anesthetics on the CBF and ICP. Isoflurane, etomidate, and the barbiturates are generally recognized as contributing substantially to reduction of $CMR_{O_2}$, affording some cerebral protection.

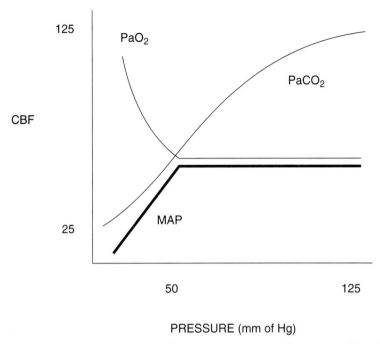

**Figure 10-1.** Alterations in CBF owing to changes in $Pa_{O_2}$, $Pa_{CO_2}$, and mean arterial blood pressure (*MAP*). Modified from Shapiro. In: Miller RD, ed. Anesthesia. 2nd ed. New York: Churchill Livingstone, 1986:1563–1620.

2.  In patients with **pre-existing elevated ICP,** further increases can result from gravitational or positional interference with the drainage of venous blood from the head. Obstruction by occlusion of the jugular veins through surgical positioning of the head or by use of a neck leash or when obtaining blood samples or placing a catheter can rapidly result in dangerous increases in the ICP. For intracranial neurosurgery, a slight elevation of the head above the level of the heart (with the neck in a neutral position) facilitates venous drainage, lowering the ICP. Extreme elevation is avoided to minimize the risk of venous air embolization.

3.  Only at **low arterial oxygen tensions** does the CBF change. When $Pa_{O_2}$ decreases below a threshold of 50 mm Hg, CBF increases (Fig. 10-1). The relationship between $Pa_{CO_2}$ and CBF, on the other hand, is linear. Cerebral blood flow increases by about 2 mL/min/100 g of brain tissue for

every 1 mm Hg increase in $Paco_2$ from 20 to 80 mm Hg. **Hyperventilation** has been used extensively in neuroanesthesia to effectively reduce CBF via cerebral vasoconstriction. This maneuver decreases tissue bulk, facilitating intracranial surgery. Although quite effective, the technique is sometimes controversial, because a potential exists for the remaining blood flow to be preferentially diverted to diseased tissues lacking autoregulation at the expense of normal brain tissue. Deliberate hyperventilation to decrease the ICP may be risky when mean arterial blood pressures are < 50 mm Hg. The ensuing ischemia could be deleterious to normal brain tissues if a **steal** of CBF diverts remaining blood flow. The rapid and substantial reduction in CBF and ICP achieved by hyperventilation makes it a valuable tool for the immediate reduction in brain bulk to facilitate intracranial surgery and reduce acute brain swelling.

4.  Although controversial, **restriction of intravenous fluids** to the volume necessary to maintain adequate circulating volume is usually recommended for neurosurgical patients with increased ICP. Excessive fluid volume has been associated with decreased venous outflow and increased risk of compounding cerebral edema. Diuretic therapy is frequently indicated in the medical management of patients with intracranial masses and elevated ICP or cerebral edema. Dextrose administration is somewhat controversial and must be individualized to the situation. Hyperglycemia is associated with adverse outcome in animals with cerebral ischemia, and cerebral edema can be exacerbated by administration of isotonic dextrose. Its use, however, decreases the incidence of seizures in patients after metrizamide myelography and is indicated in hypoglycemic seizures or hypoglycemic coma.

5.  **Glucocorticoids** are effective in the treatment of some forms of cerebral edema. Corticosteroids have been shown to be effective in reducing the increased ICP that is caused by brain tumors and hydrocephalus. Glucocorticoid therapy may be considered in the management of patients with cerebral edema associated with primary or metastatic brain neoplasia, trauma, some types of hemorrhage, and contu-

sion. Because dexamethasone administration has been shown to reduce the rate of formation of CSF in dogs, there may be some value to steroid administration in the preanesthetic management of hydrocephalic patients considered at risk of further increases in ICP. Corticosteroids are contraindicated in cases of CNS diseases for which an infectious cause is considered possible. The value of steroids in treating cranial trauma is controversial. There are conflicting reports from well-controlled studies and clinical trials on the efficacy of steroid administration after head trauma. It is likely that steroid therapy is of relatively little value once cerebral ischemia has occurred. Administration of anti-inflammatory doses of corticosteroids before a traumatic insult improves the compliance of the brain and ultimately reduces cerebral edema. The practicality of this observation is for preoperative steroid therapy (primarily with dexamethasone) as a means of reducing subsequent cerebral edema. Glucocorticosteroid therapy should optimally begin the day before surgery. Dexamethasone is recommended at 0.25 mg/kg every 8 h, with a dose of 0.25 to 1 mg/kg IV after the induction of anesthesia.

## B.    Pharmacologic Considerations

1.    *Sedatives, Tranquilizers, and Analgesics*

a.    Increased seizure activity associated with administration of the **phenothiazine (e.g., acepromazine) tranquilizers** contraindicates their use in seizure-prone patients and in patients undergoing diagnostic EEG. Control of seizures with benzodiazepine tranquilizers (e.g., diazepam, midazolam) is desirable in the management of seizure-prone patients but can obscure characteristic patterns in diagnostic EEGs.

b.    Use of **xylazine** in dogs and cats is controversial, yet clinical evidence for or against its use in the patient with neurologic disease is lacking. Dexmedetomidine, an optical isomer of medetomidine, decreases the CBF in both halothane- and isoflurane-anesthetized dogs. Medetomidine is not, however, associated with increased ICP in isoflurane-anesthetized dogs.

c.    **Opioids or neuroleptanalgesic combinations** are sometimes used in anesthetic management of patients with increased ICP. The direct effects of opioids on CBF and ICP are minimal; however, opioids may indirectly increase CSF pressure and should be used cautiously in patients with cerebral trauma, tumors, and so on. Increases in pressure within the cranium may aggravate the underlying condition. The elevation in CSF pressure is caused by the accumulation of $CO_2$, which in turn is the result of opioid-induced hypoventilation. If the patient is ventilated to prevent hypercapnia, the increase in CSF pressure does not occur when opioids are administered. When opioids are used in these cases, the respiratory status must be assessed; and when necessary, the patient should be ventilated to prevent hypercapnia. The judicious use of opioids for pain management in the postoperative period often does not cause as much respiratory depression as does pain itself. Thus opioid analgesic medication is based on the relative severity of pain in each animal.

2.    *Injectable Anesthetics*

a.    Most **injectable anesthetics** cause significant reductions in $CMR_{O_2}$, CBF, and ICP (Table 10-2). Recognition of these effects has contributed to the development of **barbiturate-coma** therapy for cerebral resuscitation after periods of cerebral ischemia, such as occurs in near-drowning and cardiopulmonary resuscitation. The value of barbiturates as a therapy for cerebral ischemia–hypoxia is controversial at best. In humans, it is likely that barbiturates are protective if administered before the insult but of relatively little value if administered after clinical signs of ischemia have developed. As with glucocorticoids, barbiturates may be of value in avoiding postoperative sequelae to surgical trauma. It must be recognized, however, that barbiturate anesthesia often prolongs anesthetic recovery. In neurosurgical patients, the CNS depression associated with residual barbiturates can seriously obscure postoperative evaluation and prevent meaningful neurologic evaluation.

     b.     The **dissociative anesthetics** represent a notable exception to the reduction in CBF, ICP, and CMRo$_2$ characteristic of most injectable anesthetics. EEG activity also increases with dissociative anesthesia. Convulsant activity, ranging from muscle twitching to seizures, occurs as an infrequent adverse effect of the dissociatives. Patients with a history of seizure-related disorders and those with intracranial masses, closed-head traumatic injuries, and other conditions potentially increasing the ICP should not receive dissociative anesthetics.

   3.    *Volatile Anesthetics*

     a.     **Volatile anesthetics** increase CBF and alter CMRo$_2$ to varying degrees (Table 10-2). Because increased CBF and ICP are also highly influenced by carbon dioxide retention, respiratory depression associated with vol-

### Table 10-2. Effects of Anesthetics and Anesthetic Adjuncts

| Agent | CBF | ICP | BP | CPP |
|---|---|---|---|---|
| Halothane | ↑↑ | ↑↑ | ↓ | ↓ |
| Isoflurane | ↑ | ↑ | ↓ | ↓ |
| Thiobarbiturates | ↓↓ | ↓↓ | ↓ | ⇌ |
| Fentanyl | ↓ | ↓ | ↓ | ⇌ |
| Morphine | ↓ | ⇌ | ⇌ or ↓ | ⇌ |
| Droperidol | ↓ | ↓ | ↓ | ⇌ |
| Atracurium | ⇌ | ⇌ | ⇌ | ⇌ |
| Succinylcholine | ↑ | ↑ | ⇌ | |
| Diazepam | ↓ | ⇌ or ↓ | ↓ | ⇌ |
| Midazolam | ↓ | ⇌ | ⇌ | ⇌ |
| Ketamine | ↑↑ | ↑↑ | ↑ | ↓ |
| Halothane-thiopental | ⇌ | ⇌ | ↓ | ⇌ or ↓ |

*BP,* blood pressure; *CPP,* cerebral perfusion pressure.

atile anesthesia can be responsible for increases in ICP that are clinically significant for neurosurgical patients. There is evidence that regional changes in the distribution of CBF result from administration of the volatile anesthetics so that our understanding of cerebrovascular effects may not be accurately predicted based on global estimates of CBF in animals.

b.  Among the volatile anesthetics clinically used in veterinary medicine, **halothane dramatically blocks autoregulation,** increasing CBF and ICP. Methoxyflurane, enflurane, and isoflurane all interfere with autoregulation to a more limited extent than does halothane. At 1.1 minimum alveolar concentration (MAC) levels of anesthesia, cerebral blood flow increases almost 200% with halothane but by only about 40% with enflurane and is unchanged with isoflurane. Higher concentrations of isoflurane cause increases in CBF. The loss of cerebral autoregulation with halothane is implicated in the greater degree of brain swelling noted during neurosurgery with this anesthetic. The increase in CBF occurs rapidly with halothane administration and occurs independent of changes in arterial blood pressure, implicating halothane's direct cerebrovascular effects.

c.  Fortunately, **modest hyperventilation,** reducing arterial carbon dioxide to about 30 mm Hg, eliminates the volatile anesthetic-induced increase in CBF. Hyperventilation is rapidly effective in reducing CBF and ICP and in preventing their rise in patients at risk. It is easy, rather cost-free, and the safest method available. In light of the respiratory depression of general anesthesia and the potential rise in CBF and ICP, modest hyperventilation should be incorporated into the anesthetic technique for animals with intracranial masses or other disorders of autoregulation.

d.  **Nitrous oxide** has substantial cerebrovascular effects. Although there are conflicting reports and a minority opposing opinion, the adverse effects of nitrous oxide for neurosurgical patients have been well documented in animals. Nitrous oxide causes the most profound increase in both CBF and ICP of all the inhalant anesthetics. Owing largely to the limited potency of nitrous oxide in veterinary patients, its use is primarily in combination with other general anesthetics. The combination of volatile anesthetic gases and nitrous oxide can produce greater increases in CBF and ICP. In rabbits, nitrous oxide administration produced a consistent increase in CBF and ICP regardless of whether it was combined with halothane, isoflurane, or fentanyl-pentobarbital. Furthermore, these potentially adverse effects were not blocked by hyperventilation. In dogs, nitrous oxide increases $CMRo_2$ by 11%. In animal models of regional cerebral ischemia, the use of nitrous oxide worsens the neurologic outcome. The **disadvantages of nitrous oxide appear to be substantial** for the neurosurgical patient.

## C.     Anesthetic Management of Specific Neurologic Problems

1. *Myelography and Intervertebral Disc Disease*

     a.     For the relatively common surgical procedures to decompress cervical or thoracolumbar **intervertebral disc herniation,** anesthetic management should address protection from possible seizures and other potential complications associated with the administration of myelographic contrast agents, perioperative pain relief, maintenance of adequate spontaneous ventilation, and management of concurrent disorders (e.g., urinary incontinence) or other factors predisposing the patient to adverse recovery.

     b.     **Radiographic contrast myelography** is frequently performed in the immediate preoperative period to localize lesions and identify the proper sites for surgical decompression. Because these procedure are often performed during the same anesthetic period, patient management is designed to optimize the conditions for both the diagnostic (radiographic) and the therapeutic (surgical) procedures. Dural puncture for sampling of CSF and/or for administration of myelographic contrast agent requires a depth of anesthesia at less than a surgical plane but adequate to prevent patient movement with subsequent trauma.

---

**Table 10-3. Anesthetic Management for Myelography and Surgical Decompression of Intervertebral Disc Disease**

---

Benzodiazepine tranquilization (e.g., diazepam 0.4 mg/kg IM, IV)

Low-dose opioid or partial-agonist opioid (analgesia without marked respiratory depression)

Anticholinergics, if indicated

Intravenous induction with propofol or thiopental; inhalational induction with desflurane, halothane, or isoflurane; or induction by mask with sevoflurane

Avoid hyperextension of neck in patients with cervical trauma, instability, and disc disease

Maintenance of protected airway and spontaneous ventilation (for recognition of side effects of myelography and to minimize vertebral sinus blood flow during surgery)

Fluid therapy with dextrose for metrizamide myelography

Positioning to avoid venous occlusion

Postoperative analgesics, as needed

Considerations for an anesthetic protocol suitable for spinal cord surgery are listed in Table 10-3.

c. **Avoidance of potent respiratory depressants** and a light surgical plane of anesthesia will optimally maintain spontaneous ventilation during myelography. Among the less frequent complications associated with myelography are respiratory depression, respiratory arrest, and cardiac arrhythmias. Respiratory depression is probably the result of the effects of the contrast agent at the level of brainstem and medullary respiratory centers. As such, respiratory effects are most likely to be associated with high myelograms, typically those showing contrast agent ascending to the brain and brainstem. The incidence of seizure activity and other potential adverse side effects of myelography appears to be greatly reduced with use of the newer contrast agents iopamidol and iohexol rather than metrizamide. Hyperflexion of the cervical spine for cisternal CSF collection and cervical administration of myelographic contrast can easily kink most endotracheal tubes, resulting in airway obstruction. Armored or spiral wire–containing endotracheal tubes are quite resistant to kinking.

Metal or other radiopaque reinforcement in the armored tubes makes them unsuitable for use in cervical and cranial radiographic studies. Close attention to the adequacy of the airway and spontaneous ventilation is of paramount importance.

d.   In addition to the precautions and considerations appropriate for thoracolumbar disc disease, cervical disc disease can be associated with an **increased risk of cardiac arrhythmias.** Increased vagal stimulation during ventral approaches to the cervical spine may occur with retraction of the carotid sheath. There is often greater postoperative pain with cervical than with thoracolumbar surgical repair. Patients that have lost deep pain perception are surgical emergencies. Rapid-sequence induction, using intravenous general anesthetics rather than inhalation anesthesia is indicated if the animal has or may have a full stomach. Additional management related to the emergent nature of the patient's distress may be indicated. The fact that these animals do not feel painful stimuli of the rear limbs suggests that these areas can be used preferentially for injection and intravenous catheter sites without contributing additional stress to an already highly stressed patient.

2.   *Intracranial Masses and Elevated ICP*
Patients with **intracranial masses,** dysfunctional CBF autoregulation, and/or increased ICP are at risk of rapid deterioration under anesthesia, as described earlier. Anesthetic monitoring should address the physiologic variables associated with altered ICP. Venous and arterial pressures and airway or arterial sampling for $CO_2$ analysis should be included, if possible. Optimal anesthetic management can substantially improve patient status and the outcome of intracranial surgical procedures. A recommended anesthetic technique is summarized in Table 10-4.

3.   *Management of Seizures in the Perianesthetic Period*
**Seizures** are most commonly observed in animals with other signs of brain disease. An animal that displays seizure activity before anesthesia should be medically treated using the standard recommendations before anesthesia is at-

tempted. Development of the hepatic microsomal enzymes and renal function in the neonate is immature in most species. Thus concurrent medication with other drugs may cause unexpected interactions or changes in elimination, necessitating careful patient monitoring and alteration of the anticonvulsant dosage regime. **Phenothiazine tranquilizers** have been shown to augment epileptiform activity on the EEG of dogs. Intrathecal injection of radiographic contrast agents is frequently associated with seizures; therefore, acepromazine and other phenothiazine tranquilizers should be avoided in animals with pre-existing seizures and in animals undergoing myelography (Table 10-5).

4. *Anesthesia for Electrodiagnostic Techniques*

a. **Electrodiagnostic procedures** involve recording spontaneous or evoked electric activity from tissues or organs. Although consistent with the definition, ECG is usually not considered under this rubric. In veterinary medicine, clinical electrodiagnostic techniques are used to record potentials taken from muscle, peripheral nerves, spinal cord, brainstem, cortex, and retina in animals. In humans, these procedures are performed without the use of general anesthetics, tranquilizers, or analgesics. With adequate instruc-

---

**Table 10-4. Anesthetic Management for Intracranial Surgery and Patients with Elevated CBF or ICP**

Preanesthetic critical care management and stabilization (including glucocorticosteroid and diuretic therapy as indicated)

Fluid therapy limited to minimize cerebral edema but adequate to support circulation

Avoid potent respiratory depression, jugular venous occlusion, and coughing at induction of anesthesia and during recovery

Avoid dissociatives, halothane, enflurane, and nitrous oxide

Intravenous propofol or barbiturate induction of anesthesia

Minimal concentration of desflurane, isoflurane, or sevoflurane supplemented with opioids, propofol, or barbiturates for maintenance of anesthesia

Modest hyperventilation to reduce CBF and ICP

Postoperative critical care with support of ventilation and circulation, as indicated

---

**Table 10-5. Anesthetic Management for Seizure-Prone Patients and for Diagnostic EEG**

I. Control of Seizures

    Treatment or avoidance of hypoglycemia

    Avoid phenothiazine tranquilizers (e.g., acepromazine)

    Benzodiazepine tranquilization (diazepam 0.4 mg/kg IM, IV) or barbiturate sedation (phenobarbital 2–5 mg/kg IM)

    Intravenous induction with propofol or thiopental but not methohexital

    Inhalational induction with desflurane, halothane, isoflurane, or sevoflurane but not enflurane

    Avoidance of increases in CBF and ICP

II. Diagnostic EEG

    Avoid preanesthetic tranquilizers and sedatives

    Intravenous induction with propofol or thiopental

    Maintain light plane of anesthesia with desflurane, halothane, sevoflurane, or incremental thiobarbiturate, if necessary to prolong duration

    Infiltration of temporal muscles with lidocaine as an alternative to general anesthesia

---

tion, most adults will tolerate some degree of discomfort or boredom to achieve good test results. A few of the procedures, such as nerve conduction studies or electromyography (EMG), cause some pain; whereas others, such as visual or auditory evoked potentials, may simply require human patients to concentrate or refrain from movement. A fundamental problem encountered in the use of electrodiagnostic techniques in veterinary medicine, however, is that of patient cooperation. Even during procedures in which the stimulus is innocuous, artifacts caused by movement may render the technique ineffective. Therefore, many of the procedures are performed on anesthetized or tranquilized animals. This approach is usually less stressful to the animal, ensures a minimum of recording artifacts, and often gives the examiner an opportunity to collect more useful data. The obvious trade-off is a nervous system that has been chemically altered to some degree.

    b.    The effects of anesthetics on the **outcome** of electro-diagnostic procedures range from insignificant to dramatic. In some instances, the use of anesthetic agents altogether precludes recording certain types of potentials. The order of increasing anesthetic effects on recordings is peripheral nerve and skeletal muscle, spinal cord and retina, brainstem, and cerebral cortex. Even so, as long as the effects are understood, the benefits of the recordings still outweigh the alterations induced by anesthetics. Today, intraoperative monitoring has become standard practice in humans when the physician needs direct and prompt feedback about neural function during a surgical procedure. The use of intraoperative electrodiagnostic monitoring in veterinary medicine is not widespread, but many electrodiagnostic laboratories judiciously use anesthetics for procedures. Certainly, the precautions vary among animal species and the physical condition of the patient. Published reports underscore the importance of this area.

5.    *Electroencephalogram and Electromyography*

    a.    Two procedures record electric activity from spontaneously, reflexively, or volitionally active tissue: **EEG** records activity produced by the cerebral cortex, and **EMG** records electric activity produced by skeletal muscle. Most other electrodiagnostic procedures require a stimulus to evoke activity from excitable tissue. The evoking stimulus may be electric, visual, auditory, or mechanical.

    b.    Anesthetic effects on the EEG depend on the type of drug and depth of anesthesia. Anesthesia initially causes an increase in the voltage and a decrease in the frequency of cortical potentials compared to those of an awake, alert dog. Spikes and spindles may also riddle the EEG of lightly anesthetized dogs and cats. As anesthesia deepens, the overall voltage begins to diminish. A dose–response decrease in $CMR_{O_2}$ accompanies the use of isoflurane in dogs and causes the EEG to become isoelectric at an end-expired concentration of 3%. The same type of cortical alteration of electric activity, sometimes referred to as burst suppression, has been reported in other species. Isoflurane anesthesia may thereby interfere with the acquisition of diagnostic information. A recommended anesthetic technique for diagnostic EEG evaluation and for procedures other than EEG in seizure-prone patients is summarized in Table 10-5.

c.     Dose–dependent CNS depression of EEG activity by most anesthetics is characteristic and has led to the development of EEG-based **anesthetic monitoring techniques** (bispectral analysis; BIS monitor). Use of computer-analyzed quantitative EEG in isoflurane-anesthetized dogs has been reported. Enflurane anesthesia can be accompanied by increased EEG activity that extends to seizures, particularly if the patient is hyperventilated and hypocarbic. Alterations in the normal $Pa_{CO_2}$ are associated with significant changes in the quantitative EEG of dogs during halothane anesthesia. Methoxyflurane and halothane anesthetics cause a progression of cerebral depression in dogs; and the latter is more likely to promote burst suppression than is the former. Similar results in dogs have been reported for sodium pentobarbital. In dogs, barbiturate anesthesia was accompanied by reduced EEG amplitude and burst suppression.

# IV. RENAL DISEASE

*Stephen A. Greene*

The kidneys have three primary functions: **filtration, reabsorption, and secretion.** To accomplish these functions, they receive about 25% of the cardiac output. The renal tubules and collecting ducts reabsorb up to 99% of filtered solutes, indicating that the total filtration volume is much greater than is the daily urine production. Neurohumoral substances and physiologic factors that affect reabsorption of the filtered water and sodium include aldosterone, antidiuretic hormone (ADH), arterial blood pressure, atrial natriuretic factor, catecholamines, prostaglandins, renin–angiotensin, and stress.

## A.    Renal Blood Flow

**Renal blood flow** (RBF) is regulated by extrinsic nervous and hormonal control and by intrinsic autoregulation. Renal vasculature is highly innervated by sympathetic constrictor fibers originating in the T4–L1 spinal cord segments. The kidneys lack sympathetic dilator fibers and parasympathetic innervation. Intrinsic autoregulation of RBF is defined by a constant flow when mean arterial blood pressure ranges from 80 to 180 mm Hg. When the mean arterial blood pressure is between 80 and 180 mm Hg, the kidney is able to control blood flow by altering resistance in the renal afferent arterioles. Although the exact mechanism of renal autoregulation is not known, the significance of this phenomenon relates to protection of glomerular capillaries during hypertension and preservation of renal function during hypotension. Even within the range of blood pressure described for the function of renal autoregulation, however, extrinsic forces (e.g., neural, hormonal, pharmacologic) may cause alterations in RBF and the glomerular filtration rate (GFR). The renal vascular anatomy is unique in its distribution to cortical and medullary zones. Because of this vascular dichotomy, local tissue ischemia and hypoxia may occur even though total organ blood flow is normal. Experimental evidence indicates that the medullary thick ascending loop of Henle is selectively vulnerable to hypoxic injury.

### B.  Anesthetic Effects on Renal Function

1.  **Effects of anesthetics on RBF** can be generally summarized as follows: All anesthetics are likely to decrease the rate of glomerular filtration. Anesthetics may directly affect RBF, or they may indirectly alter renal function via changes in cardiovascular and/or neuroendocrine activity. Most anesthetics decrease the GFR as a consequence of decreased RBF (Table 10-6). Inhalation anesthetics tend to decrease RBF and the GFR in a dose–dependent manner. Light planes of inhalation anesthesia preserve renal autoregulation of blood flow, whereas deep planes are associated with depression of autoregulation and decreases in RBF. Although isoflurane has little effect on RBF, it decreases the GFR and urine output. Thiobarbiturates increase systemic vascular resistance but decrease renal vascular resistance with no net change in RBF. In contrast, ketamine increases RBF and renal vascular resistance. Most anesthetics cause less disruption of renal autoregulation of blood flow at lower doses (lighter anesthetic planes). Renal responses to

| Table 10-6. Effects of Anesthetics on RBF and GFR | | |
|---|---|---|
| **Drug** | **RBF** | **GFR** |
| Diethyl ether | Decrease | Decrease |
| Desflurane | No change | ? |
| Enflurane | Decrease | Decrease |
| Etomidate | No change | No change |
| Halothane | Slight decrease | Decrease |
| Isoflurane | Slight decrease | Decrease |
| Ketamine | Increase | Decrease or no change |
| Methoxyflurane | Decrease | Decrease |
| Thiopental | No change | No change or slight decrease |

anesthetics depend on the pre-existing hydration status and the quantity of perioperative fluids administered.

2. **Renal ischemia** may occur during anesthesia owing to systemic hypotension or renal vasoconstriction. Systemic hypotension may be caused by excessive depth of inhalation anesthesia, because all potent halogenated anesthetics cause peripheral vasodilation. Inhalant anesthetics also depress myocardial contractility and cardiac output in a dose–dependent manner. Hypotension may also be induced by phenothiazine or butyrophenone tranquilizers. Dopamine receptor blockade by acepromazine premedication may prevent dopamine-induced increases in RBF during surgery.

3. Anesthesia and the **stress** associated with surgery cause release of aldosterone, vasopressin, renin, and catecholamines. Thus RBF and GFR (and, therefore, urine production) are generally decreased with surgery in any patient. For most patients, the effects of inhaled anesthetics on renal function are reversed at the termination of anesthesia. Some patients, however, may not regain the ability to regulate urine production for several days.

4. $\alpha_2$-**Agonists** can dramatically increase urinary output and reduce urinary osmolality. Xylazine is believed to decrease

ADH concentration, accounting, in part, for the increased urine production. Medetomidine-induced diuresis has also been reported. Because they can induce diuresis, $\alpha_2$-agonists should not be used in animals with urethral obstruction. The antidiuresis seen after morphine administration in animals has been attributed to an increased release of ADH.

5. **Methoxyflurane** is the only anesthetic known to cause nephrotoxicity as a consequence of biotransformation to oxalate and free fluoride ion (Fig. 10-2). Dogs appear to

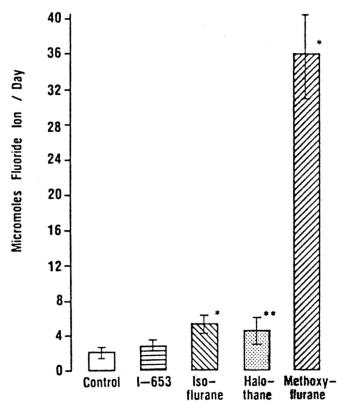

**Figure 10-2.** The 24-h excretion of fluoride ion in urine of rats pretreated with phenobarbital and anesthetized with 1.6 MAC desflurane (I-653), isoflurane, halothanes, or methoxyflurane for 2 h. Reprinted with permission from Koblin DD, Eger EI, Johnson BH, et al. I-653 resists degradation in rats. Anesth Analg 1988;67:534.

| Table 10-7. Potential Nephrotoxins in the Perianesthetic Period | |
| --- | --- |
| Aminoglycoside antibiotics | Iodinated radiographic contrast agents |
| Amphotericin B | Methoxyflurane |
| Bilirubin | Myoglobin |
| Fluoride ion | Nonsteroidal anti-inflammatory agents |
| Hemoglobin | Oxalate |

be more resistant to fluoride-induced renal toxicosis than are humans. In addition, nephrotoxic activity of other drugs used during anesthesia may be enhanced by methoxyflurane (Table 10-7). Methoxyflurane anesthesia combined with flunixin meglumine precipitates renal failure in dogs. Administration of aminoglycoside antibiotics also enhances renal toxicity of methoxyflurane. Sevoflurane is transformed by soda lime (and to a greater extent by Baralyme) in the carbon dioxide absorber of the anesthesia machine. A product of this reaction (identified as compound A) is potentially renal toxic in laboratory rats. A minimum oxygen flow rate of 2 L/min when using an adult circle rebreathing system reduces sevoflurane exposure to the $CO_2$ absorbent and is recommended for eliminating the production of compound A.

## C. Renal Insufficiency and Anesthesia

**Azotemia** in the patient with renal insufficiency will alter the response to anesthetics. Azotemia may be associated with changes in the blood–brain barrier, leading to increased CNS drug sensitivity. Patients with renal insufficiency may be acidotic, which increases the fraction of unbound barbiturate and other injectable drugs in the plasma. Increased unbound fraction of any injectable anesthetic will increase drug activity. Thus lower doses of highly protein-bound injectable anesthetics are required in acidotic patients.

1. **Hyperkalemia** may be present in animals with renal insufficiency, obstructed urethra, or rupture of the urinary bladder. Acidosis may be associated with a concurrent increase in serum potassium. Patients in renal failure with hypocal-

cemia are at even greater risk, because hypocalcemia potentiates the myocardial toxicity of hyperkalemia. **As a rule, patients with a serum potassium concentration > 5.5 or 6.0 mEq/L should not be anesthetized.** The resting membrane potential of cardiac muscle depends on permeability and extracellular concentration of potassium (Fig. 10-3). During hyperkalemia, the membrane's resting potential is raised (partially depolarized) and fewer sodium channels are available to participate in the action potential. As the serum potassium concentration increases, repolarization occurs more rapidly and automaticity, conductivity, contractility, and excitability are decreased. These changes produce the classic electrocardiographic appearance of a peaked T wave with a prolonged PR interval, progressing to wide QRS complexes and loss of P waves.

If hyperkalemia is acute or electrocardiographic abnormalities are noted, treatment should be initiated before induction of anesthesia. **The most rapid treatment for the cardiac effects associated with hyperkalemia is 10% calcium chloride (0.1 mg/kg IV).** Calcium will increase the membrane's threshold potential, resulting in increased myocardial conduction and contractility. Because increased serum potassium concentration causes the

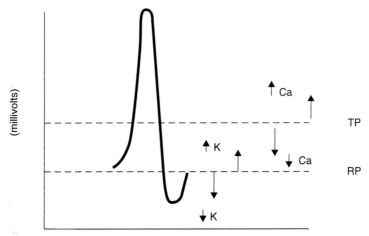

**Figure 10-3.** Relationship between extracellular concentrations of potassium and calcium and the resting potential (*RP*) and threshold potential (*TP*). An action potential is generated when there is sufficient depolarization to reach the TP. Increased extracellular potassium results in a raised (less negative) RP, whereas increased extracellular calcium results in a raised TP.

resting potential to be less negative (partially depolarized), the calcium ion–induced increase in threshold potential temporarily restores the normal gradient between resting and threshold potentials (Fig. 10-3). It should be recognized that administration of calcium will not affect the serum potassium concentration; therefore, its effects will be short-lived. Regimens to decrease the serum potassium concentration by shifting potassium intracellularly include bicarbonate administration and combined infusion of glucose and insulin.

2.  Patients in **chronic renal failure** are frequently anemic because of bone marrow suppression and decreased erythropoietin production. In response to anemia, the cardiovascular system may become hyperdynamic in an attempt to maintain oxygen delivery. Chronic renal disease may be associated with hypertension and increased cardiac output but reduced cardiac reserve. Patients undergoing anesthesia should have a red blood cell transfusion if the hematocrit is < 18% (cat) or 20% (dog).

3.  In dogs and cats with **mild renal insufficiency,** a rapid intravenous induction of anesthesia may be accomplished with thiobarbiturates, diazepam-ketamine, or diazepam-opioid combinations. Depressed patients can be mask induced with desflurane, isoflurane, sevoflurane, or halothane. Medications that are potentially nephrotoxic should be avoided.

4.  **Urine production** is an indirect monitor of renal perfusion. Normal urine output for the dog is 0.5 to 1 mL/kg/h. Intravenous fluids should be administered during anesthesia at the rate of 20 mL/kg for the first hour. A rate of 10 mL/kg/h is used thereafter. The choice of intravenous fluid is based on the individual animal's particular electrolyte and acid–base status. In general, animals with mild to moderate renal insufficiency that are well prepared for surgery or anesthesia are given lactated Ringer's solution. Measurement of arterial blood pressure is advised to detect systemic hypotension and prevent renal hypoperfusion. The mean arterial blood pressure should be maintained

above 70 mm Hg. Normal central venous pressure (CVP) should be between −3 and +5 cm $H_2O$. If the CVP rises more than 10 cm $H_2O$, fluid administration should be slowed or stopped. If the CVP falls in response to stopping the fluids, they may be resumed at a slower rate.

### D.  Tests of Renal Function

Measurements of the GFR and renal tubular function such as **urine specific gravity** and **BUN** are not specific for renal disease; however, BUN concentrations > 50 mg/dL nearly always indicate renal insufficiency. Serum creatinine is a specific indicator of the GFR, but it may be eliminated via nonrenal routes. Thus patients with mild renal insufficiency may not have elevated serum creatinine. In the absence of proteinuria or casts, normal BUN, creatinine, and urine-concentrating ability may be present with up to 67% loss of renal parenchyma.

### E.  Postoperative Oliguria

**Postoperative oliguria (< 0.5 mL/kg/h)** should be investigated. If the animal does not have congestive heart failure or pulmonary edema, a fluid challenge of 5 mL/kg of isotonic saline may be given. If urine production resumes, the animal was hypovolemic and fluids should be continued. If not, dopamine may be initiated as an infusion at a rate of 1 to 3 µg/kg/min. Dopamine improves renal function when used at low doses by increasing the RBF, GFR, urine output, and sodium excretion and by decreasing renal vascular resistance. At moderate doses (5 to 10 µg/kg/min), dopamine activates β-adrenoceptors, which may dilate renal arterial beds and increase cardiac output. Recall that in patients medicated with acepromazine, dopamine may be ineffective at increasing RBF because of dopaminergic receptor blockade.

The use of diuretics in the perioperative period is controversial. Furosemide is used to promote diuresis in patients with pulmonary edema but should not be used when the patient is known to be hypovolemic. In hypovolemia, furosemide will increase nephrotoxicity of other drugs by increasing their contact time in the renal tubules. Mannitol can be given at 0.25

to 0.5 mg/kg to prevent pulmonary edema or hyponatremia if the patient does not respond to fluid administration.

### F.   Urethral Obstruction

Patients with **urethral obstruction** become hyperkalemic, azotemic, acidotic, and hyperphosphatemic. Selected species (e.g., cats) may also develop hyperglycemia, hypocalcemia, and hyponatremia. Hyponatremia is associated with leakage of urine into the peritoneal cavity. Any metabolic abnormalities should be evaluated and corrected before anesthesia. Hyperkalemia is the primary concern in most cases of urethral obstruction.

   **Anesthesia** may be induced using injectable or inhalation anesthetics. In many animals, distension of the urinary bladder is associated with increased heart rate. Cats that are chamber-induced with an arrhythmogenic inhalation anesthetic, such as halothane, should be preoxygenated and tranquilized before exposure to high concentrations of the anesthetic. Chamber induction with isoflurane is preferred over halothane for small animals with urethral obstruction. Ketamine has been used in obstructed cats, even though active metabolites of the drug are excreted by the kidney. The rationale is that once the obstruction is relieved, excretion of the anesthetic will proceed normally. Cats with a long duration of urethral obstruction, however, may develop metabolic disturbances and renal insufficiency so that elimination of drugs is slowed even after removal of the obstruction. Thus it is recommended that low doses of ketamine (2 mg/kg IV) in combination with acepromazine (0.05 mg/kg IV) be used in these circumstances.

### G.   Ruptured Urinary Bladder

Rupture of the urinary bladder is an emergency situation. Animals may become hyperkalemic, hyponatremic, hypochloremic, and acidotic after rupture of the urinary bladder. Intravenous fluids, such as isotonic saline, should be given to aid in correcting electrolyte imbalances. Potassium enters the abdominal cavity from the ruptured bladder and is reabsorbed into the circulation, causing an increased serum potassium concentration. Hyperkalemia (serum $[K^+] > 5.5$ mEq/L) should be treated before anesthesia. Isoflurane is commonly used because of its minimal myocardial depressant action and its minimal potentiation of catecholamine-induced cardiac arrhythmias.

| Table 10-8. Effect of Inhaled Anesthetics on Hepatic Blood Flow | | |
|---|---|---|
| **Agent** | **Portal Vein** | **Hepatic Artery** |
| Desflurane | Decrease | No change |
| Halothane | Decrease | Decrease or no change |
| Isoflurane | Decrease | Increase |
| Methoxyflurane | Decrease | Decrease |
| Nitrous oxide | No direct effect | No direct effect |

## V.  HEPATIC DISEASE

*Stephen A. Greene*

About **20% of cardiac output is delivered to the liver.** The hepatic artery supplies 30% of the blood flow and 90% of the oxygen, and the remainder is supplied by blood flowing through the portal vein. Anesthetics may affect hepatic blood flow by altering vascular tone in the hepatic artery, the portal vein, or both (Table 10-8). Decreased blood flow may occur in cirrhotic livers or patients with portocaval shunt syndrome. Significant decreases in blood flow may be associated with decreased hepatic extraction and, ultimately, decreased elimination of drugs.

### A.  Determination of Hepatic Insufficiency

1.  **Clinical signs of hepatic insufficiency** include ascites, depression, seizures, jaundice, and petechial hemorrhage. Tests of substrate metabolism may give an indication of hepatic function. Low values for plasma proteins and albumin, urea nitrogen, and cholesterol are associated with poor hepatic function. Coagulation defects, such as prolonged prothrombin time and increased fibrinogen values, may also indicate decreased hepatic function. Bilirubin is formed by metabolism of degraded hemoglobin by macrophages and carried by albumin to the liver for conjugation.

2.  **Blood ammonia** concentration and retention of dyes such as sulfobromophthalein (BSP) or indocyanine green

(ICG) indicate liver dysfunction as evidenced by the liver's inability to eliminate these substances in a normal manner. The dyes, like bile acids, are more sensitive indicators of liver dysfunction than is a change in bilirubin concentration.

3. Normal fasting **bile acid concentrations** are < 5 mmol/L for the cat and < 10 mmol/L for the dog. Marked increases in postprandial bile acid concentration indicate decreased hepatic function or the presence of a portal–caval vascular shunt. Normal 2-h postprandial concentrations of bile acids are < 15 mmol/L in the cat and < 25 mmol/L in the dog.

4. Tests of **cell membrane integrity** (i.e., alanine aminotransferase, $\gamma$-glutamyltransferase, sorbitol dehydrogenase, lactate dehydrogenase, and serum alkaline phosphatase) indicate hepatocellular damage but may not reflect hepatic function.

## B.   Pharmacologic Considerations

1. **Acepromazine, droperidol,** and $\alpha_2$-**adrenergic agonists** should be avoided in patients with moderate to severe liver disease. Hypotension may occur after administration of phenothiazine (acepromazine) or butyrophenone (droperidol) tranquilizers because of peripheral vasodilation mediated by $\alpha$-adrenergic blockade. Dysrhythmias, such as bradycardia or heart block, and alterations of plasma glucose concentration may occur after administration of $\alpha_2$-agonists. Diazepam is generally considered safe when used in doses < 0.2 mg/kg IV because it causes minimal changes in cardiovascular function. Diazepam may not consistently tranquilize the healthy young animal but frequently produces tranquilization in animals with liver disease. When diazepam is administered intravenously, it should be injected slowly to decrease irritation and prevent hypotension associated with the propylene glycol carrier.

2. **Morphine** and **meperidine** can cause release of histamine, which may cause a decrease in total hepatic blood flow. Morphine also constricts the sphincter of Oddi, which

could be of significance in obstructive biliary disease. Opioid-induced bradycardia will decrease cardiac output and should be prevented by administration of an anticholinergic agent. Butorphanol is associated with less respiratory depression than are other opioid agonists and is a reasonable choice for the patient with hepatic disease.

3. **Thiobarbiturates** should be used in low doses or avoided altogether in patients with liver disease. A single, intubating dose of thiobarbiturate is not necessarily contraindicated because it will be redistributed from the brain to less well perfused tissues, terminating the anesthetic effect. Liver disease, however, may affect the duration and depth of thiobarbiturate induced-anesthesia because of increased sensitivity of the CNS, hypoalbuminemia, or decreased protein binding of the anesthetic. Anesthesia should not be maintained by re-dosing thiobarbiturates in patients with liver disease. Methohexital should be avoided in patients with hepatic encephalopathy.

4. **Propofol** is an alkylphenolic compound used for induction of anesthesia that is supplied in a lecithin emulsion, giving it a milky white appearance. Redistribution and metabolism of propofol after a single injection are extremely rapid. The total body clearance of propofol exceeds hepatic blood flow, indicating sites other than the liver (probably the lung) may play a role in its elimination. The major advantage over a thiobarbiturate is the rapid rate of propofol elimination, which is not totally hepatic dependent.

5. **Etomidate** is an imidazole compound used for induction of anesthesia. Etomidate does not decrease hepatic perfusion. It has a short duration of action, primarily because of rapid redistribution from the brain to the muscle tissue. Etomidate is metabolized by the hepatic microsomal enzyme system as well as by plasma esterases. The total body clearance rate for etomidate is five times as fast as for thiopental. Etomidate has been shown to cause adrenocortical suppression with repeated administration. The importance of etomidate's effect on steroidogenesis after single bolus administration in the patient with hepatic disease is unknown. In both humans and dogs, etomidate

infusion has been associated with hemolysis. Hemolysis appears to be caused by the propylene glycol vehicle in which etomidate is formulated. Etomidate is a reasonable drug choice for induction of anesthesia in patients with cardiac and/or hepatic disease.

6. **Dissociative anesthetics,** such as tiletamine and ketamine, are generally acceptable for induction of anesthesia in patients with hepatic disease. Intravenous administration is preferred to minimize the dose required for intubation. In the dog, these drugs are largely metabolized by the liver, so maintenance of anesthesia should be with an inhalant. Dissociative anesthetics may induce seizures in dogs or cats. In the cat, ketamine is metabolized to a small extent by the liver to form norketamine, which has about 10% of the activity of ketamine.

7. **Zolazepam,** the benzodiazepine tranquilizer in Telazol, has been suspected of causing prolonged recovery after intramuscular injection in the cat. Zolazepam's effect in the cat is antagonized by flumazenil, a benzodiazepine antagonist, providing an alternative to the apparently slow hepatic metabolism of the benzodiazepines in this species.

8. **Inhalation anesthetics** are good choices for maintenance of anesthesia. Although it is recommended that halothane be avoided if possible in patients with liver disease. The presence of hepatic disease does not necessarily result in increased hepatotoxicity when the patient is subsequently exposed to an unpredictable hepatotoxin such as halothane. Precautions should be taken when using halothane (or any other anesthetic) to ensure adequate blood pressure, flow, and oxygen delivery during anesthesia. Prevention of hepatic hypoxia during inhalation anesthesia is probably more important than the choice of anesthetic in preventing the occurrence of postanesthetic hepatopathy.

   a.  Less than 1% of inhaled **isoflurane** is metabolized. It has not been associated with hepatic or renal toxicity. The higher cardiac output associated with isoflurane anesthesia is likely to maintain better hepatic perfusion and oxygen delivery than will halothane. Thus isoflurane appears to be the best choice for maintenance of anesthesia in patients with hepatic disease.

b. **Nitrous oxide** has been used in patients with hepatic disease in an effort to decrease the amount of volatile anesthetic required for anesthesia. There are no reports of direct hepatic injury caused by exposure to nitrous oxide as used in clinical practice.

9. **Nondepolarizing muscle relaxants,** such as pancuronium and vecuronium, are metabolized by the liver. Effects of these relaxants may be prolonged in patients with hepatic disease. Concurrent administration of aminoglycoside antibiotics with nondepolarizing muscle relaxants may also prolong neuromuscular blockade. Because atracurium undergoes plasma degradation via a metabolic pathway (Hofmann elimination) that primarily depends on plasma pH and temperature and not hepatic degradation, atracurium seems to be a good choice.

## C. General Guidelines for Patients with Hepatic Disease

1. **Most anesthetics are metabolized by the liver,** so elimination may be significantly slowed in animals that are hypothermic. Use of heated circulating water blankets and administration of warm intravenous or irrigation fluids is advised.

2. **Glucose metabolism** is frequently affected by hepatic disease. Homeostasis of glucose can be maintained with loss of up to 80% of functional liver mass. Nevertheless, patients with severe hepatic disease that are stressed by anesthesia and surgery may become hypoglycemic. Hypoglycemia is present in 35% of dogs with portal–caval shunts. For this reason, blood glucose concentration is routinely determined, and glucose (e.g, $D_5W$) is administered when indicated.

3. **Ascitic fluid** may impede lung expansion and pulmonary function. Ascitic fluid should be removed before anesthesia. Rapid removal of a large quantity of fluid may result in a fluid shift from the vascular space to the abdominal cavity as the formation of ascites continues. When removing

massive amounts of ascitic fluid, intravenous fluids should be simultaneously administered to avoid cardiovascular collapse. Hypoalbuminemia is often present in patients with liver disease. When albumin concentration is < 1.5 g/dL, the plasma oncotic pressure is decreased so that pulmonary edema may occur after intravenous fluid administration. Arterial blood pressure may be difficult to maintain when plasma oncotic pressure is significantly decreased. Replacement of albumin and plasma proteins is indicated in these cases. If matched plasma from a donor animal is not available, dextran 70 (up to 20 mL/kg) or hetastarch may be administered. Although exogenous colloids will aid in re-establishing plasma oncotic pressure, their duration of effect is not as great as that of plasma.

4. **Seizures** resulting from hepatic encephalopathy may require treatment. Diazepam or phenobarbital is commonly used to control seizures. Avoid the use of anesthetics that may induce seizure activity, such as enflurane, ketamine, tiletamine (Telazol), and methohexital. There is increased cerebral sensitivity to γ-aminobutyric acid (GABA) in some patients with hepatic disease. This increased sensitivity to GABA-ergic inhibition within the CNS may enhance the depressant effects of the barbiturates and benzodiazepine tranquilizers.

5. **Local anesthetics** of the ester class (e.g., procaine, tetracaine) are metabolized by plasma cholinesterases produced by the liver, whereas the amide class (lidocaine, mepivacaine, bupivacaine) is directly metabolized by the liver. For this reason, the generalized effects of local anesthetics may be prolonged in patients with severe hepatic disease long after local analgesia has waned. This is unlikely to be a major deterrent for their clinical use.

6. The **coagulation profile** should be evaluated before surgery in patients with hepatic disease. If coagulopathy exists, clotting factors or whole blood should be administered.

## D.   Portal–Caval Shunt

1. Anesthetic management of the dog with portal–caval shunt should be based on presenting clinical signs and physical

status (Table 10-9). Signs of **hepatic encephalopathy and hypokalemia** may be present. Hypokalemia in animals with portal–caval shunt may be caused by gastrointestinal (vomiting and diarrhea) upset or urinary loss (diuresis). Hypokalemia ($[K^+]$ 3.5 mEq/L) should be corrected before anesthesia. Intravenous potassium administration should not exceed the rate of 0.5 mEq/kg/hour.

2. **Chronic hepatic dysfunction** may be associated with increased GABA-ergic sensitivity and permeability of the blood–brain barrier. The effect of anesthetics and anesthetic adjuncts may be greater than expected and unpredictable. Diazepam is frequently used as preanesthetic medication in dogs with portal–caval shunt. Antagonists of the benzodiazepine receptor, such as flumazenil, have been reported to ameliorate signs of encephalopathy in a woman and in animal models.

3. **Hepatic insufficiency** may be present in animals with portal–caval shunt. When termination of action depends highly on drug hepatic metabolism (e.g., ketamine, acepromazine, xylazine) such drugs should be avoided. Drugs that are highly protein bound (e.g., barbiturates) will be more active in animals with hypoalbuminemia. Drugs such as methohexital and ketamine that may induce seizure activity are contraindicated in animals with hepatic encephalopathy. Halothane may cause hepatopathy in animals with poor hepatic perfusion and oxygenation and, therefore, should be used cautiously in patients with portal–caval

---

**Table 10-9. Problems Associated with Portal–Caval Shunt**

| Problem | Significance |
| --- | --- |
| Weight loss | May affect drug dose or disposition |
| Hypoalbuminemia | May affect drug dose, disposition, or plasma oncotic pressure |
| Hepatic shunt | Loss of hepatic metabolism of drugs |
| Low bile salts | Increased absorption of intestinal endotoxin |
| Portal hypertension | May require second surgery and CVP monitoring |

shunt. Isoflurane is the preferred anesthetic in patients with this condition. Mask induction and maintenance with isoflurane is frequently used. Opioids may be used as analgesic supplements before or after anesthesia for surgical correction of the shunt.

4.  **Arterial blood pressure** should be monitored during portal–caval shunt surgery. Hypoalbuminemia predisposes the patient to hypotension, which may be revealed by isoflurane-induced peripheral vasodilation. Judicious use of plasma or dextran 70 (10–20 mL/kg given over 1 h) or other colloid substitute to aid in maintenance of plasma oncotic pressure may be indicated. Hypotensive patients with portal–caval shunt may fail to respond to catecholamine infusions, such as dobutamine or dopamine. Surgical retraction of the liver or compression of the caudal vena cava may further decrease venous return, cardiac output, and arterial blood pressure.

5.  In normal dogs, **portal pressure** is reported to be between 6 and 15 cm $H_2O$, whereas portal pressure in dogs with portal–caval shunt is usually lower. After surgical correction of the shunt, portal venous pressure should not be more than 9 cm $H_2O$ above baseline measurement, or a maximum of 20 cm $H_2O$. Intraoperative measurement of central venous pressure is a useful method for estimating portal resistance and for predicting the development of postoperative portal hypertension. A decrease in central venous pressure after ligation of a single portal–caval shunt indicates decreased transit of blood from the intestine to the vena cava. Central venous pressure should not decrease by more than 1 cm $H_2O$ from baseline measurement at 3 min after ligation to avoid postoperative portal hypertension.

## VI.  GASTROINTESTINAL DISEASE
*Stephen A. Greene*

Fractures of the **mandible, maxilla, or temporomandibular joint** may not permit examination to determine the range of jaw motion. **Temporal myositis** may prevent opening of the mouth even while the patient is anesthetized. Anesthetic management of these conditions should be initiated by preparing for placement of a tracheostomy tube. In the dog, a combination of acepromazine (0.05 mg/kg IM) and oxymorphone (0.2 mg/kg IV) will induce neuroleptanalgesia, permitting the mouth and jaw to be examined without inducing apnea or severe respiratory depression. Owing to oxymorphone-induced vagal bradycardia, premedication with an anticholinergic is recommended. In dogs weighing > 20 kg, a maximum dose of 3 mg oxymorphone is suggested to prevent excessive respiratory depression. In the cat, a low dose of ketamine (4 mg/kg IM) combined with acepromazine (0.05 mg/kg) usually permits examination of the oral cavity. Intramuscular or subcutaneous administration of xylazine or medetomidine in the dog or cat may cause emesis. Dogs and cats with oral or pharyngeal masses are at high risk for aspiration pneumonia, so xylazine, morphine, and other drugs that induce emesis should be avoided. In the cat, the proximal two-thirds of the esophagus has a striated muscle layer, whereas in the dog, the entire esophagus contains striated muscle. Skeletal muscle relaxation of the esophagus to facilitate removal of esophageal foreign bodies may be improved with a short-acting muscle relaxant (e.g., atracurium; 0.2 mg/kg IV). Administration of atracurium must be accompanied by tracheal intubation and support of ventilation.

### A.    Anesthesia for Dogs with Gastric Dilation or Volvulus

1.  **Canine gastric dilation or volvulus** is associated with multiple system problems, resulting in a high mortality rate (40 to 60%) (Table 10-10). The distended stomach severely restricts ventilation and decreases cardiac function. Metabolic alkalosis may develop from gastric sequestration of hydrogen ions. Later in the course of the disease, metabolic acidosis may occur from decreased cardiac output and poor ventilation, resulting in tissue hypoxia and lactate production.

2.  **Cardiac arrhythmias,** such as sinus tachycardia and ventricular premature contractions, are frequently observed. Cardiac arrhythmias should be identified and treated before induction of anesthesia. Lidocaine (4 mg/kg IV, then 20 to 80 mg/kg/min) and procainamide (0.5 to 2 mg/kg IV, then 20 to 40 mg/kg/min) separately or in combination have been used for treating premature ventricular contractions and ventricular tachycardia. A

| Table 10-10. Problems Associated with Gastric Dilatation–Volvulus | |
| --- | --- |
| **Problem** | **Significance** |
| Acidosis or alkalosis | pH should be measured |
| Cardiac arrhythmias | Attempt correction before anesthesia |
| Gastric necrosis | May cause arrhythmias |
| Hypokalemia or hyperkalemia | K⁺ should be measured |
| Impaired venous return | Correct by decompressing stomach; treat shock |
| Respiratory impairment | Correct by decompressing stomach; ventilate |
| Peritonitis | Begin antibiotics; poor prognosis |
| Shock | Correct underlying problems |

continuous lidocaine infusion may be prepared by adding 25 mL of 2% lidocaine to each 500 mL of fluid given at a daily maintenance rate of 66 mL/kg/day.

3. Because the **metabolic status** is difficult to predict, it is suggested that serum electrolytes, blood pH, and plasma bicarbonate concentration be measured before anesthesia. Electrolyte abnormalities, acid–base imbalance, fluid losses, and gastric distension should be corrected as soon as possible. It has been suggested that restoration of circulating plasma volume should be initiated first using isotonic saline (90 mL/kg IV) and colloidal preparations (e.g., 6% hetastarch) before decompression to minimize the hemodynamic consequence of released vasoactive substances from the spleen and gastric tissues.

4. Administration of **oxygen** via face mask should be begun before induction of anesthesia. Large doses of arrhythmogenic agents, such as thiobarbiturates and halothane, should be avoided. $\alpha_2$-Agonists decrease intestinal motility and may prolong recovery of normal gastrointestinal function after correction. Neuroleptanalgesic combinations, such as Innovar-Vet (0.5 mL/20 kg IV) and diazepam (0.2 mg/kg IV) with oxymorphone (0.1 mg/kg IV), are good choices for induction of anesthesia in dogs with unstable cardiovascular function. Opioids may decrease

intestinal motility, but this effect is usually of minor clinical significance. Diazepam-ketamine has also been suggested as a good choice for induction of anesthesia. For maintenance of anesthesia, isoflurane and sevoflurane are good choices. Nitrous oxide is contraindicated before gastric decompression.

5. If a **neuromuscular blocking agent** is used in the anesthetic management of gastric dilation or volvulus, it should be a nondepolarizing drug, such as pancuronium or atracurium.

6. **Reperfusion injury** has also been implicated as a factor associated with the high mortality from this condition. Iron-chelating drugs, such as deferoxamine (Desferal) are currently being evaluated for their ability to decrease injury in anoxic tissues that are subsequently reperfused.

## B.   Disorders of the Pancreas

1. **Acute pancreatitis** in dogs and cats is frequently associated with vomiting, anorexia, and abdominal pain. Classic laboratory findings associated with pancreatitis (increased amylase and lipase activity) may not be observed. Conversely, increased pancreatic enzyme activity is not specific for pancreatitis. Acute pancreatitis has been induced by drugs, including corticosteroids, nonsteroidal anti-inflammatory agents, organophosphates, thiazide diuretics, sulfonamides, tetracycline, valproic acid, furosemide, and estrogen. Thus it is likely that animals with acute pancreatitis are anesthetized for reasons unrelated to diagnosis or treatment of pancreatitis. Iatrogenic pancreatitis may also occur after abdominal surgery. The incidental finding of acute pancreatitis at necropsy of many patients with an unknown cause of death is not uncommon.

2. The **choice of anesthetics** for use in the patient with pancreatitis is often based on other complicating factors identified for the patient. Intravenously administered $\alpha_2$-adrenergic agents have a hyperglycemic effect owing to inhibition of insulin release by the $\beta$ cells in the islets of Langerhans. It is unknown whether the $\alpha_2$-adrenergic ef-

fects on the pancreas are of clinical significance in patients with pancreatitis. A conservative approach to anesthetic management of these patients, however, generally avoids use of these drugs. Opioid analgesics (oxymorphone, buprenorphine, butorphanol) are a suitable alternative for providing sedation and analgesia before induction of anesthesia. In humans, epidural administration of morphine is preferred for treatment of pain associated with pancreatitis, because of better pain relief with fewer side effects (spasm of the sphincter of Oddi). Maintenance of anesthesia with isoflurane or sevoflurane is preferred.

## C.  Obesity

1.  **Obese patients** often have underlying physiologic problems in addition to the condition for which anesthesia is required. Drug dose should be adjusted to the patient's lean weight to avoid overdosing with anesthetic drugs. Isoflurane is a good inhalation anesthetic for an obese animal, because of its minimal biotransformation and low tissue solubility.

2.  **Preoperative hypoxemia (Pickwickian syndrome)** is a common feature of obesity in humans and is markedly worsened by anesthesia. Obesity decreases the ventilatory capacity of the patient during anesthesia, owing to decreased chest wall compliance. Hypoventilation may occur because of limited diaphragmatic excursion from the increased weight of the abdominal contents. The increased mass of the pharyngeal tissues and tongue may lead to upper airway obstruction after premedication with tranquilizers or during induction of anesthesia. Obese patients given sedatives or tranquilizers before anesthesia should be continuously observed for airway obstruction. Rapid control of the airway at induction and positive pressure ventilation during anesthesia are recommended. During recovery from anesthesia, obese patients should be kept intubated until they will no longer tolerate the endotracheal tube. Obese animals must regain normal muscle function to maintain an adequate tidal volume and a patent airway after extubation.

## VII. ENDOCRINE DISEASE
*Robert R. Paddleford and Ralph C. Harvey*

### A.    Diabetes Mellitus

**Insulin** is essential for normal cellular function. The effects of insulin on normal cellular function include inhibition of glycogenolysis, inhibition of gluconeogenesis, inhibition of lipolysis, stimulation of glucose uptake into cells, stimulation of potassium transport into cells, and suppression of ketogenesis.

1.    **Clinical signs** include a recent history of polyuria, polydipsia, weight loss, or rapid onset of cataracts; dehydration, weakness, collapse, mental dullness, hepatomegaly, and/or muscle wasting; and/or increased rate and depth of respiration and a sweet acetone odor to the breath. Diabetes mellitus occurs more frequently in female dogs and male cats. These clinical signs should alert the clinician to the possibility of diabetes mellitus in a patient. The presence of glucose and ketones in the urine is diagnostic. A resting blood glucose of > 250 mg/dL with ketonemia is a common finding.

2.    The key to the **anesthetic management** of a diabetic is to use preanesthetic and anesthetic agents that result in the shortest anesthetic recovery time with the least amount of drug hangover. Drugs that can be antagonized (narcotics, $\alpha_2$-agonists, benzodiazepine tranquilizers) or are readily eliminated from the patient (propofol, etomidate, inhalant anesthetics) should be considered. The goal is to get the patient awake as soon as possible so that it can resume its normal feeding schedule. The procedure should be scheduled early in the morning after the administration of the patient's normal dose of insulin. Preoperative and serial intraoperative and postoperative blood glucose levels should be determined. Ideally, the blood glucose should be maintained between 150 to 250 mg/dL. During the procedure, 5% dextrose in a balanced electrolyte solution should be administered to prevent hypoglycemia. Depending on the blood glucose values, the dextrose drip may need to be continued after the procedure. A rate of 11 to 15 mL/kg/h is usually adequate. As soon as the patient

starts eating, it is probably not necessary to maintain the dextrose drip.

**B.　Hypoadrenocorticism (Addison Disease)**

Hypoadrenocorticism is a deficiency of aldosterone and/or glucocorticoids resulting from adrenal cortex dysfunction. As with the diabetic, the patient with hypoadrenocorticism should be stabilized and regulated before anesthesia and surgery.

1.　Primary **idiopathic hypoadrenocorticism** is the most common cause of hypoadrenocorticism in dogs and may be immune mediated. It is characterized by an acute necrosis of the adrenal cortex. Other diseases that may cause destruction of the adrenal glands include systemic mycosis, metastatic tumors, hemorrhagic infarction, amyloidosis of the cortices, and canine distemper as well as therapy for hyperadrenocorticism that may inadvertently produce a selective deficiency of glucocorticoids caused by destruction of the zona fasciculata.

2.　**Decreased corticotropin secretion** may also lead to hypoadrenocorticism. Adrenocorticotropic hormone (ACTH) directly controls glucocorticoid secretion and is secreted by the pituitary gland. Decreased ACTH secretion may develop with diseases or tumors of the pituitary gland or with decreased secretion of corticotropin-releasing factor (CRF) owing to hypothalamic lesions. Prolonged negative feedback from exogenous corticosteroid therapy also results in decreased ACTH secretion and atrophy of the adrenal cortex. Decreased ACTH secretion usually produces glucocorticoid insufficiency, although mineralocorticoid secretion often remains normal.

3.　The **clinical signs** of hypoadrenocorticism depend on the particular adrenal hormone (aldosterone, glucocorticoids) most affected by the disease. Aldosterone's primary function is to stimulate absorption of sodium in the distal renal tubules and promote the excretion of potassium. Aldosterone deficiency produces hyponatremia and hyperkalemia. Hyponatremia with concurrent water loss can produce lethargy, nausea, impaired cardiac output, hypovolemia, hypotension, and/or impaired renal perfusion. Hyperkalemia will produce muscle weakness, decreased cardiac conduction and excitability and bradycardia.

4. **Glucocorticoid deficiency** can result in significant problems. Cortisol stimulates gluconeogenesis, increases blood glucose, enhances extravascular fluid movement to the intravascular compartment, stabilizes lysosomal membranes, and counteracts the effects of stress. Cortisol depletion impairs renal excretion of water and energy metabolism, decreases stress tolerance, and can cause anorexia, vomiting, and/or diarrhea.

5. **Diagnosis of hypoadrenocorticism** is made by measuring serum cortisol. Plasma cortisol levels are the most accurate method of diagnosing hypoadrenocorticism. Hypoadrenocorticism should be suspected in any dog with a history of anorexia, vomiting, diarrhea, and lethargy when there are clinical findings of muscle weakness, dehydration, and bradycardia. Electrolyte imbalance may suggest hypoadrenocorticism. Serum sodium levels are often < 135 mEq/L, and serum potassium levels may be > 5.5 mEq/L. The Na:K ratio may be < 25:1 (normal is 33:1). The CBC reflects dehydration, and decreased cortisol will cause eosinophilia and lymphocytosis. The BUN may be elevated owing to prerenal uremia or renal failure. The ECG may show evidence of hyperkalemia.

6. The **anesthetic protocol** used in a patient with hypoadrenocorticism is not as critical as the medical management before anesthesia. A patient with hypoadrenocorticism must be stabilized. The treatment objectives are to correct the dehydration and treat the hypovolemic shock, return renal function to normal, correct electrolyte imbalances, and supply glucocorticoids. Addisonian patients have decreased stress tolerance. The key is to provide adequate intravenous fluid volume replacement during and after surgery and to provide exogenous glucocorticoids. A balanced electrolyte solution should be administered intraoperatively at a rate of 15 to 22 mL/kg/h. Glucocorticoids should be given concomitantly with initiation of the anesthetic regimen. Preoperatively, 2 to 4

mg/kg dexamethasone should be given intravenously or subcutaneously. Intraoperatively, a rapid-acting glucocorticoid, such as prednisolone sodium succinate (Solu-Delta-Cortef) at a dose of 11 to 22 mg/kg IV or prednisolone calcium phosphate (Cortisate-20; 11 mg/kg IV), should be given and repeated as necessary. Postoperatively, additional glucocorticoids are given as needed.

### C. Hypothyroidism

A hypothyroid patient often has a **decreased metabolic rate.** This can prolong the effects of many preanesthetic and anesthetic drugs. Any anesthetic drug should be used in low doses and ideally should require minimal or no metabolism or can be readily antagonized. Narcotics, low doses of tranquilizers, propofol, and inhalants are the preferred preanesthetic and anesthetic drugs. A hypothyroid patient is often obese and may suffer from anemia. This may cause ventilatory problems under anesthesia caused by the excess amounts of abdominal and intrathoracic fat. Assisted or controlled ventilation may be necessary in these patients to keep them adequately ventilated. Anemia may range from subclinical to severe. If the anemia is severe, whole blood transfusion should be considered before anesthesia and surgery.

### D. Hyperthyroidism

Patients with thyroid adenomas or adenocarcinomas may exhibit evidence of hyperthyroidism. A thyroid tumor may place mechanical pressure on the trachea, causing a partial obstruction and interfering with respiration.

1. Hyperthyroid patients may develop a **thyroid storm** during the procedure as a result of excessive thyroid hormone production. This is precipitated by catecholamine release and is characterized by an increased heart rate, increased blood pressure, cardiac dysrhythmias, elevated body temperature, and shock. There is increased oxygen and glucose demand, and increased carbon dioxide production.

2. **Preanesthetic and anesthetic agents** that decrease catecholamine response and myocardial irritability are preferred. Low doses of acepromazine or an $\alpha_2$-agonist can be used as a preanesthetic in hyperthyroid patients. Acepromazine

decreases myocardial irritability and blocks α-adrenergic receptors; thus it may help counteract hypertension. An opioid can be combined with acepromazine, because opioids generally slow the heart rate and decrease myocardial oxygen consumption.

3.  Anesthesia may be induced with **low-dose thiopental, propofol, etomidate, or an inhalant** by mask. Isoflurane is the inhalant of choice, because cardiac output is better maintained and the drug has minimal dysrhythmic properties.

# Chapter 11

---

## Anesthesia for Special Procedures and Patients

*Some patients require attention to factors not commonly encountered when planning anesthetic protocols for healthy adult patients. Those factors may have to do with the presence of specific diseases or organ malfunction, unusual physiologic alterations, or the extremes of age. This chapter discusses the physiologic alterations and pharmacologic considerations commonly encountered when contemplating induction and maintenance of anesthesia in patients undergoing ocular surgery, cesarean section surgery, surgical repair of severe trauma, and in patients at the extremes of age (neonates and geriatrics).*

### Introductory Comments

**Ocular Patients**
**Cesarean Section Patients**
**Trauma Patients**
**Neonatal Patients**
**Geriatric Patients**

---

## I.   OCULAR PATIENTS

The requirement for deep general anesthesia when performing ophthalmic surgery increases risk. Primary objectives for safe anesthetic management of ophthalmic patients are central globe position, the maintenance of normal intraocular pressure, pupillary dilation for intraocular surgery and adequate cardiopulmonary function.

476

### A. Intraocular Pressure

1. **Intraocular pressure** (IOP) normally ranges from 10 to 26 mm Hg in dogs and cats. Pressures exceeding these values should be considered abnormal. Coughing or straining can result in a pressure increase of > 40 mm Hg. Tracheal intubation can increase IOP without any outward clinical signs.

2. **Obstruction of ocular outflow** induced by coughing, retching, or manual restraint of the head and neck can dramatically increase IOP. A sudden rise in IOP of patients with an ocular penetrating wound or an open anterior chamber can easily result in extrusion of vitreous and permanent loss of vision. Some physiologic factors and drugs associated with alterations in IOP are presented in Table 11-1.

### B. The Oculocardiac Reflex

1. The oculocardiac reflex (OCR) occurs most often in **younger patients.** This reflex is more likely to occur when there is inadequate relaxation of the extraocular muscles and hypercapnia is present. Dysrhythmias associated with the OCR include atrioventricular block, bradycardia, bigeminy, and ectopic beats.

2. **Stimuli** that can activate the OCR include traction on the ocular muscles, enucleation, direct pressure on the globe, and other ocular manipulations. The afferent–efferent pathway of the OCR is trigeminal–vagal.

3. The **best prevention** is gentle manipulation of the eyeball. Preoperative intramuscular atropine injection and controlled ventilation help decrease the incidence of OCR activation.

4. Should the OCR be triggered, **eyeball manipulation should cease.** If bradycardia persist, intravenous atropine (0.02 mg/kg) should be given immediately.

### Table 11-1. Factors Altering Intraocular Pressure

| Factors | Change | Comments |
|---|---|---|
| Blockade of aqueous outflow | ↑ | Caused by acute venous congestion and increased choroidal congestion |
| Acute increase in arterial pressure | ↑ | Sudden increase in blood pressure causes only a transient increase in IOP |
| Hypoventilation, airway obstruction, hypercapnia, choroidal vessel dilation | ↑ | |
| Hyperventilation, hypocapnia | ↓ | |
| Endotracheal intubation | ↑ | Resulting from coughing, straining, or vomiting; prevented with laryngeal lidocaine spray |
| Eyeball pressure | ↑ | Face mask, orbital tumors, ocular muscle traction, retrobulbar traction |
| Anesthetic drugs | | |
|   Barbiturates | ↓ | May depress central centers controlling IOP or promote aqueous outflow |
|   Propofol | ↓ | May prevent the increase in IOP associated with tracheal intubation, appears to suppress the increase in IOP induced by depolarizing muscle relaxants |
|   Etomidate | ↑ | Etomidate-induced myoclonus appears to be responsible in large part for the increase in IOP |
|   Ketamine | ↑ or ↓ | Controversial; in properly premedicated patients (e.g., with a benzodiazepine), there probably is little or no effect |
|   $\alpha_2$-agonists | ↓ | Induced bradycardia, may promote initiation of the OCR; decreases IOP directly |
|   Benzodiazepines | ↓ | The decrease in IOP appears to be in response to a central relaxing action of these drugs on the ocular muscles |
|   Acepromazine | ↓ | Decreases arterial blood pressure, suppresses retching and vomiting |

*Continued*

| Factors | Change | Comments |
|---------|--------|----------|
| Opioids | ↓ | Sudden increases can occur with retching and vomiting and should be preceded by administration of a tranquilizer |
| Muscle relaxants | | |
| Depolarizing | | |
| Succinylcholine | ↑ | Increase is transient; minimal effect when given in stage III anesthesia |
| Nondepolarizing | | |
| Pancuronium | ↓ | Either decreases or has no effect; IOP may |
| Vecuronium | | increase during intubation of lightly |
| Atracurium | | anesthetized patients |
| Other drugs | | |
| Acetazolamide | ↓ | Carbonic anhydrase inhibitor; decreases formation of aqueous humor; acts within 2 min after IV injection; may produce metabolic acidosis and compensatory hyperventilation |
| Hypertonic solutions (Mannitol) | ↓ | Increases plasma osmotic pressure, decreasing formation of aqueous humor and IOP |
| Phenylephrine | ↑ or ↓ | Depends on dose; 1.5 mg IV or 5 mg SC should not be exceeded; for topical application, 1 drop of 2.5% per hour should not be exceeded |
| Epinephrine | ↑ or ↓ | Depends on dose; a topical dose of 0.5 mg for humans has been recommended |

## C. Preanesthetic Medication

1. **Preanesthetic medication** should relieve anxiety, suppress coughing, prevent vomiting, and provide analgesia in the perioperative period. The drugs selected should have minimal effect on IOP. Preanesthetics most frequently used are anticholinergics, tranquilizers, sedatives, and opioids (Table 11-1).

2. The **cornea** is one of the most enervated tissues in the body, and corneal or intraocular surgery may cause intense pain. Control of pain to improve the patient's comfort and minimize self-trauma is essential.

3. **Topical anesthesia** can be used to perform a number of diagnostic and therapeutic procedures, including tonometry, third eyelid examination, corneal scraping, flushing of the nasolacrimal duct, conjunctival biopsy and electroretinography, and grid keratotomy.

4. **Proparacaine** (0.5%) is the most commonly used topical anesthetic. Analgesia occurs within several seconds and may persist for 10 to 20 min after topical application. Excessive application into an open ocular wound should be avoided. Topical anesthetics should not be used to control ocular pain over a long period of time, because they can damage corneal epithelium and delay healing.

5. **Tear production** decreases during general anesthesia in most species. Although the administration of an anticholinergic has been used to decrease tearing, general anesthesia with inhalants will nearly abolish production. Ocular lubrications to prevent corneal drying are commonly administered in small animals.

## D. Anticholinergics

**Atropine** or **glycopyrrolate** can be used to decrease salivary and airway secretions and relieve bradycardia. Atropine (0.04 mg/kg IM or SC) or glycopyrrolate (0.02 mg/kg IM or SC) administered 20 min before surgery may prevent activation of the OCR. Anticholinergics appear to have little or no effect on IOP when administered systemically. **Topical administration** is associated with mydriasis, filtration angle closure, and increases in IOP.

## E. Tranquilizers, Sedatives, and Opioids

1. **Vomiting** may occur after premedication with an opioid or $\alpha_2$-agonist in dogs and cats. Gagging and vomiting can usually be prevented if the opioid is administered after the

onset of action of a tranquilizer (e.g., acetylpromazine 0.1 to 0.2 mg/kg IV). Acepromazine premedication has been shown to decrease IOP.

2. **Diazepam** (0.2 to 0.4 mg/kg IV) or **midazolam** (0.1 to 0.2 mg/kg IV or IM) may be safely used in dogs and cats scheduled for ocular surgery. Benzodiazepines enhance ocular muscle relaxation and promote smooth recovery.

3. **Morphine** causes **miosis** in dogs and rabbits and mydriasis in cats, rats, mice, and monkeys. Opioid preanesthetic medication in dogs may prevent mydriasis necessary for cataract surgery. The pupil should be dilated and immobile for cataract extraction.

## F. Induction of Anesthesia

1. All commonly used injectable **anesthetics decrease IOP** (Table 11-1). Gentle handling and restraint of the patient is important to avoid excitement and struggling. Tight-fitting leashes will result in increased jugular venous pressure and should not be used for restraint during induction. When using a nose cone for administration of oxygen or inducing anesthesia, direct pressure on or around the eye should be avoided.

2. **Thiobarbiturate, propofol,** or **ketamine** may be used to induce anesthesia. Thiobarbiturates and propofol decrease cardiac output, lower blood pressure, relax extraocular muscles, and promote aqueous outflow. Ketamine may increase or have no effect on IOP when given alone but when combined with a benzodiazepine may decrease IOP.

3. **Lidocaine** given intravenously (1.0 mg/kg) or by topical application to the larynx following the onset of unconsciousness may help suppress the cough reflex during tracheal intubation.

## G. Maintenance of Anesthesia

1. **Halothane, isoflurane,** and **sevoflurane** all decrease arterial blood pressure. The decrease is proportionate to the depth of anesthesia and is reflected in a proportionate decrease in IOP. Decreases in IOP may range from 35 to 55%. In all species, high-flow inhalation anesthetic techniques are recommended over low-flow techniques, so that the alveolar concentration more nearly reflects vaporizer concentration output, thus ensuring an adequate depth of anesthesia.

2. **Unexpected nystagmus** and **sudden body movement** are more likely to occur with low-flow techniques, unless depth of anesthesia is closely and continuously monitored, which is sometimes made difficult during ophthalmic surgery.

3. **Guarded endotracheal tubes** to prevent kinking should be used, and all connections must be well secured before draping of the head is begun.

4. **Nitrous oxide** is not commonly used in ocular patients. Its administration is contraindicated after air injection into the anterior chamber of a closed eye. Nitrous oxide will diffuse into an intraocular bubble faster than air can diffuse out, causing air bubble expansion and increased IOP. During retinal reattachment surgery, when an expandable gas is injected into the vitreous to expand the globe, nitrous oxide will rapidly diffuse into the bubble, increasing IOP.

5. **Renal tubular necrosis** has been reported in dogs after flunixin meglumine administration and methoxyflurane anesthesia. Although it is not approved by the FDA for use in these species, flunixin meglumine (0.25 to 0.5 mg/lb) before surgery is commonly used as a preoperative anti-inflammatory drug in ocular patients. Its use with methoxyflurane is discouraged.

6. **Nondepolarizing muscle relaxants** (i.e., pancuronium, vecuronium, atracurium) are commonly used in dogs and

cats to ensure complete immobility of the eye. In birds, muscle relaxants are required to induce mydriasis for lens extraction, because birds have striated musculature of the iris rather than smooth muscle, as in mammals.

7. **Peripheral muscle relaxants** require controlled ventilation for prevention of hypercapnia and increases in IOP. At completion of surgery, the patient must be weaned from the ventilator; and if spontaneous ventilation does not ensue, antagonism of the nondepolarizing muscle relaxant's' paralytic action is necessary for timely recovery. Intravenous atropine (0.02 mg/kg IV) followed by neostigmine (0.02 to 0.04 mg/kg IV) is commonly used. These drugs are not associated with increases in IOP.

## II. CESAREAN SECTION PATIENTS

The ideal anesthetic protocol for cesarean section surgery provides ample analgesia, muscle relaxation, and sedation for optimal operating conditions without endangering mother or fetus. Anesthetics, analgesics, tranquilizers, and sedatives must of necessity cross the blood–brain barrier. The physicochemical properties that allow drugs to cross the blood–brain barrier also enable their placental transfer.

### A. Implications of Physiologic Alterations

Because **cardiac reserve** diminishes during pregnancy, the potential for cardiac decompensation or failure increases. Likewise, pregnant patients are prone to hypoventilation, hypoxia, and hypercapnia as a result of altered pulmonary function. Inhalation and local anesthetic requirement are decreased, thus increasing the likelihood of a relative overdose and excessive depression. Vomition and aspiration can occur if induction is not followed immediately by rapid control of the airway. Because of the physiologic alterations induced by pregnancy, parturients are a greater anesthetic risk than for healthy nonparturient patients.

### B. Perinatal Pharmacology

1. The effects of pregnancy on **drug biotransformation** and excretion are variable and not fully understood. Inhalation anesthetic dose (minimum alveolar concentration;

MAC) is decreased. Hepatic biotransformation of barbiturates appears to be decreased in pregnancy. As a result of decreased plasma cholinesterase concentrations, succinylcholine metabolism is minimally decreased. The increase in renal blood flow and glomerular filtration should favor renal excretion of drugs.

2. **Placental transfer** of drugs can occur by several mechanisms, but by far the most important is simple diffusion. The placenta does not appear to metabolize anesthetics. The amount of drug crossing the placenta and entering the fetal circulation is described by the **Fick equation:**

$$Q/t = KA(C_m - C_f)/D$$

where $Q/t$ is amount of diffused substance per unit time; $K$ is the diffusion constant of a given substance; $A$ is the surface area available for diffusion; $C_m$ is the concentration of the substance in the maternal blood perfusing the placenta (uterine artery concentration); $C_f$ is the concentration of the substance in the fetal blood perfusing the placenta; and $D$ is the thickness of the (placental) membrane.

3. The **maternal blood concentration** of drug depends on the total dose, site and route of administration, rate of distribution and uptake of the drug by maternal tissues, and maternal metabolism and excretion. Thus drugs with rapidly declining plasma concentration after administration of a fixed dose (e.g., thiopental, propofol, and succinylcholine) result in a short period of exposure to high maternal blood drug concentration.

4. **Fetal drug concentration** is the result of passive diffusion across the placenta and is altered by fetal redistribution, metabolism, and protein binding. The concentration of drug in the umbilical vein is not necessarily available to the fetal organs (brain, heart, and other vital organs); as much as 85% of umbilical venous blood initially passes through the fetal liver, where the drug may be sequestered or metabolized. In addition, umbilical venous blood containing the drug enters the inferior vena cava via the ductus venosus and mixes with drug-free blood returning from the lower extremities and pelvic viscera (Fig. 11-1).

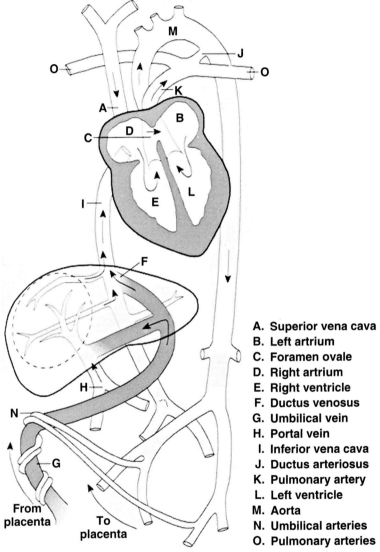

**A. Superior vena cava**
**B. Left artrium**
**C. Foramen ovale**
**D. Right artrium**
**E. Right ventricle**
**F. Ductus venosus**
**G. Umbilical vein**
**H. Portal vein**
**I. Inferior vena cava**
**J. Ductus arteriosus**
**K. Pulmonary artery**
**L. Left ventricle**
**M. Aorta**
**N. Umbilical arteries**
**O. Pulmonary arteries**

**Figure 11-1.** The direction of blood flow in the fetal vascular system (*arrows*) and the path of the umbilical blood (*darkened*) as it flows into the liver and inferior vena cava via the ductus venosus. Blood flow through the foramen ovale and ductus arteriosus provides a direct path to the arterial system, bypassing the lungs. In the neonate, the ductus arteriosus and foramen ovale close shortly after birth, which results in blood flowing through the neonate's lungs, where it is arterialized as in the adult.

### C.  Drug Selection

Drugs that induce **sedation** and/or **tranquilization** include the barbiturates, phenothiazines, butyrophenones, benzodiazepines, and $\alpha_2$-adrenoceptor agonists. All of these drugs rapidly cross the placenta, resulting in neonatal depression.

1. **Phenothiazine** and **butyrophenone tranquilizers** are frequently used as preanesthetics and are often used in conjunction with opiates. Phenothiazines potentiate opioid-induced depression. They induce hypotension via $\alpha$-adrenergic blockade as well as central depression. This results in respiratory depression and decreased ability to regulate body temperature. The use of tranquilizer-sedative drugs should be restricted to the markedly apprehensive or excited parturient and then only in doses sufficient to induce a calming effect.

2. **Benzodiazepines** can induce neonatal lethargy, hypotonus, and hypothermia. It has been suggested that these effects can be minimized by administering $< 0.14$ mg/kg IV. Residual benzodiazepine-induced lethargy and muscle relaxation in either the mother or neonate can be antagonized with flumazenil. A ratio of $1:15$ (flumazenil:diazepam or midazolam) is a reasonable initial dose.

3. **$\alpha_2$-Agonists** are potent sedative-hypnotics with significant analgesic properties. These drugs rapidly cross the placenta, however, inducing both maternal and fetal respiratory and circulatory depression. When used in conjunction with ketamine, there are significant cardiopulmonary changes resulting in decreased tissue perfusion in healthy dogs. Thus use of $\alpha_2$- or $\alpha_2$-ketamine combinations should be avoided in patients presented for cesarean section.

4. **Opioids** rapidly cross the placenta and can cause neonatal respiratory and neurobehavioral depression that may last up to 24 h. Fetal elimination may require 2 to 6 days. The most commonly used opioids are fentanyl, meperidine, oxymorphone, and morphine in order of increasing dura-

tion of action. The most effective antagonist is naloxone (0.04 mg/kg).

5. **Opioid antagonists** rapidly cross the placenta. Maternal administration before delivery has been advocated to reverse opioid-induced neonatal depression. This technique deprives the mother of analgesia at the time when it is needed most. Therefore, these agents should be administered directly to the neonate. Because of its short action, re-narcotization may occur when naloxone is metabolized and excreted.

6. **Ketamine** can be given intravenously to induce anesthesia for intubation rather than a barbiturate. Because effective induction doses for these drugs are higher in dogs and cats than in humans, some neonatal depression is more likely to be associated with their use.

7. **Propofol** rapidly induces basal narcosis for intubation. Recovery from propofol is prompt and smooth, owing to rapid redistribution and metabolism. Metabolism occurs primarily in the liver, but extrahepatic metabolism also occurs. Because of the extensive distribution and metabolism of propofol, recovery is rapid. Propofol is rapidly cleared from the neonatal circulation. Apnea is common on induction. The advantages of propofol are fast onset and rapid smooth termination of action. In dogs and cats, the induction dose of propofol is 6 to 8 mg/kg IV in unpremedicated patients. Supplemental doses are 0.5 to 2.0 mg/kg IV given to effect.

8. **Muscle relaxants** cross the placenta to a limited degree and induce little effect on the neonate when used in clinical doses. These drugs are useful in balanced anesthesia techniques for cesarean section.

9. **Inhalation anesthetics** readily cross the placenta with rapid fetal and maternal equilibration. Thus the degree of neonatal depression is proportional to the depth of anesthesia induced in the mother. Deep levels of maternal anesthesia cause maternal hypotension, decreased uterine blood flow, and fetal acidosis.

10. **Nitrous oxide** can be used to potentiate the more potent volatile agents. If nitrous oxide is administered at 60%, fetal depression is minimal and neonatal diffusion hypoxia does not occur on delivery.

11. **Maternal oxygen administration** can result in a significant increase in fetal oxygen content. Therefore, oxygen administration is indicated regardless of the anesthetic protocol. Inspired oxygen concentrations of 50% or more during general anesthesia often result in more vigorous neonates.

12. **Local anesthetics** are frequently used in combination with other drugs or as the sole anesthetic for regional techniques. Amide derivatives (e.g., lidocaine, mepivacaine, bupivacaine, and etidocaine) are metabolized by hepatic microsomal enzymes. Neonatal blood concentrations in excess of 3 µg/mL lidocaine or mepivacaine cause neonatal depression at delivery. These concentrations rarely occur after epidural administration but can occur when excessive volumes of drug are used for local infiltration.

13. **Anticholinergics** such as atropine or glycopyrrolate should be administered to most parturient patients to decrease salivation and inhibit excessive vagal tone when traction is applied to the uterus.

D. **Anesthetic Techniques for Cesarean Section**

1. Advantages of **general anesthesia** include speed and ease of induction, reliability, reproducibility, and controllability. General anesthesia provides optimum operating conditions with a relaxed immobile patient. Tracheal intubation ensures control of the maternal airway, thereby preventing aspiration of vomitus. In addition, it provides a route for maternal oxygen administration, thereby improving fetal oxygenation. There are many satisfactory protocols for induction of general anesthesia for cesarean section in dogs and cats (Table 11-2).

2. **Regional anesthesia** for cesarean section is a well-established technique. Local infiltration or field block may

Table 11-2. Drugs Used for Anesthesia for Cesarean Section in Canines and Felines

| Species/Drug or Technique | Dosage | Comments |
|---|---|---|
| **ELECTIVE CESAREAN SECTION** | | |
| Canines | | |
| I. Lidocaine (epidural) | 1 mL/3–5 kg | Assistant required for restraint; |
| Oxymorphone | 0.05–0.2 mg/kg | oxygen administered by face mask; glycopyrrolate given as needed |
| II. Droperidol-fentanyl | 1 mL/20–30 kg IV | Supplemental dose of droperidol- |
| (Innovar-Vet) | 0.01 mg/kg | fentanyl or fentanyl may be |
| Glycopyrrolate | to effect | needed; inhalant given in low |
| Isoflurane[a] | 0.5–1.0% | dosage until delivery; $N_2O$ |
| Halothane[a] | 0.35–0.75% | probably should not be given before umbilical vein clamp to prevent diffusion hypoxia in the neonate when initial breathing of room air ensues |
| III. Propofol | 5–8 mg/kg IV to effect | |
| Felines | | |
| I. Ketamine | 1–3 mg/kg IV | Fetal depression occurs with ex- |
| Isoflurane[a] | to effect | cessive doses; lidocaine (0.25 |
| Halothane | 0.5–1.0% | mL) applied to arytenoid carti- |
| | 0.35–0.75% | lages reduces likelihood of laryngospasm |
| II. Propofol | 5–8 mg/kg IV to effect | |
| **EMERGENCY CESAREAN SECTION**[b] | | |
| Canines | | |
| I. Diazepam | 0.2 mg/kg IV | Opioids used to keep dose of in- |
| Ketamine | 5.5 mg/kg IV | halant low; large doses may |
| Isoflurane[a] | 0.5–1.0% | result in excessive ion trapping; |
| Oxymorphone | 0.05–0.1 mg/kg IV | patient may decompensate with excessive dose of inhalant |
| II. Diazepam | 0.2 mg/kg IV | Supplemental doses of oxymor- |
| Oxymorphone | 0.05–0.1 mg/kg IV | phone may be needed |
| III. Diazepam | 0.2 mg/kg IV | |
| Etomidate | 1.5–3.0 mg/kg IV | |

*Continued*

| Table 11-2. *(continued)* | | |
| --- | --- | --- |
| **Species/Drug or Technique** | **Dosage** | **Comments** |
| Felines | | |
|   I. Diazepam | 0.2 mg/kg IV | Topical lidocaine to larynx facili- |
| Ketamine | 1–2 mg/kg IV | tates intubation |
| Oxymorphone | 0.05 mg/kg IV | |
| Isoflurane[a] | 0.05–1.0% | |
|   II. Diazepam | 0.2 mg/kg IV | |
| Etomidate | 1.5–3.0 mg/kg IV | |

[a]Inhalant anesthetics are used in low concentrations, and only if necessary, before the fetuses are delivered.
[b]Techniques listed for emergencies are also suitable for elective cesarean sections.

be used, but it has several disadvantages when compared to the epidural technique. Infiltration requires larger amounts of local anesthetic, which when absorbed can depress the fetus. The field block must often be supplemented with heavy sedation or tranquilization.

3. **Epidural anesthesia** provides good muscle relaxation and analgesia. Disadvantages include hypotension secondary to sympathetic blockade. Nausea and vomiting can occur during the procedure as a result of hypotension and visceral manipulation. The hypotension induced by epidural anesthesia can be readily offset by concurrent fluid and catecholamine administration.

### E.    Care of the Newborn

1. The **umbilical vessels** should be milked toward the fetus to empty them of blood, clamped 2 to 5 cm from the body wall, and severed from the placenta. The head is cleared of membranes and the oropharynx of fluid. The neonate can then be gently rubbed with a towel to dry it and stimulate breathing. It may also help to gently swing the neonate in a head down position to help clear the respiratory tree of

fluid. The head and neck should be supported to avoid a whiplash action and prevent injury.

2. **Doxapram** can be used to stimulate breathing in the neonate. For pups, the dosage is 1 to 5 mg (1 to 5 drops from a 20- to 22-gauge needle); and for kittens, the dosage is 1 to 2 mg (1 to 2 drops) administered topically to the oral mucosa or injected intramuscularly or subcutaneously. Before doxapram administration, the airway must be clean of tissue and fluid.

3. Newborns are susceptible to **hypothermia** and should be kept warm.

## III. TRAUMA PATIENTS
*David D. Martin*

Upon the patient's arrival, assessment of circulation, ventilatory, and neurologic function should be made repeatedly during the initial treatment period. A trauma score can be used to quantify the patient's prognosis during the initial treatment period (Table 11-3). Severely traumatized patients are subject to a variety of complications that may manifest themselves in the first few days. These complications may not be directly related to the initial trauma but reflect overall tissue destruction, immune suppression, and metabolic imbalances.

### A. Complications

A global activation of cytokine mediators that results in a generalized increase in vascular permeability, neutrophil infiltration, and capillary microemboli has been termed the **systemic inflammatory response syndrome** (SIRS). Early signs of SIRS or septic shock include brick-red mucous membranes, tachycardia, high cardiac output (in euvolemic patients), normal or low blood pressure, and low vascular resistance. Definitions of SIRS for dogs and cats based on the presence of various key clinical signs have been proposed (Table 11-4). All organs may be affected. In cats, lung function owing to rapid fluid accumulation appears to be most often disrupted early in the course of SIRS. In dogs, the order of organ dysfunction is commonly gastrointestinal tract, followed by liver and kidney. Persistent **microcirculatory perfusion failure** may lead to sludging of blood and increased platelet

**Table 11-3. Method to Determine Prognosis in Severely Traumatized Animals**

| Trauma | Value | Points | Score |
|---|---|---|---|
| I. Respiratory rate per minute | 10–20 | 4 | |
| Number of respirations | 20–30 | 3 | |
| in 15 s, multiplied by four | > 30 | 2 | |
| | < 5 | 1 | I ____ |
| II. Respiratory effort | | | |
| Normal | | 1 | |
| Shallow or labored | | 0 | II ____ |
| III. Systolic blood pressure | > 90 | 4 | |
| Systolic cuff pressure, either | 70–90 | 3 | |
| by auscultation or palpation | 50–69 | 2 | |
| | < 50 | 1 | III ____ |
| IV. Capillary refill | | | |
| Normal, refill in 2 s | | 2 | |
| Delayed > 2 s | | 1 | |
| None, no refill | | 0 | IV ____ |
| V. CNS function scale | | | |
| A. Eye opening | | | |
| Spontaneously | | 4 | |
| To voice | | 3 | |
| To pain | | 2 | |
| Will not open | | 1 | VA ____ |
| B. Mentation | | | |
| Alert | | 4 | |
| Stuporous | | 3 | |
| Comatose | | 2 | VB ____ |
| C. Motor responses | | | |
| Obeys commands | | 5 | |
| Purposeful movement (pain) | | 4 | |
| Withdraws (pain) | | 3 | |
| Flexion (pain) | | 2 | |
| No response | | 1 | VC ____ |
| | | | V total ____ |
| *Total score*[a] | | | _____ |

[a]A low score indicates severe trauma and a poor prognosis.

aggregation. Along with the release of inflammatory mediators, these conditions result in enhanced coagulation and propagation of the inflammatory response. If oxygen delivery to tissues is chronically impaired, the systemic inflammatory state can result in **multiple organ dysfunction (MODS),** traditionally defined as irreversible shock.

### B.    Treatment

An algorithm for **SIRS management** is given in Figure 11-2. Early intervention and cardiovascular resuscitation to supernormal levels are recommended (Table 11-5). A list of 20 parameters to be assessed twice daily has been proposed to improve the clinical management of SIRS (Table 11-6). Therapeutic agents and doses used in the treatment of various metabolic derangements associated with SIRS are given in Tables 11-7 and 11-8. The primary goal is to **optimize tissue perfusion and oxygen delivery** to all vital organ systems.

### C.    Anesthetic Considerations

Anesthesia should not be undertaken until vital organ function has been stabilized. In cases with a history of severe trauma, the

---

| Table 11-4. Proposed Definitions of SIRS in Canines and Felines |
|---|

Canines
    The presence of two or more of the following clinical conditions:
        Body temperature > 40° or < 38°C
        Heart rate > 120 bpm in calm, resting dog
        Hyperventilation of $Paco_2$ < 30 mm Hg
        White blood count > 18,000 or < 5000/mL or > 5% immature (band) forms
Felines
    The presence of two or more of the following clinical conditions:
        Body temperature > 40° or < 38°C
        Heart rate > 140 bpm in calm, resting cat
        Respiratory rate > 20 breaths/min or $Paco_2$ < 28 mm Hg
        White blood cell count > 18,000 or < 5000/mL or > 5% immature (band) forms

Reprinted with permission from Hardie EM. Life threatening bacterial infection. Compend Contin Ed 1995; 17:763–777.

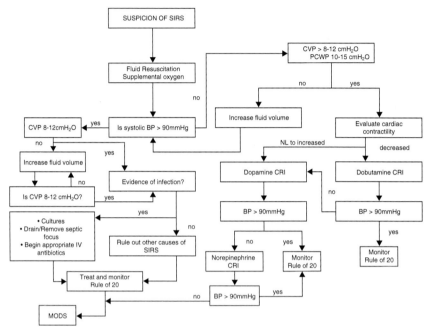

**Figure 11-2.** Algorithm for managing the SIRS patient. *CVP,* central venous pressure; *PCWP,* pulmonary capillary wedge pressure; *NL,* normal; *CRI,* continuous rate of infusion; *BP,* blood pressure (implies systolic). Reprinted with permission from Purvis D, Kirby R. Systemic inflammatory response syndrome: septic shock Vet Clin North Am Small Anim Pract 1994; 24:1225–1247.

| Table 11-5. Cardiovascular Resuscitation Goals for Animals with SIRS | |
|---|---|
| **Variable** | **Goal** |
| Mixed venous oxygen tension, $Pvo_2$, mm Hg | > 40 |
| Pulmonary artery pressure, mm Hg | > 25/10 |
| Pulmonary wedge pressure, mm Hg | < 18 |
| Systemic vascular resistance, $dyn/s/cm^5/m^2$ | > 1450 |
| Pulmonary vascular resistance, $dyn/s/cm^5/m^2$ | 45–250 |
| Oxygen extraction, % | 22–30 |
| Cardiac index, $L/min/m^2$ | > 4.5 |
| Oxygen delivery, $mL/min/m^2$ | > 600 |
| Oxygen consumption, $mL/min/m^2$ | > 170 |

Reprinted with permission from Hardie EM. Life threatening bacterial infection. Compend Contin Ed 1995; 17:763–777.

patient should always be considered a likely candidate for developing some type of shock.

1. **Anaphylactic and neurogenic shock** are characterized by relative hypovolemia and hypotension resulting from acute increases in vascular capacitance. Hypovolemic and neurogenic shock are typically observed in the acutely traumatized patient, whereas septic shock (SIRS) develops after the initial insult. Spinal shock is a common sequela to spinal cord injury or blunt trauma, which can cause a mechanical disruption of sympathetic nervous system outflow. The patient's extremities will feel warm (peripheral vasodilation), and even though hypotension is present, heart rate is slow because of sympathetic denervation. If arterial pressure is low and the pulse cannot be palpated, mixed inotropic and vasoconstrictor-type drugs should be

---

**Table 11-6. SIRS Treatment Checklist**[a]

☐ Fluid balance
☐ Blood pressure and perfusion
☐ Cardiac function and rhythm
☐ Albumin
☐ Oncotic pull
☐ Oxygenation and ventilation
☐ Glucose
☐ Electrolytes and acid–base balance
☐ Mentation and intracranial pressure
☐ Coagulation
☐ RBC and hemoglobin
☐ Renal function and urine output
☐ Immune state, WBC, and antibiotic level
☐ Gastrointestinal motility and integrity
☐ Drug metabolism and dosages
☐ Nutrition
☐ Pain control
☐ Nursing mobility and catheter care
☐ Bandage and wound care
☐ Tender loving care

Reprinted with permission from Purvis D, Kirby R. Systemic inflammatory response syndrome: septic shock. Vet Clin North Am Small Anim Pract 1994;24:1225–1247.
[a]The importance of each will vary from patient to patient.

**Table 11-7. Therapeutic Agents Used to Treat Metabolic Derangements Associated with SIRS**

| Metabolic Derangement | Dose Regimen | Use and/or Frequency |
|---|---|---|
| **HYPOVOLEMIA** | | |
| Hypertonic crystalloids | | |
|   7.5% NaCl solution | 4 mL/kg, IV | Once |
|   (70 mL 23.4% NaCl in 180 mL | | |
|     0.9% NaCl or 6% dextran 70) | | |
| Colloids | | |
|   Plasma | Maximum: 20 mL/ kg/24 h IV | As needed |
|   Hetastarch 120 | Maximum: 20 mL/kg/ first 24 h, then 10 mL/kg/24 h IV (slow infusion) | As needed |
|   Dextran 70 | Maximum: 20 mL/kg/ first 24 h, then 10 mL/kg/24 h IV (slow infusion) | As needed |
|   3% Albumin | 20 mL/kg IV | Resuscitation |
|   (12 mL 25% human albumin | | |
|     in 488 mL lactated Ringer's | | |
|     solution) | | |
| Isotonic crystalloids | | |
|   Lactated Ringer's solution | 90–270 mL/kg IV | Resuscitation |
| | 10–20 mL/kg/h IV | To meet ongoing needs |
| **ALTERED CLOTTING FUNCTION** | | |
| Heparin (low dosage) | 75–100 U/kg SC | Every 6–8 h |
| Heparin-activated plasma | 10 mL/kg IV | Every 3 h, based on clotting function |
|   (incubate 5–10 units/kg heparin | | |
|     with 1 unit fresh plasma for | | |
|     30 minutes) | | |

*Continued*

| Metabolic Derangement | Dose Regimen | Use and/or Frequency |
|---|---|---|
| **METABOLIC DYSFUNCTION** | | |
| KCl | 0.125–0.25 mEq/kg/h IV; do not exceed 0.5 mEq/kg/h | As needed |
| Glucose | 50–500 mg/kg/h IV | As needed |
| NaHCO$_3$ | Base excess × 0.3 × body weight in kg = mEq needed to correct deficit, IV (slow infusion) | As needed (pH 7.1 or less) |
| **GASTROINTESTINAL TRACT DYSFUNCTION** | | |
| Cimetidine | 5–10 mg/kg IV, IM, PO | Every 6–8 h |
| Ranitidine | 2 mg/kg IV, IM, PO | Every 8–12 h |
| Omeprazole | 0.7 mg/kg PO | Every 24 h |
| Misoprostol | 3 µg/kg PO | Every 24 h |
| Sucralfate | 250 mg (felines) PO | Every 8–12 h |
| | 500 mg (canines < 20 kg) PO | Every 8–12 h |
| | 1 gram (canines > 20 kg) PO | Every 8–12 h |
| Kaolin/pectin | 1–2 mL/kg PO | Every 6–8 h |
| Metoclopramide | 0.2–0.5 mg/kg SC | Every 6–8 h |
| **RENAL DYSFUNCTION** | | |
| Mannitol | 0.25–1 g/kg IV | Once (slow bolus) |
| Furosemide | 1–2 mg/kg IV | If no effect, repeat in 2 h and increase dose by 1 mg/kg |
| Dopamine | 1–3 µg/kg/min IV | As needed until urine production consistently > 2 mL/kg/h |

Reprinted with permission from Hardie EM. Life threatening bacterial infection. Compend Contin Ed 1995; 17:763–777.

**Table 11-8. Positive Inotropic Drugs**

| Drug (Trade Name) | Catecholamine Receptor Activation | | | | | Noncatecholamine Mechanism | Drug Dose and Infusion Schemes |
|---|---|---|---|---|---|---|---|
| | $\alpha_1$ | $\alpha_2$ | $\beta_1$ | $\beta_2$ | Dopamine | | |
| Epinephrine (Adrenalin) | +++ | +++ | ++ | ++ | – | No | 0.01–0.03 µg/kg/min (vasopressor) 0.1–0.2 mg/kg IV (cardiac arrest) |
| Isoproterenol (Isuprel) | – | – | +++ | +++ | – | No | 0.01–0.1 µg/kg/min; used primarily to increase heart rate; may cause hypotension |
| Dobutamine (Dubutrex) | Little | Little Direct and minimal indirect effects | +++ | ++ | – | No[a] | 2–10 µg/kg/min |
| Dopamine (Intropin) | ++ (high dose) | + (low dose) | ++ (low dose) Direct and indirect actions | + | +++ | No[a,b] | 2–5 µg/kg/min; renal dose 5–10 µg/kg/min; β effects 10–20 µg/kg/min; vasoconstriction |
| Dopexamine | – | – | Little | +++ | ++ | No[a] | 1–10 µg/kg/min |
| Ephedrine | + | + | + Both direct and indirect effects | + | – | No[b] | 0.1–0.25 mg/kg/min IM 0.03–0.07 mg/kg IV |
| Milrinone | – | – | – Phosphodiesterase inhibitor, ↑ cAMP in heart, peripheral vasodilator, ↑ inotropy additive to other types | – | – | Yes | 50–75 µg/kg IV bolus; oral administration possible |

+, positive effect; –, no effect; ↑, increased.
[a]Blocks reuptake of norepinephrine.
[b]Promotes release of norepinephrine from nerve terminal.

given to increase blood flow to vital organs (Table 11-8). **Clinical signs of hemorrhagic shock** most commonly encountered in the acutely traumatized patient include pallor, cyanosis, disorientation, tachycardia, cold extremities, cardiac dysrhythmias, pump failure, tachypnea, hypotension, oliguria, disseminated intravascular coagulation (DIC), and progressive metabolic acidosis.

2.  The **primary treatment of shock** is aggressive fluid therapy. When rapid infusion of large volumes of crystalloids decreases serum total solids concentration to < 3.5 g/dL, simultaneous colloid solution administration is advantageous in maintaining intravascular volume (Table 11-7). When hematocrit drops below 20%, whole blood or blood substitute, such as oxyglobin, should be given to improve blood oxygen carrying capacity. **Hypertonic saline** may be beneficial in the early treatment of hypovolemic and hemorrhagic shock in animals. Intravenous administration of small volumes (4 to 6 mL/kg) of 7.5% hypertonic saline results in beneficial cardiovascular effects in hypovolemic dogs and cats. A second potential benefit of hypertonic saline administration is minimizing the risk of cerebral edema in head trauma patients. Massive blood loss will eventually require transfusion of whole blood, packed red blood cells, or oxyglobin to replace oxygen transport capacity.

## D. Preanesthetic Evaluation

1.  *Head Trauma*

    a.  The hallmark of **closed head injury** is loss of consciousness associated with increased intracranial pressure and brain ischemia.
    b.  **Anesthetic agents** that increase cerebral blood flow (e.g., halothane, $N_2O$, ketamine) should not be used in these patients. Because barbiturates produce rapid induction and decrease cerebral metabolism ($CMRo_2$) and blood flow, they may be the preferred agents for patients with severe head injury. After acute brain injury, large doses of glucocorticosteroids (1 to 3 mg/kg dexamethasone) may help control cerebral edema.

c. **Hyperosmotic solutions** may help minimize intracranial pressure. Mannitol is an ideal drug for preventing or treating increased intracranial pressure and cerebral edema associated with global ischemia caused by cardiogenic shock or cardiac arrest. It is not, however, recommended for immediate use in patients with suspected intracranial hemorrhage (head trauma). Hemorrhage or leaking of hyperosmotic solutions into extravascular neural tissue runs the risk of increasing interstitial fluid volume and intracranial pressure.

2. *Thoracic and Abdominal Trauma*

a. **Penetrating trauma of the thorax and abdomen** is usually obvious. Blunt trauma presents a greater diagnostic challenge, because external examination may reveal nothing. A chest radiograph is essential after any type of thoracic trauma and will often require anesthesia.

b. **Severe hypoxia** often results from extensive lung contusions, and ventilatory support or oxygen therapy may be required. Pulmonary lesions tend to worsen within 24 to 36 h after injury. Chest tubes are often necessary for evacuation of air or fluids (pneumothorax and hemothorax) and will require local, regional (intercostal nerve block), or general anesthesia for placement.

c. **Lung contusions** usually resolve in 2 to 5 days. Medical management of pulmonary contusions includes oxygen, corticosteroid, analgesic, and antibiotic administration, and diuretic therapy when pulmonary edema is present.

d. Patients with **pericardial effusion** and **cardiac tamponade** manifest jugular vein distention, muffled heart sounds, and hypotension (Beck's triad) in addition to tachycardia and narrowed pulse pressure. Intravenous fluid administration, inotropic drugs, and immediate pericardial tap and drainage (pericardiocentesis) may be necessary to maintain an adequate cardiac output (Table 11-8). It is best to avoid controlled positive pressure ventilation in patients with tamponade.

e. Patients with **myocardial contusions** will often develop ventricular dysrhythmias, which require correct diagnosis and appropriate therapy with antiarrhythmic agents before and during surgery.

f. **Blunt abdominal trauma** can result in damage to several vital organs, including ruptured spleen and/or liver, bowel perforation, kidney and urinary bladder rupture, and the perforation of large abdominal vessels.

g. **Hypovolemic shock** caused by organ or vessel rupture and/or septic shock resulting from septicemia are common sequelae. Abdominal compression may reduce abdominal hemorrhage. Urinary catheterization will help evaluate urinary tract injury and renal function.

3. *Thermal and Burn Trauma*

a. If the patient is **apneic,** is in stridor, or has a burned face or the history indicates inhalation of steam, smoke, or toxic fumes, the trachea should be intubated immediately after sedation. Inhalation of carbon monoxide can result in severe hypoxia, because carbon monoxide has 200 times more affinity for hemoglobin than oxygen. Oxygen administration is the treatment.

b. **Fluid loss** owing to increased capillary permeability, protein loss into the interstitial tissues, and evaporative losses can be extensive, especially within the first 12 to 24 h after the accident. It has been suggested that only crystalloid solutions be administered during this time, because colloid solutions would likely rapidly extravasate. Patients should be carefully observed for **myoglobinemia** and **renal failure** as well as neurologic deficits.

c. **Volume replacement** should be closely monitored by measuring urine output and hemodynamic variables regularly.

d. Burn patients are **hypermetabolic** and will often have increased temperatures, increased catabolism, and increased oxygen requirements. **Parenteral** solutions commonly administered to fulfill nutritional requirements include 50% dextrose, 20% lipid, 8.5% amino acid with electrolytes, vitamin B complex, and lactated Ringer's.

e.   **Opioids** (e.g., fentanyl patches) should be considered with any technique to enhance preoperative and postoperative analgesia. Patches must be placed on a nonburned skin area.

## E.   Anesthetic Management

All classes of anesthetic agents may be used in the trauma patient; however, dosage requirement is usually reduced. Endogenous release of enkephalins, endorphins, and other amino peptides to reduce pain and stress may produce mild sedation and analgesia, reducing subsequent anesthetic agent requirement.

1.   *Premedication*
Analgesics and/or sedatives can be given to help alleviate pain, fear, and apprehension. Some clinicians have used fentanyl patches. Butorphanol (0.2 mg/kg IV) or oxymorphone (0.05 mg/kg IV) may be given in small incremental doses. When further CNS depression is desirable, diazepam (0.2 mg/kg IV) or midazolam (0.2 mg/kg IV or IM) can be combined with the opioid. If shock and/or severe blood loss are not of concern, acepromazine (0.05 mg/kg) can be combined with butorphanol or oxymorphone to induce neuroleptanalgesia. In cats, Demerol (1 to 2 mg/kg IM) has proven to be a good short-duration sedative-analgesic.

2.   *Induction*

a.   **Barbiturates** cause venodilation and usually decrease venous return, cardiac output, and blood pressure. The degree of myocardial depression induced is a function of dose and rate of injection. Barbiturates are highly bound to proteins, and normal pharmacokinetics are influenced by the patient's acid–base status, albumin content, and concurrent drug administration. Trauma victims are often acidotic and hypoproteinemic, so the induction dose requirement may be greatly decreased and should be anticipated by the clinician. Because barbiturates are arrhythmogenic when given rapidly, they should be used cautiously in patients with pre-existing arrhythmias.

b. **Propofol** induces similar hemodynamic depressive effects to those of thiopental. Accordingly, propofol is not recommended as a primary induction agent in trauma patients unless cardiovascular stability has been reinstated.

c. **Inhalation agents** are equally hypotensive compared to barbiturates and are only safer as induction agents because homeostatic mechanisms have longer to compensate for the depressant effects of the anesthetic during induction. Isoflurane is least depressant to cardiac output at equipotent (e.g., 1.5 MAC) concentrations. If the traumatized dog or cat is alert and likely to struggle, induction with an inhalation agent alone is not recommended.

d. **Ketamine** is one of the few anesthetic agents with indirect cardiovascular stimulant properties. In healthy patients, it raises blood pressure secondary to increased sympathetic activity, heart rate, and cardiac output; however, it also induces a direct myocardial depressant effect in patients whose sympathetic system is maximally stressed by hemorrhagic shock. This is often the case in severely traumatized patients. In patients with hypertrophic or restrictive cardiomyopathy (e.g., cats with idiopathic cardiomyopathy and normal left ventricular contractility), ketamine is contraindicated because it may induce tachycardia and decrease preload further. In contrast, in large- or giant-breed dogs suffering from cardiogenic shock and myocardial failure as defined by poor contractility (dilated cardiomyopathy), ketamine may be a good choice for inducing anesthesia. Because of their propensity to increase intracranial pressure, dissociatives are not recommended for patients with severe closed head injury or open eye injury. **Diazepam** (0.2 mg/kg IV) and **ketamine** (2 to 3 mg/kg IV) can be given in rapid sequence to induce anesthesia in either the traumatized dog or cat. If the patient is not sufficiently depressed after diazepam-ketamine administration, delivery of low concentrations of halothane or isoflurane (0.5 to 1.0%) by face mask will complete the induction.

e.  In depressed trauma victims, **oxymorphone** is commonly given intravenously in small increments (0.05 mg/kg) along with **diazepam** (0.2 mg/kg) until intubation is possible. Alternatively, **midazolam** (0.2 mg/kg) and **oxymorphone** (0.1 to 0.2 mg/kg) can be administered intramuscularly. Because opioids and benzodiazepines given together do not cause myocardial depression or vasodilation, they make a good induction combination in the patient who is hypovolemic or dehydrated or in cardiogenic or septic shock.

f.  **Etomidate** (0.5 to 2.0 mg/kg) produces minimal hemodynamic alterations and cardiac depression. Etomidate preserves hemodynamic function in dogs with experimentally induced hypovolemia. Adrenal cortical suppression may follow induction of anesthesia, but this is of limited concern when etomidate is given as a single bolus. Etomidate is a safe induction agent for patients in compensated or decompensated (congestive) heart failure, whether caused by acquired chronic atrioventricular valvular disease or myocardial failure (dilated cardiomyopathy).

3.  *Maintenance*

a.  **Opioids,** such as oxymorphone (0.1 mg/kg IV), fentanyl (0.01 mg/kg IV), and ketamine, can be given in small aliquots with diazepam or midazolam to maintain short periods of anesthesia. Ketamine should be repeated at an approximate dosage of 1 to 2 mg/kg IV every 20 to 30 min or as necessary to keep the patient anesthetized. Diazepam or midazolam can also be repeated (0.2 mg/kg IV) every 30 to 60 min or as necessary to provide adequate muscle relaxation.

    b.    **Isoflurane** is equally hypotensive as halothane but does not sensitize the myocardium to the arrhythmogenic effects of catecholamines to the same extent as does halothane. It is less depressant to the myocardium and a more potent vasodilator. Consequently, isoflurane is preferred in patients with congestive heart failure or with severe arrhythmias but not in patients in hypovolemic shock before they receive volume replacement. If blunt thoracic trauma is suspected and pneumothorax or hemothorax is present, nitrous oxide is contraindicated. Similarly, in patients with a distended abdomen or diaphragmatic hernia resulting in respiratory compromise, nitrous oxide should be avoided.

4.   *Regional Anesthesia*

    a.    **Epidural or spinal blocks** are contraindicated in trauma patients with severe hemorrhage. The profound sympathetic blockade induced by these techniques when using local anesthetics may result in acute hypotension.

    b.    Superficial lacerations and wounds of the extremities can be managed with **infiltration of local anesthetic** or by performing **peripheral nerve blocks. Intercostal nerve blocks** (0.5 to 1.0 mL per site) using 2% lidocaine or 0.5% bupivacaine can be used to control postoperative thoracotomy pain as well as pain associated with fractured ribs. **Interpleural administration** of local anesthetics (2% lidocaine or 0.25 to 0.5% bupivacaine) is also effective for thoracotomy and cranial abdominal pain associated with pancreatitis or diaphragmatic hernia repair. A bupivacaine dosage of 1.5 mg/kg for dogs and 0.75 mg/kg for cats to bathe the pleural surfaces can be used.

    c.    **Epidural or intrathecal administration of opioids** (0.1 mg/kg morphine or oxymorphone diluted with 1 mL saline per 4.5 kg of body weight) or low doses of $\alpha_2$-agonists may prove to be effective alternatives to local anesthetics in providing analgesia without sympathetic blockade.

## F.    Patient Support

1.    *Fluid Support*

a.    A **physiologic salt solution,** such as lactated Ringer's, restores and expands intravascular volume to help maintain cardiac output. In general, patients should be administered 20 to 40 mL/kg solution intravenously before anesthetic induction. Patients in hypovolemic shock can generally be given one blood volume of isotonic electrolyte solution in the first hour. **Replacement solutions** should be isotonic, but not all isotonic solutions are optimal. Although $D_5W$ and lactated Ringer's with 2.5% dextrose are isotonic, once glucose is metabolized, the remaining fluid is hypotonic and contains either all (5% dextrose) or half (2.5% dextrose) free water, which rapidly leaves the vascular compartment. In general, even optimal isotonic physiologic salt solutions remain intravascular for only 30 to 60 min before redistributing throughout the entire extracellular space. To **prolong the initial improvement** seen with isotonic fluids or hypertonic saline, blood (if PCV is < 20%), conventional fluids, or the addition of colloids should be considered. One suggested protocol combines bolusing a synthetic colloid solution (7 mL/kg) with a replacement crystalloid solution (15 mL/kg). The dose of colloid solution should not exceed 20 mL/kg within the first 24 h.

b.    **Colloid solutions** maintain intravascular volume for 2 to 5 h but may have associated complications (Table 11-7). **Dextran solutions** can cause bleeding disorders and allergic reactions and must be stored at stable temperatures (25°C) to prevent precipitate formation. **Protein solutions** can impair pulmonary function if they extravasate into damaged lung. **Hydroxyethyl starch** (6% solution in normal saline) is a glucose polymer that has proven useful when the dose is limited to < 20 mL/kg. If membrane permeability is normal, fluids containing colloids (albumin, dextran, hydroxyethylstarch) expand plasma volume rather than interstitial fluid volume or intracellular volume.

c.  When extreme blood loss occurs, **fresh whole blood** (< 6 h old) is given. Whole blood is preferred over packed red blood cells. In acute trauma, the large majority of clotting disorders are secondary to large volume fluid replacement, resulting in dilutional thrombocytopenia. If possible, surgery and anesthesia should be delayed until the packed cell volume can be increased to above 20%. When ongoing losses and replacement are occurring simultaneously, the best method of assessing adequate blood volume replacement is to assess urine output (1 to 2 mL/kg/hr is optimal), serial hematocrits, and total protein.

d.  **Rapid fluid loading** is often associated with dilutional thrombocytopenia, hypoglycemia, and/or hypokalemia; and fluids should be supplemented to maintain serum levels within normal ranges.

e.  **Survival** is correlated with a tissue oxygen delivery ($Do_2$), that is at least 600 mL $O_2$/min/m$^2$ (Table 11-5). To implement $Do_2$ goal-oriented fluid resuscitation, cardiac output, hemoglobin content, and oxyhemoglobin saturation must be continually monitored.

f.  **Sodium bicarbonate** should be reserved for cases of severe nonrespiratory acidosis. Rapid sodium bicarbonate administration may in fact be detrimental in treating lactic acidosis, because it depresses both arterial pressure and cardiac output. More important measures in treating metabolic acidosis are fluid resuscitation, adequate ventilation, and rewarming.

2.  *Inotropic Support*

    **Dopamine and dobutamine** have short half-lives and require constant infusion administration. **Dopexamine** may be the preferred dopaminergic agent, because it does not activate $\alpha$-receptors (Table 11-8). In refractive cases, inotropic doses of dopamine and dobutamine may be supplemented with the coadministration of ephedrine to reduce vascular compliance and improve preload and stroke volume.

3. *Temperature and Renal Support*

a. **Hypothermia** should be treated vigorously, because it is associated with reduced kidney function, poor platelet activity, low glucose use, shivering and increased oxygen consumption by nonvital tissues, metabolic acidosis, and decreased metabolism of anesthetics. **Warming fluids and blood** before administration helps maintain body temperature, reduces blood viscosity, and improves tissue blood flow. Warm water blankets and heat lamps may help prevent further heat loss but will not rewarm the patient, because of inadequate body surface area contact. The operating room should not be cold.

b. To prevent **acute oliguric renal failure** every effort should be made to maintain normal renal function in severely traumatized patients. Unfortunately, there is no way to predict the degree of hypoperfusion that will result in renal failure in a given patient. Myoglobinemia must be treated by vigorous diuresis after muscle crush or electrocution. Once fluid volume and blood pressure have been normalized, furosemide (1 mg/kg) and dopamine (2 to 5 µg/kg/min) can be used together to increase renal blood flow and water and solute excretion.

c. In critically ill patients **dopamine's natriuretic action** is not always apparent, as antinatriuretic factors (antidiuretic hormone, aldosterone) may be present to induce sodium conservation. With lower than normal levels of GFR, low doses of **dopamine** become less effective. This lack of response may be caused by exhaustion of the renal reserve system, by which low renal blood flow may have already caused a shift of blood flow to the inner cortex in an adaptive response to loss of nephron renal function. Consequently, the routine administration of dopamine in the severely traumatized patient should be carefully considered in the perioperative period. There is no correlation between the amount of urine volume produced and histologic evidence of acute tubular necrosis, GFR, creatinine clearance, BUN levels, and creatinine levels in burn patients, trauma patients, or shock states.

    d.    **Redistribution of renal blood flow** is designed to protect the vulnerable medullary oxygen supply and demand balance at the expense of urine formation. Reduced GFR may reduce medullary tubular workload and oxygen consumption. Oliguria may be viewed in some circumstances (e.g., low blood volume or anesthesia) as a sign of normal protective compensatory mechanisms at work. **Inadequate urine production** (output < 0.5 mL/kg/hr) may reflect a variety of factors independent of inadequate glomerular filtration. Reduced urine output during the anesthetic period in euvolemic patients is usually of little consequence to long-term renal function.

## IV.  NEONATAL PATIENTS

### A.   Physiology

**Neonatal animals** gradually develop normal (adult) physiologic responses and function by 6 to 8 weeks (Table 11-9). By 12 weeks, the majority of circulatory, ventilatory, thermoregulation, hepatic, and renal functions are well developed.

    1.    **Cardiac output** in neonates is more rate dependent than in adults. Slowing of the heart rate results in larger decreases in cardiac output. An adult can increase cardiac output by 300%, whereas the neonate can only increase output by 30%.

    2.    **Sympathetic stimulation** results in minimal increases in rate and contractility. Sympathetic immaturity also manifests itself in poor vasomotor control and greater susceptibility to hypothermia. Rapid or excessive fluid administration may result in pulmonary edema.

    3.    Neonates have a **high oxygen consumption** because of their high metabolic rate. Their minute ventilation is, therefore, higher than that of an adult and is achieved through

higher breathing rates. Neonates are especially susceptible to hypoxia during apnea or airway obstruction.

4. Neonates are susceptible to **hypothermia,** because of their high body surface to mass ratio and limited ability to vaso-constrict to conserve heat.

5. **Body fat** is low in the neonate as opposed to the adult, such that adipose tissue does not comprise a significant compartment for redistribution.

6. **Renal function** is not fully developed at birth and does not reach full function in most species until 1 to 2 months. This also contributes to prolonged tissue levels of drug. Glomer-ular filtration rate requires at least 14 days in puppies to reach adult levels, whereas tubular secretion reaches adult levels in 4 to 6 weeks.

**Table 11-9. Physiologic Characteristics of Neonates**

Low myocardial contractile mass
Low ventricular compliance
High cardiac index
Low cardiac reserve
Fixed stroke volume
Cardiac output rate dependent
Immature sympathetic nervous system
Poor vasomotor control
High oxygen consumption and minute volume of ventilation
High closing volume
Thermoregulation limited
Permeable blood–brain barrier
Low body fat and muscle tissue
Low protein binding of drugs
High body water content, large extracellular fluid compartment
Immature hepatic microsomal enzyme system
Immature kidney function

### B. Pharmacology

1. Large **extracellular fluid volume** results in a greater apparent volume of distribution of drugs that are highly ionized in plasma or relatively polar (e.g., nonsteroidal anti-inflammatory drugs, nondepolarizing neuromuscular blockers). Volume of distribution is also affected by lower protein binding and decreased rates of metabolism and excretion.

2. The most important factor during early life is the **deficiency of hepatic microsomal enzyme function** during the first 4 weeks, and especially during the first week. The relative inability to metabolize drugs leads to prolonged tissue levels of drugs if adult dosages are used.

3. The **blood–brain barrier,** because of the open tubocisternal endoplasmic reticulum of cerebral endothelial and choroid plexus epithelial cells, allows drugs greater access to the brain. Accordingly, sedative and anesthetic dosages should be reduced for at least the first 4 weeks of life.

## V. GERIATRIC PATIENTS

### A. Physiology

1. **Aging** is an all-encompassing multifactorial process, resulting in decreased capacity for adaptation and producing a decrease in functional reserve of organ systems. There is little correlation between chronologic and physiologic age. The effect of age per se on perioperative morbidity and mortality is related to the decreased physiologic reserve of the various organ systems that occur with aging (Table 11-10).

2. **Cardiovascular changes** result in gradual deconditioning. Myocardial fiber atrophy results in decreased pump function and cardiac output. The geriatric patient is more **dependent on preload** and is not as tolerant of volume depletion as is the younger patient. Heart rate may be affected if pacemaker cells are involved. Fibrosis of the endocardium and valves leads to decreased compliance. Valvular incom-

| Table 11-10. Physiologic Characteristics of Geriatric Patients |
| --- |

Decreased elasticity and compliance of the vasculature
Increased blood pressure
Increased left ventricular mass
Decreased responsiveness to catecholamines
Increased incidence of dysrhythmias
Increased incidence of conduction abnormalities
Cardiac output is preload dependent
Decreased ventilatory volumes
Decreased efficiency of pulmonary gas exchange
Decreased liver mass
Decreased total hepatic blood flow
Decreased renal mass
Decreased muscle mass
Increased body fat as a percent of total body weight
Decreased total body water
Decreased intracellular and blood volume
Decreased albumin
Decreased basal metabolic rate

petence may accompany valvular fibrosis and calcification. The vascular tree gradually loses elasticity, resulting in decreased distensibility, increased impedance to left ventricular output, and progressive hypertrophy of the ventricle. Maximum coronary perfusion decreases as coronary artery elasticity and caliber decrease.

3. **Pulmonary changes** associated with aging include decreased ventilatory volumes and efficiency of gas exchange. Vital capacity, total lung capacity, and maximum breathing capacity decrease as the intercostal and diaphragmatic muscles gradually waste and the thorax becomes more rigid and less compliant. Age-related parenchymal changes in the lung resemble those of emphysema. As a result, $Pao_2$ decreases with age.

4. A **decreased requirement for anesthetic** compared to young adults has been documented. This appears to be the

result of an age-related decrease in resistance to loss of consciousness. Factors thought to be involved in this increased sensitivity to anesthetics include the continual loss of neurons associated with aging, decreased receptors and affinity of the receptors for neurotransmitters, and reduced synthesis of neurotransmitters.

5. **Loss of kidney mass** occurs in the aged, primarily in cortical tissue. As a result, GFR decreases, making the patient more susceptible to acute renal failure after nephrotoxic or ischemic episodes. Tubular function is also decreased, and the renin–angiotensin system becomes less responsive in aged patients. The ability to correct fluid, electrolyte, and acid–base disturbances and to tolerate hemodynamic insults is reduced.

6. **Basal metabolic rate** decreases with age, as does the ability to maintain body temperature. Geriatric patients tend to become more hypothermic than do younger patients, delaying recovery.

## B.   Pharmacology

1. **Hepatic clearance** of drugs decreases with age as the mass of the liver decreases. In elderly people, the liver mass as well as hepatic blood flow may be decreased by 40 to 50%. Metabolism of lipid soluble drugs, particularly anesthetics, is decreased.

2. Age-related **changes in body composition** include a decrease in skeletal muscle, an increase in body fat as a percentage of total body weight, and a loss of intracellular water. A loss of total body water occurs as a result of decreased intracellular water and a reduction in blood volume (20 to 30%). Intravenous injection of anesthetic drugs into this contracted blood volume results in an increased plasma concentration. Because of the increased adipose content of the body, there is increased sequestration of fat-soluble drugs, which slows their elimination.

3. **Protein binding of drugs** is reduced in the elderly because of decreased concentrations of albumin in the blood and

qualitative changes in protein. Drugs that are normally
highly bound to protein may have an exaggerated clinical
effect.

4.  The **"to effect" administration of anesthetics** to achieve
    CNS depression commensurate with the anesthetic re-
    quirements of the aged patient is advocated (Table 11-11).
    When possible, the use of local and regional anesthetic
    techniques in combination with sedation or neuroleptanal-
    gesia may prove safer than general anesthesia.

**Table 11-11. Anesthetics Commonly Used in Small Animal Geriatric Patients**

| | Dose, mg/kg | |
|---|---|---|
| Drug | Canine | Feline |
| **PREANESTHETICS** | | |
| Anticholinergics | | |
| Atropine[a] | 0.01–0.02 | 0.01–0.02 |
| Glycopyrrolate[a] | 0.005–0.01 | 0.005–0.01 |
| Sedatives and analgesics | | |
| Midazolam[a] | 0.1–0.3 | 0.1–0.3 |
| Diazepam[b] | 0.2–0.4 | 0.2–0.4 |
| Oxymorphone[a] | 0.1–0.2 | 0.1–0.2 |
| Butorphanol[a] | 0.2–0.4 | 0.2–0.4 |
| Buprenorphine[a] | 0.005–0.01 | 0.005–0.01 |
| **INDUCTION DRUGS** | | |
| Fentanyl–diazepam | 0.1/0.2 | |
| Oxymorphone–diazepam | 0.1/0.2 | 0.1/0.2 |
| Ketamine–diazepam | 3–5/0.2 | 3–5/0.2 |
| Etomidate | 0.5–1.5 | 0.5–1.5 |
| Isoflurane (mask) | 2–3% | 2–3% |
| **MAINTENANCE** | | |
| Inhalant: isoflurane | 1–2% | 1–2% |
| Muscle relaxant: atracurium | 0.1 | 0.1 |

[a]IM or IV administration is appropriate.
[b]Not recommended for IM use and should be given slowly when administered IV.

# Chapter 12

---

## Anesthetic Emergencies and Accidents

Introductory Comments

*In many veterinary practices, after the induction of anesthesia, no one is assigned the task of anesthetist to monitor anesthesia and be vigilant to the occurrence of untoward events that might result in morbidity and mortality. Sometimes this practice leads to anesthetic accidents or emergencies. As with most unwanted events, anticipation of possible problems and having a plan of action already mentally prepared will go a long way toward successful resolution. Because the onset of general anesthesia upsets the physiologic equilibrium of the patient and can bring it closer to the threshold of harmful events, preparation to manage these problems is critical. Table 12-1 lists a variety of complications associated with anesthesia practice and their management.*

**Definitions**
**Hypoxia**
**Aspiration**
**Respiratory Insufficiency**
**Cardiovascular Emergencies**
**Hemorrhage**
**Cardiac Dysrhythmias**
**Cardiac Arrest**
**Temperature Monitoring**
**Malignant Hyperthermia**
**Injuries During Anesthesia**
**Epidural Analgesia**

---

*A. T. Evans*

**Table 12-1. Management of Complications Associated with Anesthesia**

| Complication | Treatment | Trade Name | Dosage and Route of Administration | Side Effects |
|---|---|---|---|---|
| Excitement, delirium | Acepromazine | PromAce | 0.02–0.2 mg/kg IV, IM | Prolonged recovery |
| | Diazepam | Valium | 0.25–0.5 mg/kg IV | Hypothermia |
| | Midazolam | Versed | 0.05–0.2 mg/kg IV, IM | |
| Hypoventilation | Oxygen | | | Respiratory depression |
| | Ventilation | | | Resisting mask |
| Laryngospasm | Lidocaine spray | Xylocaine 2% | | |
| | Lidocaine jelly | | | |
| Dyspnea | Oxygen | Portex | | Hyperventilation |
| | Tracheostomy | | | |
| | Ventilation | | | |
| Pneumothorax | Oxygen | | | Infection |
| | Chest tubes | | | Hyperventilation |
| | Ventilation | | | |
| Cardiac dysrhythmias | | | | |
| Tachycardia | Lactated Ringer's | | 10–20 mL/kg/h | Bradycardia |
| | Propranolol | Inderal | 0.05–0.1 mg/kg IV | Hypotension |
| | Increase anesthesia | | | Bradycardia |
| Bradycardia | Atropine | | 0.02 mg/kg IV | Tachycardia |
| | Glycopyrrolate | Robinul V | 0.005 mg/kg IV | |
| Ventricular | Lidocaine | Xylocaine | Canines: 0.5 mg/kg IV | Bradycardia |
| dysrhythmias | | | Felines: 0.2 mg/kg IV | Convulsions |

| Condition | Treatment | Trade name | Dosage | Complications |
|---|---|---|---|---|
| Hypotension | Procainamide | Pronestyl | 10–20 mg/kg IM | Hypotension |
| | Fluids (lactated Ringer's) | | 10–20 mg/kg/h IV | |
| | Dopamine | Intropin | 3–5 µg/kg/min | Dysrhythmias |
| | Dobutamine | Dobutrex | 3–5 µg/kg/min | Tachycardia, hypertension |
| Blood or fluid loss | Fluids (lactated Ringer's) | | 40–90 mL/kg/h IV | Pulmonary edema |
| | Blood | | 20–40 mL/kg IV | Allergic reaction |
| Hypothermia | Warmed fluids | | 5–10 mL/kg/h IV | Over hydration |
| | Water heating pad | Gaymar | | |
| Hypoglycemia | D₅₀W | | 1–2 mL/kg IV | Hyperosmolality |
| Metabolic acidosis | Sodium bicarbonate | | 1–2 mEq/kg IV every 10 min | Metabolic alkalosis, hypokalemia, hyperosmolality |
| | THAM | | $mL = $ body weight (kg) × base deficit (mEq/L) × 1.1 | Coagulation time increased in canines |
| Hyperkalemia | Sodium bicarbonate | | 0.5–1.0 mEq/kg IV | Coagulation increased in canines |
| | 0.9% sodium chloride | | 10–40 mL/kg/h | |
| | Calcium chloride | | 10 mg/kg IV | Tachycardia |
| Hyperpyrexia | Oxygen | | | |
| | Fluids (lactated Ringer's) | | 5–10 mL/kg IV | |
| | Tranquilizers | PromAce | 0.4 mg/kg IM | |
| | Dantrolene sodium | | 2–4 mg/kg IV | |
| Prolonged recovery | Doxapram | Dopram V | 1–2 mg/kg IV | Excitement |
| | Yohimbine | Yobine | 0.5 mg/kg IV | |
| | Atipamezole | Antisedan | 0.04 mg/kg IM | |
| Postoperative pain | Morphine sulfate | | 0.02–1.0 mg/kg IM | Respiratory depression |
| | Buprenorphine | Buprenex | 0.01 mg/kg IV, IM | Slow recovery |
| | Butorphenol | Torbutrol | 0.2–0.4 mg/kg IM | Slow recovery |
| | Oxymorphone | | 0.06–0.1 mg/kg IV, IM | Slow recovery, respiratory depression |

## I. DEFINITIONS

**Apnea** is a transient or longer cessation of breathing.

**Apneic threshold** is the $Paco_2$ level at which ventilation becomes zero and spontaneous ventilation effort ceases and is generally 5 to 9 mm Hg below the resting $Paco_2$.

**Aspiration** as it pertains to anesthesia is the act of sucking in material, solid or liquid from the mouth into the pulmonary system.

**Asystole** is complete ventricular arrest; no P waves, QRS complexes, or T waves are seen.

**Atelectasis** is a collapsed or airless state in part or all of the lung.

**Barotrauma** is injury of certain organs owing to a change in atmospheric pressure.

**Bicarbonate** is an alkalinizing agent indicated in the treatment of metabolic acidosis.

**Cardiac pump** describes a theory of how blood is moved during cardiopulmonary resuscitation (CPR). According to this theory, compression of the chest wall mechanically compresses the heart.

**Closing volume** is the volume of the lung during expiration at which small airways begin to close; small amounts of disease in distal airways can increase the closing volume.

**Electrical mechanical dissociation** is a form of pulseless ventricular rhythm that has no relationship between the electrical rhythm and the strength of contraction.

**End-tidal carbon dioxide** is the carbon dioxide in the expired gas; can be used to monitor effectiveness of CPR.

**Functional residual capacity** is the normal amount of air remaining in the lung after a normal expiration.

**Hypoxia** is an abnormally low $Pao_2$ in tissues.

**Interposed abdominal compression** is a technique of compressing the abdomen counterpoint with thoracic compressions during CPR; purported to increase venous return.

**Regurgitation** is the return of food from the stomach to the mouth without the ordinary efforts at vomiting.

**Silent regurgitation** is the return of food from the stomach to the esophagus. This type of regurgitation is not noticed by the anesthetist.

**THAM,** or tromethamine, is an alkalinizing agent used for correction of severe acidosis. There is no increase in $CO_2$ levels when tromethamine is administered.

**Thoracic pump** describes a theory of blood flow during CPR by which cardiac output is the result of an increase in intrathoracic pressure, which squeezes the heart.

**Ventricular fibrillation** is when the ECG demonstrates jagged and irregular baseline undulations with no coordinated pattern.

**Ventricular premature contractions** are beats caused by spontaneous depolarization of electrically unstable ventricular myocardial or conduction system cells.

## II.  HYPOXIA

**Hypoxia** can be caused by decreased inspired oxygen (i.e., airway obstruction), hypoventilation (depression of ventilation by drugs), mismatching of ventilation–perfusion and increases in right-to-left intrapulmonary shunt. Diffusion block is possible but not common. Cyanosis begins to occur when the $Po_2$ drops below 60 mm Hg.

1. **Apnea** and **airway obstructions** leading to hypoxia commonly occur during induction of anesthesia. Depressant effects of anesthetics contribute to the occurrence of apnea, and animals with redundant tissue in the pharyngeal area are liable to develop physical obstructions to breathing during the induction and recovery periods. Individually, some patients develop increased mismatching of ventilation–perfusion and right to left shunting, which produces hypoxia that cannot be explained by other causes. Administration of oxygen by mask will help in most situations. Supplemental oxygen, however, will not raise the $Po_2$ to the same level as a normal animal if the animal has a right-to-left intrapulmonary shunt.

2. Administering oxygen by mask for 30 s will increase the amount of time before hypoxia is evident.

3. Use a speedy induction technique (thiopental, propofol) to ensure quick intubation.

4. Controlled ventilation or persistent end-expiratory pressure may improve oxygenation during mismatching of ventilation–perfusion.

5. During recovery from anesthesia, there are two possible ways to manage airway obstructions:

    a. Leave the endotracheal tube in place as long as possible to ensure a patent airway.

    b. Remove the tube early and then position the animal's head and neck so that the airway is patent. If by chance a patent airway cannot be achieved, and because the animal is still anesthetized, the endotracheal tube can be easily reinserted. As the patient slowly recovers from anesthesia, the endotracheal tube will not irritate the pharynx and/or larynx, allowing recovery without excitement.

## III. ASPIRATION

### A. Occurrence

**Aspiration** may occur as a result of **regurgitation** during anesthesia.

1. **Silent regurgitation** occurs when material is in the esophagus but does not reach the pharynx. This is thought to occur in up to 70% of human anesthesias. A similar occurrence probably occurs in anesthetized companion animals.

2. Predisposing factors include administration of preanesthetics that relax the lower esophageal sphincter, increased intra-abdominal pressure, head down positioning during surgery, and the presence of food or liquid in the stomach.

3. Irritation to the mucosa of the esophagus with acid could lead to postoperative esophageal stricture.

4. Aspirated stomach contents with a pH < 2.0 are more likely to cause pneumonitis.

### B. Prevention

1. Animals in a head down position during anesthesia may tend to regurgitate more but are less likely to aspirate.

2.  Patients should fast before surgery.

3.  If regurgitation does occur, use suction to remove material from the pharynx, esophagus, and stomach.

4.  Flush the esophagus with water or a bicarbonate solution.

5.  Keep anesthesia plane deep enough to prevent bucking and the resulting increased intra-abdominal pressure.

6.  Leave the esophageal or stomach tube in place for the remainder of the surgery.

7.  Before extubation, visually inspect the pharyngeal area for any remaining material.

## IV. RESPIRATORY INSUFFICIENCY

Respiratory insufficiency (increased $Paco_2$) is common during the course of anesthesia. Causes include the administration of opioids and other sedatives before anesthesia, the relative overdose of induction agents, positioning for surgery, respiratory effects of inhalants, surgical trauma, and the excessive use of opioids during recovery.

### A. Apnea

**Apnea** is common during the course of routine anesthesia. It occurs during induction after the administration of thiobarbiturates or propofol, during maintenance of anesthesia with ketamine, as a result of controlled ventilation, and as a consequence of deep inhalation anesthesia. **The apneic threshold** is the $Paco_2$ at which ventilation stops. As a result of apnea, the patient is often ventilated to keep the $Paco_2$ lower than that required to stimulate breathing. Isoflurane has a lower apneic threshold than does halothane; i.e., isoflurane is more of a respiratory depressant than is halothane.

### B. Functional Residual Capacity

Decreased **functional residual capacity** (FRC) during anesthesia can increase respiratory insufficiency by lowering alveolar ventilation to perfusion ratio (V/Q) When the FRC is close to or less than the **closing volume** (CV) of the lung, small airways begin to close. **Atelectasis** becomes greater, increasing the right-to-left shunt of blood through the lungs. This is more common in older animals and during deep anesthesia. Atelectasis can be prevented by using controlled ventilation or the addition of positive end-expiratory pressure (PEEP). Slightly closing the pop-off valve can add 5 to 10 cm $H_2O$ of PEEP. Using an end-tidal $CO_2$ monitor can help determine the severity of hypoventilation.

## V. CARDIOVASCULAR EMERGENCIES

Cardiovascular emergencies can be precipitated by anesthetic effects on cardiac output, arterial blood pressure, cardiac rhythm, and heart rate.

### A. Cardiac Output

**Cardiac output** is decreased by most anesthetics. All of the volatile anesthetics decrease cardiac output as a result of dose-related depression of contractility.

### B. Blood Pressure

**Blood pressure** is generally reduced during anesthesia and is anesthetic dose-dependent. Surgical manipulation can also acutely lower blood pressure by obstruction of venous return. Hypotension during anesthesia is diagnosed when systolic pressure is < 80 mm Hg, measured by the indirect oscillometric method. Ascertain if the anesthetic level is too high or if there have been extreme fluid losses either from hemorrhage or to the third space. Treatment should be directed at the cause. Hypertension is rare during anesthesia; however, it may occur as a result of surgical stimulation. Systemic hypertension can be considered when the systolic blood pressure is > 160 mm Hg and the diastolic pressure is > 95 mmHg. Increasing the depth of anesthesia will generally lower the pressure.

### C. Cardiac Rhythm

**Cardiac rhythm** can be affected by injectable anesthetics thiobarbiturates, $\alpha_2$-agonists, halothane, and surgical stimulation.

## VI. HEMORRHAGE

The incidence of life-threatening hemorrhage during surgical procedures is low. When it occurs, however, treatment must be quick and effective to prevent loss of life.

## A.    Blood Volume

**Blood volume** is approximately 8% of body weight and a loss of 10 to 20% of the blood volume should be treated with volume replacement. Besides hemorrhage, other avenues of loss include evaporation from pleural and peritoneal surfaces, continued formation of ascites and pleural effusions, loss of fluid into the bowel, and third space losses. Insidious blood loss can occur during nasal exploratories and spinal surgery, when blood is collected by suction or surgical sponges. A fully saturated 4 × 4 sponge contains 10 to 12 mL of blood. Signs of serious blood loss include decreasing packed cell volume when given large quantities of fluid, weak pulse, lower blood pressure, deeper anesthesia, and pale mucous membranes.

## B.    Replacement

Replace blood loss with crystalloid solutions, **colloid preparations,** or **whole blood.**

1.   Replace the volume of blood loss in a **3 : 1 ratio with crystalloid solution,** such as lactated Ringer's. Because of rapid equilibration across intravascular and interstitial fluid compartments, only 25% of the administered volume remains within the intravascular space after 30 min.

2.   A **packed cell volume** (PCV) > **25%** is desirable. A PCV in this range will lower blood viscosity while preserving adequate oxygen carrying capacity.

3.   **Total serum protein** levels should not be allowed to decrease to < 3.5 g/dL.

4.   In dogs, **hypertonic (7.5%) saline** will increase plasma volume 2 to 4 mL for each milliliter of solution administered. Other beneficial effects of hypertonic saline have been reported as improved cardiac output, aortic blood pressure, and interstitial fluid volume. Infuse at a rate of 2 mL/kg/min.

5.   Administration of the **natural or artificial colloids** increase intravascular colloid osmotic pressure, move water from the interstitial space to the intravascular space, and limit

water movement out of the intravascular space. They are more expensive but should be used when plasma albumin levels are < 1.5 gm/dL or serum protein levels are < 3.5 gm/dL (see Chapter 8).

6. Acute blood losses greater than 15 to 20% should be replaced with **whole blood in a 1 : 1 ratio** to blood loss.

## VII. CARDIAC DYSRHYTHMIAS

Cardiac dysrhythmias occur as a result of pre-existing medical conditions, administration of premedications, anesthesia induction and maintenance agents, and surgical stimulation. Dysrhythmias require treatment if they reduce cardiac output, cause sustained tachycardia, or are likely to initiate dangerous ventricular dysrhythmias.

### A. Drug-Induced Dysrhythmias

**Atropine or glycopyrrolate** can cause sinus tachycardia and increase myocardial work. **Phenothiazine tranquilizers** predispose the heart to sinus bradycardia, sinus arrest, and occasional first- and second-degree heart block. **Xylazine** has been implicated as causing bradycardias and decreasing the epinephrine threshold for VPCs. The μ-receptor agonist **opioids** (morphine, oxymorphone), will also precipitate a slow heart rate. The anesthesia induction agents **thiamylal, thiopental, and ketamine** have been reported to increase the likelihood of dysrhythmias from epinephrine during halothane anesthesia.

### B. Pre-Existing Conditions and Surgical Stimulation

1. Dysrhythmias after **gastric dilation–volvulus** presumably have their origin from acid–base imbalance, electrolyte disturbances, ischemic myocardium, circulating cardiac stimulatory substances, and/or autonomic nervous system imbalance.

2. **Traumatic myocardium** is also a source of dysrhythmias owing to bruising of the heart and resultant myocardial ischemia.

3. **Surgical factors** include altered $Pa_{CO_2}$, $Pa_{O_2}$, pH, reflexes from surgical manipulation, CNS disturbances, and cardiac disease.

4. **Ventricular premature contractions** (VPC) may follow the use of thiopental (bigeminal rhythm), halothane, surgical stimulation, and increases in $Pa_{CO_2}$ or decreases in $Pa_{O_2}$. Premature contractions should be treated when there are > 20 per min, pairs or runs of VPCs are present, or they are coming from multiple sites in the conduction system.

## C. Heart Rate

1. **Bradycardia** (heart rate below baseline or < 70 bpm in dogs and 160 in cats) can develop after administration of acepromazine, renal toxicity, CNS disease, hypothermia, and the use of the $\alpha_2$-agonist agents xylazine or medetomidine. Well-conditioned dogs may also exhibit sinus bradycardia during anesthesia. Sinus arrhythmia is common in dogs that have not received atropine or glycopyrrolate. Treat severe bradycardias with atropine 0.02 mg/kg IV or glycopyrrolate 0.01 mg/kg IV. To diminish $\alpha_2$-agonist induced bradycardias, use atropine intramuscularly 10 min before administration.

2. **Sinus tachycardia** can be a response to surgical stimulation, hyperthermia, lowered cardiac output, hyperthyroidism, anemia, infection, and pheochromocytoma. Normal heart rates are affected by breed and age; however, tachycardia can be considered if the rate exceeds 160 bpm in the average dog, 180 in toy breeds, and 220 in puppies. The normal heart rate should be < 240 bpm in cats. Treatment depends on the cause (surgical stimulation, hyperthermia, etc.). If treatment is required a low dose of intravenous acepromazine (0.01 mg/kg) can be helpful.

## D. Treatment

Because most perioperative dysrhythmias do not seriously affect cardiac output, **treatment can be discrete**. Changing to a different inhalation anesthetic or increasing the depth of anesthesia may eliminate the dysrhythmia. Other treatments for controlling ventricular dysrhythmias include giving a small dose (0.01 mg/kg) of acepromazine intravenously, correcting blood gas abnormalities, and administering a small quantity (0.5 mg/kg) of intravenous lidocaine. For gastric dilation–volvulus dysrhythmias, correct physiologic abnormalities and administer lidocaine, procainamide, or quinidine (either singly or in combination). Lidocaine and quinidine may also be effective for traumatic myocardial dysrhythmias.

## VIII. CARDIAC ARREST

### A.   The Problem

1.   The central problem in a cardiac arrest is **inadequate oxygenation** and its consequences. The goal of treatment should be to provide enough oxygenated blood flow to preserve the tissues until adequate spontaneous circulation returns.

2.   In people, the scope of the underlying problem has been found to be a major factor in the success or failure of CPR.

   a.   **Factors associated with poor outcome** are long down times before resuscitation efforts begin and long periods of ineffective resuscitation (closed chest massage) during the CPR effort.

   b.   In general, **CPR must be started within 4 min of the arrest** to be successful.

   c.   If the animal has **ventricular fibrillation,** direct current defibrillation should take precedence over other resuscitative measures.

3.   Successful resuscitation rates are **10 to 20% for intact neurologic survival** in people; a similar rate is probably present in small animals.

### B.   Diagnosis

Successful treatment of cardiac arrest requires early diagnosis. The brain is the organ most susceptible to hypoxia–ischemia, because serious injury develops after only 4 or 5 min of cardiac arrest. Once the diagnosis of cardiac arrest has been confirmed, all efforts must be toward developing effective blood flow and reestablishing a heartbeat. CPR with external cardiac massage appears to be ineffective in protecting the brain from injury and should be part of only the initial resuscitation protocol and should not be continued for long periods of time.

1. Signs of cardiac arrest include no palpable pulse, no palpable heartbeat, apnea, no muscle tone, and dilated pupils (later). Expressions of cardiac arrest are **asystole, ventricular fibrillation,** and a pulseless ventricular rhythm termed **electrical mechanical dissociation** (EMD).

## C.   Treatment

**Treatment of cardiac arrest** follows the traditional **ABCD** protocol (airway, breathing, cardiac massage, drugs or definitive therapy) (Fig. 12-1).

1. **A**irway: a patent airway should be confirmed via endotracheal intubation.

2. **B**reathing: initiate ventilation at a rate of 4 to 5 breaths per minute at an inspiratory pressure sufficient to create a normal-appearing thoracic excursion. This is equivalent to a tidal volume of 10 mL/kg. If an overdose of inhalation anesthetic has contributed to the cardiac arrest, the breathing rate should initially remain higher than 4 or 5 breaths per minute to help remove the remaining anesthetic.

3. **C**ardiac massage: either external or internal.

    a. **External cardiac massage** should be instituted at the first sign of cardiac arrest. With the animal in right lateral recumbency, stand at its dorsum and compress the thorax by placing one hand on top of the other or by using one hand between the table and the thorax to supply countersupport to the compressions made with the top hand. Small animals such as cats can be massaged with the thumb and first two fingers. Blood flow occurs as the result of one or both of two mechanisms. The **cardiac pump** mechanism pro-

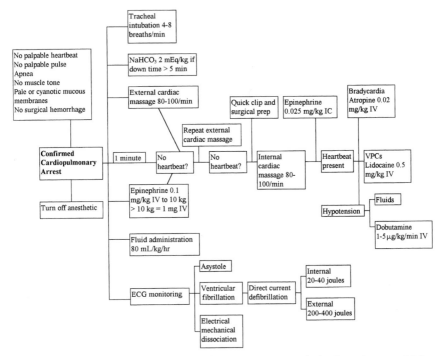

**Figure 12-1.** An algorithm for CPR to be used to resuscitate animals that have the potential for surviving cardiac arrest. Because early restoration of brain perfusion is the most important goal, a quick decision for internal cardiac massage is required. *IC,* intracardiac; *VPCs,* ventricular premature contractions.

duces blood flow by means of mechanical compression of the heart between the two lateral thoracic walls. This mechanism may account for blood flow in smaller animals or animals with narrow side-to-side thoracic wall conformation. Observations that coughing could produce blood pressure coupled with other studies of physiologic measurement of intrathoracic pressure raised questions about the cardiac pump theory. To explain these observations the alternative **thoracic pump** theory was developed.

b.  An adjunct to external thoracic compressions, **interposed abdominal compression** CPR was developed to facilitate venous return to the thorax and enhance the production of an A-V gradient required for blood flow. With this technique, the abdomen is compressed counterpoint with the thorax. Although this technique improves cerebral blood flow in dogs, the full value of the procedure awaits future study.

c.   The recommended **rate of compression** is 80 to 100 bpm.

d.   A **square wave pattern of compression,** hesitating momentarily at the compression point and the relaxation point, may improve cardiac output with the thoracic pump mechanism.

e.   **Higher survival rates** may be obtained if external thoracic massage is practiced for no longer than 2 min, after which time internal cardiac massage is initiated.

f.   Open thoracic, or **internal CPR,** is more effective at perfusing the heart and brain during the critical beginning minutes of CPR. Higher blood pressures and cardiac outputs can be achieved with internal CPR. Most veterinary practices are well equipped to perform internal CPR, because controlled ventilation and thoracotomy can be performed. The limiting factor will probably be the surgical experience of the attending veterinarian. Clip the hair from the left thorax at the fifth interspace. Spray or wipe the area with an antiseptic solution and incise the skin starting 2.5 cm (1 in) from the spine to within 2.5 cm (1 in) of the sternum. With surgical scissors, continue the incision through the various tissue layers, avoiding the internal thoracic artery near the sternum. Bluntly penetrate the pleura, extend the incision, and spread the ribs. Reach into the thorax and begin cardiac massage at 80 to 100 bpm.

4.   **Definitive** or drug therapy: recommendations start with the immediate use of epinephrine. Epinephrine has been shown to increase cerebral and myocardial blood flow through the mechanisms of prevention of arterial collapse and by producing vasoconstriction, which prevents sequestration of blood in noncritical areas. Some conflicting studies have shown that during CPR, epinephrine may increase the intrapulmonary shunt, possibly through the β-adrenergic receptor attenuation of hypoxic pulmonary vasoconstriction. Methoxamine, a pressor devoid of β-adrenergic activity, has been recommended as a substi-

tute for epinephrine. Additional studies are needed to clarify the conflicting evidence.

a.  Historically, **epinephrine remains the drug of choice** and should be given early in the treatment protocol, preferably into a central vein. Use a bolus of saline to move drugs from a peripheral vein to a central vein. Because access to a central vein may be difficult, epinephrine may alternatively be administered intrabronchially or directly into the left ventricle. For intrabronchial administration, use a flexible plastic catheter wedged into a distal bronchus. For intracardiac placement, use a 22-gauge needle inserted at the left fourth thoracic interspace and costochondral junction. A long spinal needle may be needed for larger dogs. This technique is presently discouraged.

b.  For intravenous use, **a dose of 0.05 to 0.1 mg/kg** is used, whereas bronchial administration requires 0.05 to 0.1 mg/kg diluted to 5 to 6 mL volume with saline. The dose for intracardiac epinephrine is 0.025 to 0.05 mg/kg. Even though intracardiac epinephrine seems appealing as a way of efficiently delivering the drug to the heart, the technical difficulty of positioning the needle in the chamber of the left ventricle when the heart cannot be palpated along with the potential for myocardial injury makes this technique the least advantageous.

c.  Because the goal of CPR is to revive the patient's heart as soon as possible, **early administration of epinephrine is crucial** and should be given immediately after diagnosis of cardiac arrest.

d.  **Atropine and glycopyrrolate** are important drugs to administer during CPR, because reflex bradycardia may have contributed to the initial cardiac arrest. In addition, bradycardia often occurs after a heartbeat has been established. Atropine at 0.02 to 0.04 mg/kg or glycopyrrolate at 0.01 mg/kg intravenously will protect against bradycardia.

e.  **Metabolic acidosis from hypoxia and ischemia** and respiratory alkalosis as a result of ventilation during treatment of cardiac arrest commonly occur during resuscitation. The immediate use of **bicarbonate** or **THAM** is controversial, because metabolic acidosis is slow to develop during CPR and is somewhat neutralized by an ensuing respiratory alkalosis. Generally, sodium bicarbonate or THAM will not be required immediately after the onset of cardiac arrest, unless an existing nonrespiratory acidosis contributed to the arrest. In addition, acid–base abnormalities do not necessarily correlate with successful resuscitation. Sodium bicarbonate is administered at 1 mEq/Kg IV and repeated at 10-min intervals (better guided by blood gas determinations). THAM is supplied in 500-mL bottles, and the recommended dose for treatment of cardiac arrest is 3.5 to 6.0 mL/kg IV.

f.    **Lidocaine** is used after resuscitation if ventricular dysrhythmias are compromising cardiac output. The use of lidocaine during ventricular fibrillation to improve the results of electric defibrillation is being re-evaluated. Lidocaine is usually given as an intravenous bolus at a dose of 0.5 mg/kg.

g.    If **ventricular fibrillation** is present, clip the hair from a small area from each side of the thorax. After applying electrode gel to each paddle, firmly apply the paddles to the thorax and **administer a shock of approximately 2 to 5 J/kg** (W/s/kg). Sequential discharges of increasing energy may be more effective at converting fibrillation. Internal defibrillation requires a smaller electric discharge, a total of 10 to 50 J.

## D.    Assessing Circulation During CPR

1.    Traditional assessment of productive CPR includes **palpation of pulses** and monitoring the end-organ effects of circulation, such as pupillary size. Palpation of a peripheral pulse and **constricting pupils** may indicate a good prognosis, but not always.

2.    Measuring **end-tidal carbon dioxide** ($ETco_2$) to determine the adequacy of blood flow during CPR may become a monitoring standard. The $ETco_2$ during cardiac arrest has been shown to vary directly with cardiac output (pulmo-

nary blood flow) and can predict successful resuscitation outcome. As more veterinarians upgrade their anesthesia monitoring, the measurement of $ET_{CO_2}$ could become commonplace.

## IX.  TEMPERATURE MONITORING

### A.    Heat Loss and Gain

The potential for **accidental heat loss** during surgery depends on the size of the animal, length of surgery, exposure of body compartments to ambient temperature, natural insulation (fat, hair coat), and anesthetic inhibition of thermoregulation. **Hyperthermia** can be caused by sepsis, iatrogenic overheating, high ambient temperature in the operating suite, and thick hair coat. Accidental hyperthermia must be differentiated from malignant hyperthermia. Anesthetized animals often behave as if poikilothermic until the core temperature reaches a new set point.

### B.    Responses to Temperature

The **responses to cold** include vasoconstriction, nonshivering thermogenesis, shivering, piloerection, puffing of feathers, and lowering of body temperature. **Warm** thermoregulatory effector mechanisms consist of vasodilation, sweating, panting, and salivation.

### C.    Hypothermia

Heat loss is generally through **convection and radiation** from the skin and surgical incision. Inhalation anesthetics lower the threshold for response to hypothermia in people to ~ 34.5°C, and presumably the same trend occurs in animals. Accidental hypothermia can be limited by cocooning with warm water blankets and warming intravenous crystalloid fluids if large amounts are used. Forced warm air systems have been effective in preventing hypothermia. (Baer system). The use of electric blankets is potentially dangerous because of inadequate control of heat output.

## X.    MALIGNANT HYPERTHERMIA

**Malignant hyperthermia (MH)** has been documented in animals. The term *malignant hyperthermia* was used in 1966 to describe a syndrome in humans that includes muscle rigidity, tachycardia, and fever. The use of volatile anesthetics and succinylcholine caused affected subjects to undergo an increase of aerobic and anaerobic metabolism, resulting in abnormal production of heat, carbon dioxide, and lactate. As a consequence, the whole body's acid–base balance was affected. Pigs inbred for muscle development (e.g., landrace, pietrain, Poland China) provide an animal model for studying this syndrome. The greyhound and possibly other sighthounds may be susceptible to this syndrome, although there are no studies to support this notion.

### A. Clinical Presentation

The **clinical presentation** of MH is characterized by an increasing $ET_{CO_2}$, acidosis, muscle rigidity, rhabdomyolysis, hyperkalemia, tachycardia, tachypnea, dysrhythmia, and death. Temperature elevation is a late sign of MH.

### B. Anesthetic Drugs

**Drugs** used during anesthesia reported to trigger MH include all of the inhalants except nitrous oxide and succinylcholine. No other drugs appear to be triggers including propofol and ketamine.

### C. Treatment

The essential points of **treatment** of MH are discontinuation of trigger agents, hyperventilation, administration of dantrolene in doses of 2 mg/kg, cooling by all routes available, and treatment of hyperkalemia. Sequelae include disseminated intravascular coagulation and myoglobinuric renal failure.

## XI. INJURIES DURING ANESTHESIA

Prevention of patient injuries during the anesthetic period is the responsibility of the veterinary surgeon anesthetist. It must be remembered that the anesthetized patient will not be able to respond to noxious tissue-damaging stimuli in the same manner as would an unanesthetized animal.

### A. Positional Injuries

The veterinary anesthetist must carefully observe the animal's position on the surgery table, the position of the eyes in relationship to the surface of the table, and any prominent bony protuberances that might be under pressure during the surgery. In addition, observe the position of the limbs, particularly when they are in the abducted position, to see if any nerves might be under unnecessary strain or tension. A common injury during small animal anesthesia occurs when the animal is supine (ventral-dorsal) with the legs tied to the surgery table. If the ties are tight enough to inhibit venous drainage of distal legs, the feet will become edematous.

### B.    Intubation Injuries

1.  Potential injury is also possible from **careless endotracheal intubation technique.** The use of a pointed stylet to facilitate intubation may cause injury if the stylet protrudes beyond the end of the endotracheal tube.

2.  Most new endotracheal tubes are too long for small dogs and cats. When they are advanced into the trachea, there is danger of **bronchial intubation.** New tubes should be correctly sized to the patient by comparing the length of the tube with the distance from the muzzle to the thoracic inlet when the head and neck are in the natural position (not extended or flexed).

3.  **Overinflation of the cuff,** causing tracheal epithelial injury, may not be as common as in the past owing to increased use of low-pressure cuffs. Whenever the patient is moved while an endotracheal tube is in place, however, the Y piece should be disconnected to prevent rotation of the tube within the trachea. Rotation of the tube may cause tracheal lacerations, leading to subcutaneous emphysema, pneumomediastinum, and pneumoperitoneum.

4.  High-atmospheric pressure–induced injury, or **barotrauma**, is always a possibility when semiclosed or high-oxygen-flow anesthesia systems are used. When the oxygen flow rate is > 4 to 6 mL/kg, the pop-off valve must always be open, except when controlled ventilation is being applied. To prevent barotrauma, use a commercially available **PEEP** valve in the anesthesia circuit or inflate the cuff of the endotracheal tube so that when the breathing circuit pressure > 15 to 20 mm Hg is reached, intrapulmonary pressure will be released around the cuff.

### C.    Ocular Injuries

**Ocular injuries** occur because of corneal dehydration. Anesthetics reduce or eliminate the palpebral and corneal reflex and reduce tear production, making artificial tears an important component of anesthesia protocol.

## XII. EPIDURAL ANALGESIA

The use of epidural anesthetics and analgesics for relief of pain gained new popularity after reports of successful use of epidural opioids and $\alpha_2$-agonists. The technique is easy to perform, has close to a 90% success rate, and gives the veterinary practitioner another option with which to provide intraoperative and postoperative analgesia.

**Epidural anesthesia** (use of local anesthetics such as lidocaine) can precipitate systemic toxicity owing to accidental intravenous injection, a total spinal when the anesthetic solution spreads high enough to block the entire spinal cord, and neurologic injury resulting in motor weakness. Epidural analgesia (with opioids) can potentially cause respiratory depression, pruritus, urinary retention, and decreased consciousness. To prevent accidental intravascular or spinal injection, aspirate to determine the presence of clear (spinal) fluid or blood. Other indications of correct position are a positive hanging drop sign (may give a false sign if the epidural needle is intravascular), and inject only if there is no resistance (the degree of compression of the air bubble in the syringe barrel will give an indication of resistance). Contraindications to epidural injection include sepsis, skin infection, coagulopathy, increased intracranial pressure, and hypovolemia.

# Chapter 13

---

## Euthanasia

### Introductory Comments*

*Euthanasia techniques should result in rapid unconsciousness followed by cardiac or respiratory arrest and ultimate loss of brain function. In addition, the technique should minimize any stress and anxiety experienced by the animal before unconsciousness. Stress may be minimized by technical proficiency and humane handling of the animals to be euthanatized. Emotional uneasiness, discomfort, or distress experienced by people involved with euthanasia of animals may be minimized by ensuring that the person performing the euthanasia procedure is technically proficient. Uninformed observers may mistakenly relate any animal movement with consciousness and lack of movement with unconsciousness. Although these are not adequate criteria, euthanasia techniques that preclude movement of animals are aesthetically acceptable to most people. As with many other procedures involving animals, some methods of euthanasia require physical handling of the animal. The amount of control and kind of restraint needed is determined by the animal species, breed, size, state of domestication, presence of painful injury or disease, degree of excitement, and method of euthanasia. Proper handling is vital for minimizing pain and distress in animals; to ensure safety of the person performing euthanasia; and frequently, to protect other animals and people. Table 13-1 lists the agents and methods of euthanasia employed in a variety of species. Tables 13-2 and 13-3 list conditionally acceptable and acceptable agents and methods of euthanasia, respectively. Table 13-4 lists unacceptable agents and methods.*

**General Considerations**
**Animal Behavioral Considerations**
**Modes of Action of Euthanatizing Agents**

---

*This chapter is taken with permission from the American Veterinary Medical Association from Andrews EJ, Bennett BT, Clark JD, et al. Report of the American Veterinary Medical Association Panel on Euthanasia. J Vet Med Assoc 1993;202(2):229–249.

**Inhalant Agents**
**Noninhalant Pharmaceutical Agents**
**Physical Methods**
**Adjunctive Methods**
**Zoo, Aquatic, and Poikilothermic Animals**
**Animals Raised for Fur**

## I. GENERAL CONSIDERATIONS

### A. Evaluating Methods

In evaluating methods of euthanasia, several criteria are used:

Ability to induce loss of consciousness and death without causing pain, distress, anxiety, or apprehension.
Time required to induce unconsciousness.
Reliability.
Safety of personnel.
Irreversibility.
Compatibility with requirement and purpose.
Emotional effect on observers or operators.
Compatibility with subsequent evaluation, examination, or use of tissue.
Drug availability and human abuse potential.
Age and species limitations.
Ability to maintain equipment in proper working order.

### B. Neonatal and Prenatal Animals

Euthanasia of **neonatal** or **prenatal** animals or uncommonly encountered species may be necessary. Whenever such situations arise, a veterinarian or other experienced professional should use professional judgment and knowledge of clinically acceptable techniques when selecting an appropriate euthanasia technique. Essential to the application of professional judgment is the consideration of the animal's size and its species-specific physiologic and behavioral characteristics. In all circumstances, the euthanasia method should be selected and used with the highest ethical standards and social conscience.

*Text continued on p. 543.*

| Table 13-1. Agents and Methods of Euthanasia by Species (see also Table 13-4) | | |
|---|---|---|
| **Species** | **Preferred** | **Acceptable** |
| Amphibians | Inhalant anesthetics, CO, $CO_2$, barbiturates, tricaine methanesulfonate, double-pithing, benzocaine | Pithing, gunshot, penetrating captive bolt, stunning and decapitation, decapitation and pithing |
| Birds | Inhalant anesthetics, CO, $CO_2$, barbiturates | Nitrogen, argon, cervical dislocation, decapitation |
| Cats | Inhalant anesthetics, CO, $CO_2$, barbiturates | Nitrogen, argon |
| Dogs | Inhalant anesthetics, CO, $CO_2$, barbiturates | Nitrogen, argon, electro-cution, penetrating captive bolt |
| Fish | Tricaine methanesulfonate, benzocaine, barbiturates | Stunning and decapitation, decapitation |
| Marine mammals | Barbiturates, etorphine hy-drochloride | Succinylcholine chloride and potassium chloride, gunshot |
| Mink, fox, and other animals produced for fur | Inhalant anesthetics, CO, $CO_2$, barbiturates | Nitrogen, argon, electro-cution followed by cervical dislocation |
| Nonhuman primates | Barbiturates | Inhalant anesthetics, CO, $CO_2$, nitrogen, argon |
| Rabbits | Inhalant anesthetics, CO, $CO_2$, barbiturates | Nitrogen, argon, cervical dislocation, decapitation, penetrating captive bolt |
| Reptiles | Barbiturates, inhalant anesthetics, $CO_2$ | Gunshot, penetrating captive bolt, stunning and decapi-tation, decapitation and pithing |
| Rodents and other small animals | Inhalant anesthetics, CO, $CO_2$, microwave irradia-tion, barbiturates | Nitrogen, argon, cervical dislocation, decapitation |
| Zoo animals | Inhalant anesthetics, $CO_2$, CO, barbiturates | Nitrogen, argon, penetrating captive bolt, gunshot |

**Table 13-2. Conditionally Acceptable Agents and Methods of Euthanasia**

| Agent | Classification | Mode of Action | Rapidity | Ease of Performance | Safety | Species Suitability | Efficacy and Comments |
|---|---|---|---|---|---|---|---|
| Cervical dislocation | Hypoxia owing to disruption of vital centers | Direct depression of brain | Moderately rapid | Requires training and skill | Safe | Poultry, birds, laboratory mice, and rats <1 kg | Irreversible; violent muscle contractions can occur after cervical dislocation |
| Decapitation | Hypoxia owing to disruption of vital centers | Direct depression of brain | Moderately rapid | Requires training and skill | Guillotine poses potential employee injury hazard | Laboratory rodents, small rabbits, birds, fish, amphibians, and reptiles | Irreversible; violent muscle contractions can occur after decapitation |
| Electrocution | Hypoxia | Direct depression of brain and cardiac fibrillation | Can be rapid | Not easily performed in all instances | Hazardous to personnel | Used primarily in foxes, sheep, swine, and mink | Violent muscle contractions occur at same time as unconsciousness |
| Pithing | Hypoxia owing to disruption of vital centers, physical damage to brain | Trauma of brain and spinal cord tissue | Rapid | Easily performed but requires skill | Safe | Some poikilotherms | Effective, but death not immediate unless double pithed |
| Nitrogen, argon | Hypoxic hypoxemia | Reduced $Po_2$ available to blood | Rapid | Use closed chamber with rapid filling | Safe if used with ventilation | Cats, small dogs, birds, rodents, mink, rabbits and other small species of zoo animals | Effective except in young and neonates; an effective agent, but other methods preferrable; not acceptable in most animals <4 months old |

**Table 13-3. Acceptable Agents and Methods of Euthanasia**

| Agent | Classification | Mode of Action | Rapidity | Ease of Performance | Safety for Personnel | Species Suitability | Efficacy and Comments |
|---|---|---|---|---|---|---|---|
| Barbiturates | Hypoxia owing to depression of vital centers | Direct depression of cerebral cortex, subcortical structures, and vital centers; direct depression of heart muscle | Rapid onset of anesthesia | Animal must be restrained; personnel must be skilled to perform IV injection | Safe except for human abuse potential; DEA-controlled substance | Most species | Highly effective when appropriately administered; acceptable IV and IP in small animals |
| Inhalant anesthetics | Hypoxia owing to depression of vital centers | Direct depression of cerebral cortex and subcortical structures and vital centers | Moderately rapid onset of anesthesia; some excitation may occur during induction | Easily performed with closed container; can be administered to large animals by means of a mask | Must be properly scavenged or vented to minimize exposure to personnel | Amphibians, birds, cats, dogs, fur-bearing animals, rabbits, reptiles, rodents and other small animals, zoo animals | Highly effective provided that subject is sufficiently exposed |
| Carbon dioxide | Hypoxia owing to depression of vital centers | Direct depression of cerebral cortex, subcortical structures, and vital centers; direct depression of heart muscle | Moderately rapid | Used in closed container | Minimal hazard | Small laboratory animals, birds, cats, small dogs, mink, zoo animals, amphibians | Effective, but time required may be prolonged in immature and neonatal animals |

| | | | | | | |
|---|---|---|---|---|---|---|
| Carbon monoxide (bottled gas only) | Hypoxia | Combines with hemoglobin, preventing its combination with oxygen | Moderate onset time; insidious, so animal is unaware of onset | Requires appropriately operated equipment for gas production | Extremely hazardous, toxic, and difficut to detect | Most small species, including dogs, cats, rodents, mink, chinchillas, birds, reptiles, amphibians, and zoo animals | Effective; acceptable only when equipment is properly designed and operated |
| Microwave | Brain enzyme inactivation | Direct inactivation of brain enzymes by rapid heating of brain | Very rapid | Requires training and highly specialized equipment | Safe | Mice and rats | Highly effective for special needs |
| Tricaine methane-sulfonate | Hypoxia owing to depression of vital centers | Depression of CNS | Very rapid, depending on dose | Easily used | Safe | Fish and amphibians | Effective but expensive |
| Benzocaine | Hypoxia owing to depression of vital centers | Depression of CNS | Very rapid, depending on dose | Easily used | Safe | Fish and amphibians | Effective but expensive |

**Table 13-4. Unacceptable Agents and Methods of Euthanasia**

| Agent | Comments |
|---|---|
| Exsanguination | Because of the anxiety associated with extreme hypovolemia, exsanguination should be done only in sedated, stunned, or anesthetized animals. |
| Decompression | Decompression is not a recommended method for euthanasia of animals because of the numerous disadvantages: (1) Many chambers are designed to produce decompression at a rate 15–60 times faster than that recommended as optimum for animals, resulting in pain and distress caused by expanding gases trapped in body cavities. (2) Immature animals are tolerant of hypoxia, and longer periods of decompression are required before respiration ceases. (3) Accidental recompression, with recovery of injured animals, can occur. (4) Bloating, bleeding, vomiting, convulsions, urination, and defecation, which are aesthetically unpleasant, may occur in the unconscious animal. |
| Rapid freezing | Rapid freezing as a sole means of euthanasia is not considered to be humane. If it is used, animals should be anesthetized before freezing. |
| Air embolism | Air embolism may be accompanied by convulsions, opisthotonos, and vocalization; if used, it should be done only in anesthetized animals. |
| Drowning | Drowning as a means of euthanasia is inhumane. |
| Strychnine | Strychnine causes violent convulsions and painful muscle contractions. |
| Nicotine, magnesium sulfate, potassium chloride, all curariform agents (neuromuscular blocking agents) | When used alone, these drugs all cause respiratory arrest before unconsciousness, so the animal may perceive pain after it is immobilized. |
| Chloroform | Chloroform is a known hepatotoxin and a suspected carcinogen and, therefore, hazardous to human beings. |
| Cyanide | Cyanide poses an extreme danger to personnel, and the manner of death is aesthetically objectionable. |
| Stunning | Stunning may render an animal unconscious but is not a method of euthanasia; if used, it must be followed by another method to ensure death. |

### C.   Verification

It is **imperative that death be verified** after euthanasia and before disposal of the animal. To a casual observer, an animal in deep narcosis after administration of an injectable or inhalant agent may appear dead; but the animal may eventually recover. Death should be confirmed by examining the animal for cessation of vital signs.

## II.   ANIMAL BEHAVIORAL CONSIDERATIONS

### A.   Physical Signs

The **facial expressions** and **body postures** that indicate various emotional states of animals have been described. Behavioral and physiologic responses to noxious stimuli include distress vocalization, struggling, attempts to escape, defensive or redirected aggression, salivation, urination, defecation, evacuation of anal sacs, pupillary dilation, tachycardia, sweating, and reflex skeletal muscle contractions (causing shivering, tremors, or other muscular spasms). Some of these responses can occur in unconscious as well as conscious animals. Fear can cause immobility or playing dead in certain species, particularly rabbits and chickens. This immobility response should not be interpreted as unconsciousness when the animal is, in fact, conscious.

### B.   Minimizing Distress

The need to **minimize animal distress**, including fear, anxiety, and apprehension, must be considered when determining the method of euthanasia. Distress vocalizations, fearful behavior, and release of certain odors or pheromones by a frightened animal may cause anxiety and apprehension in other animals. Therefore, whenever possible, other animals should not be present when euthanasia is performed, especially euthanasia of the same species. This is particularly important when vocalization or release of pheromones may occur during induction of unconsciousness. Gentle restraint, preferably in a familiar environment, careful handling, and talking during euthanasia often have a calming effect on companion animals. Some of these methods, however, may not be effective with wild animals or animals that are injured or diseased. When struggling during capture or restraint may cause pain, injury, or anxiety to the animal or danger to the operator, the use of tranquilizers, analgesics, and/or immobilizing drugs should be considered.

## III. MODES OF ACTION OF EUTHANATIZING AGENTS

### A. Basic Mechanisms

Euthanatizing agents cause death by three basic mechanisms: direct or indirect hypoxia, direct depression of neurons vital for life function, and physical disruption of brain activity and destruction of neurons vital for life.

### B. Hypoxia

Agents that induce death by **direct** or **indirect hypoxia** can act at various sites and can cause unconsciousness at different rates. For death to be painless and distress free, unconsciousness should precede loss of motor activity (muscle movement). This means that agents that induce muscle paralysis without unconsciousness are absolutely condemned as the sole agents for euthanasia (e.g., curare, succinylcholine, gallamine, strychnine, nicotine, magnesium and potassium salts, pancuronium, decamethonium, vecuronium, atracurium, pipecuronium, and doxacurium). With other techniques that induce hypoxia, some animals may have motor activity after unconsciousness, but this is reflex activity and is not perceived by the animal.

### C. Depression of Neurons

The second group of euthanatizing agents depress nerve cells of the brain, inducing unconsciousness followed by death. Some of these agents release **muscle control** during the first stage of anesthesia, resulting in a so-called **excitement or delirium phase,** during which there may be vocalization and some muscle contraction. These responses do not appear to be purposeful. Death follows unconsciousness and is attributable to hypoxemia after direct depression of respiratory centers and/or cardiac arrest.

### D. Disruption of Brain Activity

**Physical disruption of brain activity**, caused by concussion, direct destruction of the brain, or electric depolarization of the neurons, induces rapid unconsciousness. Death occurs because of destruction of the midbrain centers that control cardiac and respiratory activity or by adjunctive methods (e.g., exsanguination) used to kill the animal. Exaggerated muscular activity can follow unconsciousness; although this may disturb some observers, the animal is not experiencing pain or distress.

## IV. INHALANT AGENTS

### A. Concentration

Any gas that is inhaled must reach a certain **concentration in the alveoli** before it can be effective; therefore, euthanasia with any of these agents takes some time. The suitability of a particular agent depends on whether an animal experiences distress between the time it begins to inhale the agent and the time it loses consciousness. Some agents may induce convulsions, but these generally follow unconsciousness. Agents that induce convulsions before unconsciousness are unacceptable for euthanasia.

### B. Considerations

Certain considerations are common to all inhalant agents:

1. In most cases, onset of **unconsciousness** is more rapid, and euthanasia more humane, if the animal is rapidly exposed to a high concentration of the agent.

2. The **equipment** used to deliver and maintain this high concentration must be in good working order. Leaky or faulty equipment may lead to slow, distressful death and/or be hazardous to other animals and to personnel.

3. Most of these agents are hazardous to the health of personnel because of the risk of **narcosis** (e.g., halothane), **hypoxemia** (e.g., nitrogen, carbon monoxide), **addiction** (e.g., nitrous oxide), or **health effects from chronic exposure** (e.g., nitrous oxide, carbon monoxide).

4. Alveolar concentrations rise slowly in an animal with decreased ventilation, making agitation more likely during induction. Other noninhalant methods of euthanasia should be considered for such animals.

5. **Neonatal** animals appear to be resistant to **hypoxia;** and because all inhalant agents ultimately cause hypoxia, neonatal animals take longer to die than do adults. Therefore, these drugs should not be used in neonates unless the animal can be exposed long enough to ensure death. Newborn dogs, rabbits, and guinea pigs will survive a nitrogen atmosphere much longer than will adults. On the other hand, inhalants may be used to induce unconsciousness, followed by use of some other method to kill the animal.

6. **Rapid gas flows** can produce a noise that **frightens animals.** If high flows are required, the equipment should be designed to minimize noise.

7. **Animals placed together in chambers** should be of the same species and, if needed, should be restrained so that they will not hurt themselves or others. Chambers should be kept clean to minimize odors that might distress animals subsequently euthanatized.

## C. Inhalant Anesthetics

1. Inhalant anesthetics (e.g., **halothane, isoflurane, enflurane, and sevoflurane**) have been used to euthanatize many species. Halothane induces anesthesia rapidly and is the most effective inhalant anesthetic for euthanasia. Enflurane is less soluble in blood than is halothane; but because of its lower vapor pressure and lower potency, induction rates may be similar to those for halothane. At deep anesthetic planes, animals often undergo seizure when exposed to enflurane. It is an effective agent for euthanasia, but the seizure activity may be disturbing to personnel. Isoflurane and sevoflurane are potent inhalant anesthetics commonly used to induce anesthesia rapidly; however, isoflurane has a slightly pungent odor, and animals often hold their breath, delaying the onset of unconsciousness. More isoflurane or sevoflurane is needed to kill an animal than is halothane. Although isoflurane and sevoflurane are acceptable as euthanasia agents, halothane is more economical and usually preferred.

2. With **inhalant agents,** the animal is placed in a closed receptacle containing cotton or gauze soaked with the anes-

thetic. The anesthetic may also be introduced from a vaporizer, but this usually results in longer induction time. Vapors are inhaled until respiration ceases and death ensues. Because the liquid state of most inhalant anesthetics is irritating, animals should be exposed only to vapors. Also, sufficient air or oxygen must be provided during the induction period to prevent hypoxemia. In the case of small rodents placed in a large container, there will be sufficient oxygen in the chamber to prevent hypoxemia. Larger species placed in small containers may need supplemental air or oxygen.

3. **Nitrous oxide** ($N_2O$) may be used with the other inhalants to speed the onset of anesthesia, but it alone does not induce anesthesia in animals, even at 100% concentration. If $N_2O$ is used as a sole euthanasia agent, hypoxemia develops before respiratory or cardiac arrest, and animals may become distressed before unconsciousness.

4. **Occupational exposure** to inhalant anesthetics constitutes a human health hazard. Spontaneous abortion and congenital abnormalities have been associated with exposure of women to trace amounts of inhalation anesthetic agents in early stages of pregnancy. In human exposure to inhalant anesthetics, the concentration of halothane, enflurane, isoflurane, and sevoflurane should be < 2 ppm and of nitrous oxide, < 25 ppm.

5. **Advantages**

   a. The **inhalant anesthetics** are particularly valuable for euthanasia of smaller animals (under about 7 kg) or in animals in which venipuncture may be difficult.
   b. Halothane, enflurane, isoflurane, sevoflurane, and $N_2O$ are nonflammable and nonexplosive under ordinary environmental conditions.

6. **Disadvantages**

   a. **Struggling and anxiety** may develop during induction of anesthesia because anesthetic vapors may be irritating and can induce excitement.

    b.   **Nitrous oxide** will support combustion.

    c.   **Personnel** and animals can be injured by exposure to these agents.

    d.   There is a potential for **human abuse** of some of these drugs, especially $N_2O$.

7.  **Recommendations**

    a.   In order of preference, **halothane, sevoflurane, enflurane, and isoflurane,** with or without nitrous oxide, are acceptable for euthanasia of small animals (under about 7 kg). Although acceptable, these agents are generally not used in larger animals because of their cost and difficulty of administration.

## D.  Carbon Dioxide

1.  **Room air** contains 0.04% carbon dioxide ($CO_2$), which is heavier than air and nearly odorless. Inhalation of $CO_2$ in concentrations of 7.5% increases the pain threshold, and higher concentrations of $CO_2$ have a rapid anesthetic effect.

2.  At concentrations of **30 to 40% $CO_2$ in oxygen**, anesthesia is induced within 1 to 2 min, usually without struggling, retching, or vomiting. The signs of effective $CO_2$ anesthesia are those associated with deep surgical anesthesia, such as loss of withdrawal and palpebral reflexes.

3.  In **cats,** inhalation of 60% $CO_2$ results in loss of consciousness within 45 s and respiratory arrest within 5 min. Carbon dioxide has been used to euthanatize groups of small laboratory animals, including mice, rats, guinea pigs, chickens, and rabbits. Inhalation of high concentrations of $CO_2$ may be distressing to animals because of mucosal irritation and ventilatory stimulation.

4.  **Diving animals** may have physiologic mechanisms for coping with high concentrations of $CO_2$. It is necessary, therefore, to have a high enough concentration of $CO_2$ to kill

the animal by hypoxemia following the induction of anesthesia with $CO_2$.

5.  **Advantages**

    a.  Carbon dioxide is a rapid **depressant** and **anesthetic.**
    b.  Carbon dioxide may be **purchased in cylinders** or **in solid state** as dry ice.
    c.  Carbon dioxide is **inexpensive, nonflammable,** and **nonexplosive** and poses minimal hazard to personnel when used with properly designed equipment.
    d.  Carbon dioxide euthanasia does not distort **cellular architecture.**

6.  **Disadvantages**

    a.  Because **$CO_2$ is heavier than air,** incomplete filling of a chamber may permit tall or climbing animals to avoid exposure and to survive. This appears to be distressful to the animals.
    b.  Some species may have extraordinary **tolerance** for $CO_2$.

7.  **Recommendations**

    a.  Compressed $CO_2$ in **cylinders** is preferable to dry ice, because the inflow to the chamber can be regulated precisely.
    b.  If **dry ice** is used, animal contact must be avoided to prevent freezing or chilling.
    c.  Carbon dioxide generated by other methods such as from a fire **extinguisher** or from **chemical means** (e.g., Alka-Seltzer) is unacceptable.
    d.  With an animal in the chamber, an optimal flow rate should displace at least 20% of the chamber volume per minute.
    e.  Unconsciousness may be induced more rapidly by exposing animals to a $CO_2$ concentration of 70% or more by prefilling the chamber.
    f.  It is important to verify that an animal is dead before removing it from the chamber. If an animal is not

dead, $CO_2$ narcosis must be followed with another method of euthanasia.

g.    Larger animals, such as rabbits, and cats, appear to be distressed by $CO_2$ euthanasia; therefore, other methods of euthanasia are preferable.

## E. Carbon Monoxide

Carbon monoxide (CO) is a **colorless, odorless gas** that is non-flammable and nonexplosive until concentrations exceed 10%. It combines with hemoglobin to form carboxyhemoglobin and blocks the uptake of oxygen by erythrocytes, leading to fatal hypoxemia.

### 1. Advantages

a.    Carbon monoxide induces unconsciousness without pain and with minimal discernible discomfort.

b.    Hypoxemia induced by CO is insidious, so the animal appears to be unaware.

c.    Death occurs rapidly if concentrations of 4 to 6% are used.

### 2. Disadvantages

a.    Safeguards must be taken to prevent exposure of personnel.

b.    Any electric equipment exposed to CO (e.g., lights and fans) must be explosion-proof.

3.    Carbon monoxide used for individual animal or mass euthanasia is **acceptable** for small animals, including dogs and cats, provided that commercially compressed CO is used and the following precautions are taken:

a.    **Personnel** using CO must be instructed thoroughly in its use and must understand its hazards and limitations.

b.    The **CO source** and chamber must be located in a well-ventilated environment, preferably outdoors.

c.    The **chamber** must be well lit and have view ports that allow personnel direct observation of the animals.

    d.   The CO **flow rate** should be adequate to rapidly achieve a uniform CO concentration of at least 6% after animals are placed in the chamber, although some species (e.g., neonatal pigs) are less likely to become agitated with a gradual rise in CO concentration.

    e.   If the chamber is inside a room, **CO monitors** must be placed in the room to warn personnel of hazardous concentrations.

## V. NONINHALANT PHARMACEUTICAL AGENTS

**Intravenous administration** is the most rapid and reliable method of performing euthanasia with injectable euthanasia agents. It is the most desirable method when it can be performed without causing fear or distress in the animal. Sedation of aggressive, fearful, wild, or feral animals is recommended before intravenous administration of the euthanasia agent. When intravenous administration is considered impractical or impossible (e.g., in animals weighing $\geq 7$ kg), intraperitoneal administration of a nonirritating euthanasia agent is acceptable, provided that it does not contain neuromuscular blocking agents. Intracardiac administration is not considered acceptable in awake animals, owing to the difficulty and unpredictability of performing the injection accurately. Intracardiac injection is acceptable only when performed on heavily sedated, anesthetized, or comatose animals. Intramuscular, subcutaneous, intrathoracic, intrapulmonary, intrarenal, intrasplenic, intrathecal, and other nonvascular injections are not acceptable methods of administering injectable euthanasia agents. When injectable euthanasia agents are administered other than intravenously, animals may be slow to pass through stages I and II of anesthesia.

### A.   Barbituric Acid Derivatives

**Barbiturates** depress the CNS in descending order, beginning with the cerebral cortex, and unconsciousness progresses to anesthesia. With an overdose, deep anesthesia progresses to apnea, owing to depression of the respiratory center, which is followed by cardiac arrest. All barbituric acid derivatives used for anesthesia are acceptable for euthanasia. Induction of unconsciousness by barbiturates results in minimal or transient pain associated with needle puncture, thus satisfying the basic criterion for classifying an agent as acceptable for euthanasia. Barbiturates have rapid onset of action, which is a desirable characteristic for a euthanasia agent. Desirable barbiturates are those that are potent, long acting, stable in solution, and inexpensive. Sodium pentobarbital fits these criteria and is the most widely used, although others such as secobarbital are acceptable.

1. **Advantages**

   a.    A primary advantage of barbiturates is **speed of action.** This effect depends on the dose, concentration, and rate of injection.
   b.    Barbiturates induce euthanasia smoothly, with **minimal discomfort** to the animal.
   c.    Barbiturates are **less expensive** than many other injectable euthanasia agents.

2. **Disadvantages**

   a.    Intravenous injection is necessary for best results, necessitating trained personnel.
   b.    Each animal must be **restrained.**
   c.    Current federal drug regulations require strict accounting for the barbiturates, and they must be used under the supervision of personnel registered with the DEA.
   d.    An aesthetically objectionable terminal gasp may occur in unconscious animals.

3. The advantages of using barbiturates for euthanasia in small animals far outweigh the disadvantages. The intravenous injection of a barbituric acid derivative is the **preferred method** for euthanasia of dogs, cats, and other small animals. Intraperitoneal injection may be used in situations in which these approaches would cause less distress than would intravenous injection.

## B. Pentobarbital Combinations

Several euthanasia products are formulated to include a barbituric acid derivative (usually sodium pentobarbital) with added local anesthetics or drugs that metabolize to pentobarbital. Although some of these additives are slowly cardiotoxic, this pharmacologic effect is inconsequential. These combination products are listed by the DEA as schedule III drugs, making them somewhat simpler to obtain, store, and administer than are schedule II drugs, such as sodium pentobarbital. The pharmacologic properties and recommended use of combination products presently available (which combine sodium pentobarbital with lidocaine or phenytoin) are interchangeable with those of pure barbituric acid derivatives.

### C. T-61

T-61 is an **injectable nonbarbiturate, nonnarcotic mixture** of three drugs used for euthanasia. These drugs provide a combination of general anesthetic, curariform, and local anesthetic actions. T-61 has been withdrawn from the market and is no longer manufactured or commercially available in the United States, although it is available in Canada. T-61 should be used only intravenously, because there is some question about the differential absorption and onset of action of the active ingredients when administered by other routes.

### D. Unacceptable Injectable Drugs

The injectable drugs strychnine, nicotine, caffeine, magnesium sulfate, potassium chloride, and all neuromuscular blockers, when used alone, are unacceptable and are absolutely condemned for use as euthanasia agents.

## VI. PHYSICAL METHODS

Physical methods of euthanasia include captive bolt, gunshot, cervical dislocation, decapitation, electrocution, microwave irradiation, exsanguination, stunning, and pithing. Some of these procedures–namely **exsanguination, stunning, and pithing**–are not recommended as a sole means of euthanasia, but are adjuncts when used in association with other agents or methods. Some authors consider physical methods of euthanasia aesthetically displeasing; however, some of these methods cause less fear and anxiety, and may be more rapid, painless, humane, and practical than other forms of euthanasia when properly used by skilled personnel with well-maintained equipment.

## A.    Cervical Dislocation

Cervical dislocation is used to euthanatize **small birds, mice, and immature rats and rabbits.** For mice and rats, the thumb and index finger are placed on either side of the neck at the base of the skull or a rod is pressed at the base of the skull. With the other hand, the base of the tail or hind limbs are quickly pulled, causing separation of the cervical vertebrae from the skull. For immature rabbits, the head is held in one hand and the hind limbs in the other. The animal is stretched and the neck is hyperextended and dorsally twisted to separate the first cervical vertebra from the skull.

1.    **Advantages**

    a.    Cervical dislocation is a technique that can induce **rapid unconsciousness.**
    b.    It does not chemically contaminate tissue.
    c.    It is quickly accomplished.

2.    **Disadvantages**

    a.    Cervical dislocation may be **aesthetically displeasing** to personnel.
    b.    Data suggest that electric activity in the brain persists for 13 s after cervical dislocation.
    c.    Its use is limited to small birds, mice, immature rats, and rabbits.

3.    When properly executed, manual cervical dislocation is a **humane** technique for euthanasia of poultry, other small birds, mice, rats weighing < 200 g, and rabbits weighing < 1 kg. In heavier rats and rabbits, the greater muscle mass in the cervical region makes manual cervical dislocation physically more difficult; accordingly, it should be performed only with mechanical dislocation by individuals who have demonstrated proficiency euthanatizing heavier animals. This technique should be used in research settings only when scientifically justified by the user and approved by the Institutional Animal Care and Use Committee. Those responsible for the use of this technique must

determine that personnel who perform cervical dislocation techniques have been properly trained to do so.

## B.    Decapitation

Decapitation is most often used to euthanatize **rodents and small
rabbits.** It provides a means to recover tissues and body fluids
that are chemically uncontaminated. It also provides a means of
obtaining anatomically undamaged brain tissue for study. Guil-
lotines designed for decapitation in a uniformly instantaneous
manner are commercially available.

### 1.   Advantages

a.    Decapitation is a technique that may induce rapid
unconsciousness.
b.    It does not chemically contaminate tissues.
c.    It is rapidly performed.

### 2.   Disadvantages

a.    The handling and restraint required to perform this
technique may be distressful to animals.
b.    Following decapitation, electric activity in the brain
persists for 13 or 14 s.
c.    Personnel performing this technique should recognize the inherent danger of the guillotine and take
adequate precautions to prevent personal injury.
d.    Decapitation may be aesthetically displeasing to personnel performing or observing the technique.

3.   Until additional information is available to better define
the nature of the persistent EEG activity, this technique
should be used in **research settings** only when scientifically
justified by the user and approved by the Institutional
Animal Care and Use Committee. Those responsible for
the use of this technique must determine that personnel
who perform decapitation techniques have been properly
trained to do so.

### C.    Electrocution

Electrocution, using alternating current, as a form of euthanasia has been used in species such as **dogs, foxes, and mink.** Electrocution induces death by cardiac fibrillation, which causes cerebral hypoxia. Animals, however, do not lose consciousness for 10 to 30 s or more after onset of cardiac fibrillation. It is imperative that animals be unconscious before being electrocuted. Therefore, euthanasia by electrocution must be a two-step procedure. First, the animal must be rendered unconscious by an acceptable means, including electric stunning (electronarcosis). If electric stunning or narcosis is used, the electric current must pass through the brain.

1. **Advantages**

    a.   Electrocution is humane if the animal is first rendered unconscious.

    b.   It does not chemically contaminate tissues.

    c.   It is economical.

2. **Disadvantages**

    a.   Electrocution may be **hazardous** to personnel.

    b.   It is not a useful method for mass euthanasia because so much time is required per animal.

    c.   It is not a useful method for **dangerous, intractable animals.**

    d.   It is **aesthetically objectionable** because of violent extension and stiffening of the limbs, head, and neck.

    e.   It may not result in death in small animals (< 5 kg) because ventricular fibrillation and circulatory collapse do not always persist after cessation of current flow.

3. Electric stunning and euthanasia by electrocution require special skills and equipment that will ensure passage of sufficient current through the brain to induce unconsciousness followed by electrically induced cardiac fibrillation. Although the method is conditionally acceptable if the aforementioned requirements are met, its disadvantages far outweigh its advantages in most applications.

Techniques that apply electric current from head to tail or head to foot are unacceptable.

## D. Microwave Irradiation

Heating by microwave irradiation is used primarily by neurobiologists to fix brain metabolites in vivo while maintaining the anatomic integrity of the brain. Microwave instruments have been specifically designed or modified for use in euthanasia of laboratory mice and rats. The instruments differ in design from kitchen units and may vary in the maximal power output from 1.3 to 10 kW. All units direct their microwave energy to the head of the animal. The power required to rapidly halt brain enzyme activity depends on the efficiency of the unit, the ability to tune the resonant cavity, and the size of the rodent head. The manufacture's recommendation should be followed closely when using microwave irradiation instruments to euthanatize laboratory mice and rats.

### 1. Advantages

a. **Unconsciousness** occurs in < 100 ms, and **death** in < 1 s.
b. This is the most effective method to **fix brain tissue** in vivo for subsequent assay of enzymatically labile chemicals.

### 2. Disadvantages

a. Instruments are expensive.
b. Only animals the size of mice and rats can be euthanatized with commercial instruments that are currently available.

3. Microwave irradiation is a humane method to euthanatize small laboratory rodents if instruments that induce rapid unconsciousness are used. Only instruments that are designed for this use and have appropriate power and microwave distribution should be used. Microwave ovens designed for domestic and institutional kitchens are absolutely unacceptable for euthanasia.

## VII. ADJUNCTIVE METHODS

Stunning and pithing, when properly done, induce unconsciousness but do not ensure death. Therefore, these methods should be used in conjunction with other procedures, such as pharmacologic agents, exsanguination, or decapitation to kill the animal.

### A.    Exsanguination

Exsanguination can be used to ensure death after electric stunning or to otherwise unconscious animals. Because **anxiety** is associated with **extreme hypovolemia,** exsanguination must not be used as a sole means of euthanasia. Animals may be exsanguinated to obtain blood products, but only when they are sedated, stunned, or anesthetized.

### B.    Stunning

Animals may be stunned by a blow to the head, use of a nonpenetrating captive bolt, or with an electric current. With stunning, **evaluation of unconsciousness** is difficult, but it is usually associated with a loss of the menace or blink response, pupillary dilation, and a loss of coordinated movements. Specific changes in the EEG and a loss of visually evoked responses are also thought to indicate unconsciousness. In small laboratory animals, a single sharp blow must be delivered to the central skull bones with sufficient force to produce immediate depression of the CNS. When this is properly done, unconsciousness is rapid.

### C.    Pithing

Pithing may be used as an **adjunctive procedure to ensure death** in an animal that has been rendered unconscious by other means. For some species, such as frogs, with anatomic features that facilitate easy access to the CNS, pithing may be used as a sole means of euthanasia, but anesthetic overdose is a more suitable method.

## VIII. ZOO, AQUATIC, AND POIKILOTHERMIC ANIMALS

Compared with domesticated and laboratory animal species, euthanasia of zoo, wild, aquatic, and poikilothermic species has been studied very little, thus guidelines are limited. The means selected depends on the species, size, and location of the animals to be euthanatized and the safety and experience of the personnel. Anatomic differences must also be considered. For example, amphibians, fish, reptiles, and marine mammals differ anatomically from domestic species. Veins may be difficult to locate. For physical methods, access to the CNS may be difficult because the brain may be small and difficult to locate by inexperienced persons.

## A. Mammals and Birds

For **captive zoo mammals** and **birds** with related domestic counterparts, many of the means described previously are appropriate. To minimize injury to persons or animals, however, additional precautions such as handling and physical or chemical restraint are important considerations.

## B. Amphibians, Fish, and Reptiles

When euthanasia of poikilothermic animals is performed, the differences in their metabolism, respiration, and tolerance to cerebral hypoxia may preclude some procedures that would be acceptable in homeothermic animals. In addition, it is often more difficult to ascertain when these animals are dead.

## C. Drugs and Techniques

1. **Sodium pentobarbital** (60 mg/kg) or other barbiturates can he administered intravenously, intra-abdominally, intrapleurally, or intraperitoneally in most cold-blooded animals, depending on anatomic features.

2. **Tricaine methanesulfonate** (TMS, MS-222) may be administered by a variety of routes to induce euthanasia. For aquatic animals, including amphibians, this chemical may be placed in the water. Large fish may be removed from the water, a gill cover lifted, and a concentrated solution from a syringe flushed over the gills. This is an effective but expensive means of euthanasia that is not hazardous to personnel. Benzocaine hydrochloride, a compound similar to TMS, may be used as a bath or in a recirculation system for euthanasia of fish or amphibians.

3. Species such as **snakes, lizards, turtles, frogs, and toads** may be killed by overexposure to gaseous anesthetics such as halothane or methoxyflurane in a chamber or via face

mask. Carbon dioxide gas may be used for terrestrial animals. Some reptiles can stop or reduce their breathing for long periods without overt ill effects and may not die even after prolonged exposure. It has been suggested that, when using physical methods of euthanasia in poikilothermic species, cooling to 4°C will decrease metabolism and facilitate handling, but there is no evidence that it raises the pain threshold.

4. Most **amphibians, fish, and reptiles** can be euthanatized by cranial concussion (stunning) followed by decapitation or some other physical method. Decapitation with heavy shears or guillotine is effective in some species that have appropriate anatomic features. It has been assumed that stopping the blood supply to the brain by decapitation causes rapid unconsciousness. Recently, this view has been questioned because the CNS of reptiles and amphibians is tolerant to hypoxic and hypotensive conditions. Consequently, decapitation should be followed by pithing.

5. Severing the spinal cord behind the head by pithing is an effective method of killing some poikilotherms. Inasmuch as death may not be immediate unless both the brain and spinal cord are pithed, double pithing is recommended. Pithing of the spinal cord should be followed by decapitation and pithing of the brain or some other appropriate procedure. The anatomic features of some species preclude effective use of this method. Pithing requires dexterity and skill and should be done only by trained personnel.

6. **Snakes and turtles** immobilized by cooling have been killed by subsequent freezing. This method is not, however, recommended. Formation of ice crystals on the skin and in tissues of an animal may cause pain or distress. Quick freezing of deeply anesthetized animals is acceptable. Crocodilians and other large reptiles can be shot through the brain.

7. For smaller **marine mammals** (pinnipeds and cetaceans), barbiturates or potent opioids (e.g., etorphine hydrochloride and carfentanil) are recommended. An accurately placed gunshot may also be an acceptable method for euthanasia of stranded marine mammals.

## IX.  ANIMALS RAISED FOR FUR

Animals raised for fur are usually killed individually at the location where they are raised. Although any handling of these species constitutes a stress, it is possible to minimize this by euthanatizing animals in or near their cages. Details of the procedures described here were presented earlier in this chapter.

### A.  Carbon Monoxide

In the case of the **smaller species** (e.g., mink), CO appears to be an adequate method for euthanasia. Compressed CO is delivered from a tank into an enclosed cage that can be moved adjacent to holding cages. Using the apparatus outside reduces the risk to human beings; however, people using this method should still be made aware of the dangers of CO. Animals introduced into a chamber containing 4% CO lost consciousness in $64 \pm 14$ s and are dead within $215 \pm 45$ s. Only one animal should be introduced into the chamber at a time, and death should be confirmed in each case.

### B.  Carbon Dioxide

$CO_2$ is also a good euthanasia method for the **smaller species** and is less dangerous than CO for personnel operating the system. Using compressed $CO_2$ from a tank is likely to be more reliable and efficient than using solid $CO_2$. When exposed to 100% $CO_2$, mink lose consciousness in $19 \pm 4$ s and are dead in $153 \pm 10$ s. When 70% $CO_2$ is used with 30% $O_2$, the animals are unconscious in 28 s, but they are not dead after a 15-min exposure. Therefore, if animals are first stunned by 70% $CO_2$, they should be killed by exposure to 100% $CO_2$ or by some other means. Only one animal should be introduced into the chamber at a time.

### C.  Barbiturate Overdose

**Barbiturate overdose** is an acceptable procedure for euthanasia of many species of animals raised for fur. The drug is injected intraperitoneally, and the animal slowly loses consciousness. It is important that the death of each animal be confirmed after barbiturate injection. Barbiturates will contaminate the carcass; therefore, the skinned carcass cannot be used for animal food.

### D. Electrocution

Electrocution has been used for killing **foxes and mink.** The electric current must pass through the brain to induce unconsciousness before electricity is passed through the rest of the body. Use of a nose-to-tail or nose-to-foot method may kill the animal by inducing cardiac fibrillation, but the animal may be conscious for a period before death; therefore, these techniques are unacceptable. **Electric stunning** may be followed by cervical dislocation in mink and other small animals. It is recommended that cervical dislocation be done within 20 s of electric stunning.

# Index